Doing Right

Doing Right

A Practical Guide to Ethics for
Medical Trainees and Physicians

THIRD EDITION Philip C. Hébert

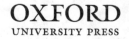

OXFORD
UNIVERSITY PRESS

OXFORD
UNIVERSITY PRESS

Oxford University Press is a department of the University of Oxford.
It furthers the University's objective of excellence in research, scholarship,
and education by publishing worldwide. Oxford is a registered trade mark of
Oxford University Press in the UK and in certain other countries.

Published in Canada by
Oxford University Press
8 Sampson Mews, Suite 204,
Don Mills, Ontario M3C 0H5 Canada

www.oupcanada.com

First Edition published in 1996
Second Edition published in 2009

Library and Archives Canada Cataloguing in Publication

Hébert, Philip C., author
Doing right : a practical guide to ethics for medical trainees
and physicians / Philip C. Hébert. – Third edition.

Revision of: Doing right : a practical guide to ethics for medical
trainees and physicians / Philip C. Hébert. – 2nd ed. – Don Mills, Ont. :
Oxford University Press, [2008], c2009.
Includes bibliographical references and index.
ISBN 978-0-19-900552-9 (pbk.)

1. Medical ethics. I. Title.

R724.H39 2014   174.2   C2013-908208-5

Cover image: Fuse/GettyImages.com

Printed and bound in Canada

6 7 8 — 18 17 16

Contents

Cases

Preface

It has now been over 15 years since the first edition of *Doing Right* was published. The reasons for this newest edition are many. As with the second edition I have updated the book with recent cases in the bioethics and jurisprudence literature that help provide directions to clinicians. I have included more material on disability, research, and cultural aspects of care. All chapters have been rewritten and revised to reflect this.

As with previous editions I have included cases that affect all health-care professionals, not just physicians. The cases and issues are shared alike by all healthcare professionals—whether medical trainees, physicians, nurses, nurse practitioners, or physician assistants. Allied health-care professionals may also find some of the cases useful and relevant for their practices. I will, in general, shy away from thinking of those we serve as "consumers," "customers," or "clients" of healthcare and instead refer to them as "patients," "partners," or "participants" in care. Call me old-fashioned, but I think the latter "p-words" better capture than the former what healthcare is all about. Those we serve are often unwell and deserve protection as well as promotion; in the country of illness, they do not need to be boondoggled and cajoled as if in a market or a *souk*.

The perspective is that of the well-intentioned healthcare professional, the "good clinician," in general. Although different healthcare profession-als will have different degrees of agency and responsibility for handling dilemmas in clinical practice, the "right way" of doing so should reflect a common "professional point of view"—best arrived at by consensus, crit-ical interprofessional discussion—and by those with an abiding commit-ment to the healing enterprise. There is an ongoing revolution in medical education in favour of patients, multidisciplinary teams, and evidence-based care, which this book, like its previous editions, mirrors, supports, and encourages. Medicine is a difficult enterprise but need not be a lonely one. When a troublesome issue must be addressed, three nostrums can be recommended: (1) *turn to the wisdom of others*; (2) *try to find someone to help you; and* (3) *turn to your best resource, the patient beside you*; he or she may know more than you realize.

There is a renewed international approach to professional medical ethics, spurred on by medical associations such as the British Medical Association and the World Medical Association.[1] Despite many large dif-ferences in culture, religion, and politics (differences that should not be minimized), the healthcare professions throughout the world share sim-ilar goals: the prevention of premature death and the treatment and pre-vention of illness and human suffering more generally. These are the good ends that the virtuous clinician strives to achieve in "doing right." These goals unite healthcare professionals across the globe and have done so ever since humans have treated illness.

Don't be overly perturbed by the seeming cacophony of language and everyday morals. Some ethicists think we are forever circumscribed and held hostage by our languages and cultures. As a result there is no "value-neutral" vantage point from which moral disputes can be resolved and so, they argue, we are left only with a moral or cultural "relativism" ("be true to yourself/your culture" pluralism). This is usually combined with an attack on the imperialism of "Western" medicine and ethics. I do not subscribe to this view. Yes, all languages and cultures may have embedded values and even worldviews. The solution isn't to seek a value-free language or throw up one's hands in despair but is to engage in dialogue with others over the common problems we face as patients and providers. Ernest Gellner, a twentieth-century anthropologist, arguing against the relativism ever so present in anthropology and ethnography, wrote that, "even if no absolute point of view is possible, fairly comfortable resting places . . . will do instead . . . We cannot but adopt some vantage point, even if only to express some doubt or to recognize some uncertainty."[2]

This approach is seen in new views of social institutions, both national and international, that do not require a heady optimism about our future[3] or an imperialist imposition of "Western" values. Diverse cultures can share rules and values to sustainably manage scarce resources such as access to water or food supplies.[4] International aid organizations, such as NGO's (non-governmental organizations) like OXFAM or MSF (Médecins Sans Frontières), would not exist if very different cultures did not share the value of human life.[5] The question is whether this value and others, such as tolerance and altruism required for just medical care, can be extended to society generally.

A seemingly "culture-friendly" relativism denies culture-independent rules of rationality and thwarts comprehensible change. But there are some things, such as healthcare, that we, as humans, need and that we can discuss across traditions and across value divides. The digital revolution and the sharing of information across and between cultures will help erode the appeal of relativism.

Dialogue and progress in ethical matters, as in medicine and society generally, do not require a common language. They do require, I think, allegiance to the core and preeminent value requisite for all professions: a respect for humans and human dignity. Thus, the abolition *across* cultures of human bondage, female degradation, childhood labour and, indeed, medical milestones such as the eradication of smallpox and soon polio, are not only definitive indicators of progress but are also the result of recognizing our shared humanity. In this book, the commitment to this value and its implications for medicine and society will be explored.

Incidentally, another word about words: I tend to use *morality* as interchangeable with *ethics*, although many would use morality to refer to the local custom and ethos, and ethics to refer to the critical reflection on diverse practices. When I write *"we,"* I am not using the word in the way Mark Twain defined it ("Only kings, presidents, editors, and people with tapeworms have the right to use the editorial 'we.'"). Instead, I usually use "we" to refer to "healthcare providers" (or "clinicians" or "healthcare professionals" or "practitioners" interchangeably) generally and sometimes to the generic members of society at large—I include myself in both groups. Finally, I use medicine interchangeably with healthcare, although the latter implies a broader scope of care.

Acknowledgments

The third edition of this book has helped me address some lacunae and limitations of earlier editions. Oxford University Press, *comme d'habitude*, patiently tolerated my ongoing failure to meet deadlines—although this time I cannot blame the surgeon's knife. I still find fault with my constitution's inability to cope with certain rigours of advancing "middle" age. For this third edition, I owe a debt of gratitude to the OUP reviewers and to my editor, Karri Yano.

This and previous editions could not have been completed without the insightful feedback and help from a tremendous number of wise and supportive family, friends, and colleagues. Thanks to those who read and commented on different editions of this book: Yusra Ahmad, Peter Allatt, the late Rob Buckman, Lisa Burzillo, David Carr, Nancy Carroll, Eoin Connolly, Russell Fleming, Rocco Gerace, Barney Giblon, Kathy Glass, Laura Hawryluck, Paul DN Hébert, Hannah Kaufman, Michael Kaufman, Nathan Kaufman, Lori Luther, Mary Rose MacDonald, Maria McDonald, Cliodhna McMullin, Ann Munro, Janice Newton, Alison Organek, Deb Selby, Linda Sheahan, Laura Sky, Polly Thompson, Frank Wagner, and Shawn Winsor. Anuradha Rose of Vellore College, India, provided a number of new cases for this edition. Thanks to Audrey Karlinsky for cases used in all editions of this book. Thanks must also go to my many teachers over the years who encouraged and facilitated my interest in philosophy and its connection with the social world: Professors Henry Laycock, Peter Landstreet, Michael Gilbert, Ian Jarvie, and Jagdish Hattiangadi. I have been helped by the many students who have read and provided feedback on this book and by my medical mentors, such as the late Dr Edward Llewellyn-Thomas, a truly remarkable Associate Dean of Student Affairs at the University of Toronto's medical school, who combined an interest in humanities and writing with medicine and engineering. Special thanks to my lifelong friend, Kristine Connidis, who took time out from her own writing to encourage mine when I was still recovering from one surgery or another. There are many other friends, colleagues, and students from medicine, the Joint Centre for Bioethics, and elsewhere who have provided support over the years, too many to mention individually. They know who they are and how grateful I am. The errors and limitations of this book remain mine.

Not surprisingly the biggest debt of gratitude I owe is, once again, to my wife, and editor-in-chief, Victoria Lee—without her unwavering support, I could not have survived and without her wise editorial advice the various editions of this book would *never* have been written. So, although saying thank you is not enough, no matter how many times I say it, to Victoria, the love of my life, I will say it thrice for three editions: thanks, thank you, and thanks again, from the bottom of my heart. To my two children who have put up with my work over the years, I also need to say thank you for helping me appreciate what matters the most: one's family and the circle of caring and understanding that, if we are fortunate enough to have, surrounds each one of us.

Philip C. Hébert MD PhD, FCFPC

Professor Emeritus
Department of Family and Community Medicine
University of Toronto
Toronto, Ontario, Canada
philip.hebert@utoronto.ca

October 2013

Introduction
A Revolution in Learning

Now, what I want is, Facts. Teach these boys and girls nothing but
Facts. Facts alone are wanted in life.

Charles Dickens, 1854[1]

The most important . . . facts are bound to transcend culture.

Sam Harris, 2010[2]

Schools for healthcare professionals traditionally emphasized the technical side of medicine and the multitude of facts the student must know. So many facts were planted in the student's brain that they threatened to choke out everything else. However, once out in the real world looking after patients, the novice healthcare trainee, as well as the seasoned practitioner, faced other less factual—but no less important and often even more important—issues, such as ethics. Ill-equipped to deal with such issues, the healthcare practitioner often managed these in ways that reflected personal or professional biases. Such attitudes and practices may have been acceptable in the time of Dickens but they will not suffice for the twenty-first century when we are able to do so much more for patients and are indeed expected by the public to do so much more.

A new medical curriculum

In the past 15 years or more since the first edition of this book was published, the traditional curriculum of all the healthcare professions has undergone, and continues to undergo, dramatic changes.[3, 4] New pedagogies of medical learning stress critical reflection and lifelong learning, rather than rote memorization and regurgitation of facts. Trainees no longer wait two years to see patients. Instead, they are in the trenches almost from day one, learning how to listen and talk to patients. Rather than days full of tedious lectures, there are subject-integrated, problem-based cases of the week whereby students learn to appreciate the many-sided aspects—physical, psychological, and social—of illness and the needs of patients. They learn what many clinicians in previous days did not: of the patient as a person, not as Disease X in Room 2, but as Ms Brown, a retired teacher with no living relatives who has been admitted to hospital because of cognitive decline and poor self-care. They learn that in Room 3 is not simply an "interesting myeloma patient with a fractured femur" but a former Olympian, Mr Yung, who is eager to know as much as possible about his condition but is also terrified about its implications for his future and for his young family.

Healthcare trainees still learn anatomy and physiology, pharmacology and cardiology, but they also learn communication skills, organizational aspects of medicine, the social determinates of illness, and how to exhibit the skills and virtues of empathy, altruism, and trustworthiness. Compared with the traditional curriculum, this has amounted to a revolution in learning. This is a revolution of which many are unaware, not everyone has accepted, and is far from completed, but it is a revolution and one, I believe, that is irreversible. Most importantly, perhaps, the nature of learning and information exchange is changing dramatically. With the advent of the Internet and the digital revolution, information (if not always expertise) is at the fingertips of not only health professionals and trainees but also patients and families. In an E-world, excluding patients from decision-making will be impossible and unwelcome.[5] This revolution in pedagogy and learning will be resistant to attempts to return to medical paternalism or authoritarianism.

As part of this revolution, entire new cadres of teachers have entered many healthcare schools: epidemiologists, information technology experts, philosophers, lawyers, theologians, sociologists, anthropologists, even poets, to name a few, in efforts to better refine and "humanize" medical teaching and care. Medicine is a human venture.[6] Becoming a better medical practitioner may be achieved not only by learning the biochemistry of the Krebs cycle or how to recognize geriatric depression but also by reading a novel such as Camus' *The Plague* or by understanding how participants in medical research should be treated. The twenty-first century medical professional must also be an expert in new technologies of information to keep up with his or her patients and know how to use them to better understand and help the plights of patients. These changes have been generally all to the good, although seen as a threat by some and a distraction by others. However, the new teaching and teachers have helped make the healthcare profession more willing *and more able to listen to patients and to each other*.[7] These are the "transcendent facts" that stand above individual cultures and can help unite patients with healthcare providers throughout the world.

Aim of book

This book aims to provide a readable introduction to modern professional medical ethics that befits the new pedagogies and curricula of healthcare. It attempts to make the complex topic of ethics more accessible to, and usable for, medical trainees and practitioners. The twentieth-century

Austrian philosopher of science Karl Popper held that anything important could and should be said clearly without obfuscation or technical language.[8] Ethics needn't be obscure and cannot be now, if it ever was, the
sole domain of an "expert" ethicist. When it comes to moral action, all
those involved in healthcare—the patient, the public, and professionals
alike—have legitimate views that deserve consideration.

One problem with this endeavour is the disarray of bioethics and the
apparent diversity of moral views and practices across cultures and across
history.[9] Although bioethicists may differ and moral practices may not be
the same the world over, increasingly, professional medical ethics, as with
medicine generally, is worldwide. This shift away from culturally based
or idiosyncratic medical practices towards an international perspective is
hastened by ready access to information everywhere and the democratic
trends this enhances. Medical regulatory authorities now meet interna-
tionally and adopt similar policies. Medical graduates everywhere must
pass similar exams of which ethics is now core material. However, an
international code of healthcare ethics seems a long way off in a world rife
with assassinations, brutal wars, mass starvation, and widespread deni-
als of basic human rights. Nonetheless, steps in the right direction can
be seen in, for example, agreements on an international code of medical
rights for patients, on rules for the proper conduct of medical research,[10]
and in widespread opposition to physicians participating in torture[11] and
in state executions, no matter how "humane."[12]

Diversity and difference over such issues in modern medicine, their lack
of resolution, are reasons for pessimism for some.[13] But they may also be
indicators of the recognition of just how difficult the work required to address
medicine's moral issues is and will be, not a mark of medicine's irreconcilable
moral divides. Certainly, we should not be complacent about the advances
that have been made and we must acknowledge the tremendous gaps that
exist in the world today between how things are and how they should be.[14]

Ethics is about right and wrong and the reasons we give for our
choices and actions. This is clearly central to medicine, since doing the
right thing for one's patients (minimizing suffering and treating illness)
has not only a factual but also an ethical dimension. Clinical ethics, the
subject of this book, is concerned with ethical problems arising out of the
care of patients.

We must often make decisions on problems that go beyond the facts
at hand. *Ethical decisions* appeal to *what we may do, should do, or ought to
do*.[15] But ethics is neither just about giving moral advice, nor an exercise
in moral indignation and finger-wagging. Ethics is about acting in ways
consistent with what we have the overall "best reasons" to do.[16] Ethics is

also about critically examining these reasons by looking at what we do every day and trying to do it better.

For example, should practitioners always inform patients fully about their condition? May confidential information about a patient be disclosed to a third party? To what extent should the odd views of an eccentric patient be respected? May desperate patients be offered medically risky research? Do parents have the right to refuse medically indicated treatment for their children? Are religious objections to brain death valid? To how much of society's resources may a patient lay claim? How far ought clinicians go in helping their patients die? As we will see, many of these dilemmas have been subject to probing thought, with a consensus of professional opinion gradually having been developed for some. There can be decisive reasons for doing one thing, as opposed to another, in medicine. But such decisive reasons do not always stand out as clear and evident choices. The goal, anyway, is not to get the "right" answer to our ethical puzzles but to recognize them as puzzles, to worry about them, in ways that are sensitive and respectful of others.

What ethics can offer

In tackling an ethical problem, if it were simply a question of the right versus the wrong path to take, there would be little doubt as to which road a morally acting person should take. Unfortunately, it is not always that easy. *Ethical dilemmas arise when there are good reasons, at least at first glance, for different ways of proceeding.* Further complicating this, their resolution sometimes requires choices involving better and worse solutions, optimal and less than optimal solutions. There are rarely unique or singular solutions to important moral dilemmas.

What medical ethics can and should offer is an expanded set of considerations to take into account when making a difficult decision. The choice in ethics is not between following clear-cut rules versus exercising individual judgment or between an "algorithmic" versus an intuitive approach. Rules and principles need not "routinize" decision-making; they can help us in exercising informed judgment. Ethics does not offer a solution but does attempt to clarify what we ought to be concerned about, why we ought to be concerned, and what we should do about it. Ethics does not and cannot replace all the other important elements, such as discernment, sensitivity, compassion, common sense, prudence, and good clinical reasoning, that go into a wise and right medical decision, the decision that seems to be the optimal (or best possible) one for the individual patient or practitioner to make.

Some have argued that ethics may not be the only source of values and factors to take into account when attempting to make a decision.[17] There are, for example, professional regulations, commitments to families or friends, availability (or not) of real alternatives, financial issues, all of which can have an impact on the decision as well as on the decision-makers. Indeed some of these less obviously "ethical" matters may be decisive. The healthcare professional will be expected to focus his or her vision on what is most important in trying to do the right thing and avoid that which is simply self-serving or distracting.

Professional ethics is different from ethics as a philosophical discipline. In the real world of healthcare, we rarely have the luxury of time for considered reflection and armchair theorizing. In caring for a patient, no matter what the uncertainties, we must have a plan of action. Resolutions to moral dilemmas are, or should be, tentative and uncertain. The wise clinician understands the importance of "triangulating" his or her decision by obtaining input from various sources, including (need-less to say!) the patient and his or her network of support. Here lies one value of interprofessional cooperation and patient-based medicine: to ensure that contentious decisions, if later called into question, have had the benefit of more than one opinion, incorporate patient preferences, and so should not invite charges of unilateral, high-handed, ham-fisted, or paternalistic decision-making.

Professional ethics is really *interprofessional* ethics. It is also *patient-based* ethics as, only by involving patients and their significant others, can a healthcare professional focus on what should be the decisive rationale for doing one thing as opposed to another. Patient-based medicine is here to stay and calls for a healthcare ethos—that of shared decision-making—to match it. (See Box I.1.) These values are relevant wherever medicine is practised, but obviously almost impossible to achieve in many regions due to crushing poverty, deprivation of liberty, and willful denial of basic human rights.

BOX I.1

Patient-based medicine:

- identifies and respects patient values;
- offers coordinated care;
- provides high-quality information;
- addresses physical and emotional needs;
- involves significant others;
- ensures continuity of care;
- provides access to care.[18]

Two trends in ethics

One of the tools needed to address ethical problems is ethical theory. Traditionally, there have been two broad schools of ethics: deontology and consequentialism. Deontology deems certain duties and/or rights to be fundamental, whereas consequentialism makes certain consequences or outcomes (either to be avoided or sought after) to be basic. Deontology treats rights and duties as the foundation of ethics, regardless of the state of affairs that results, while consequentialism treats the resulting state of affairs as the yardstick for ethics. Thus, for example, a deontologist would say it is intrinsically wrong to tell a lie, no matter what the circumstances and results. (The Bible's Ten Commandments are an example of a deontological view.) A consequentialist would say it is wrong to cause suffering and right to relieve it, no matter what act leads to that result. So, for some, one does right by following certain rules, laws or duties; for others, one does right by encouraging or avoiding certain states of affairs.

Deontology is best represented by the eighteenth-century Prussian philosopher, Immanuel Kant, and consequentialism by the nineteenth-century English philosopher, John Stuart Mill. Mill's philosophy of utilitarianism is the most famous form of consequentialism. In his wonderful 1859 book *On Liberty*, Mill explained: "I regard utility as the ultimate appeal on all things ethical, but it must be utility in the largest sense, grounded on the permanent interests of man as a progressive being."[19] (By considering utility "in the largest sense," Mill was trying to avoid the simplistic utilitarian collapse of morality into the tyranny of the welfare of the many over the few.[20])

By contrast, Kant saw ethics as arising out of self-set universal laws (maxims) of reason. To wit: "A deed is right or wrong in general insofar as it is in accordance with or contrary to duty . . . The categorical imperative, which in general only expresses what an obligation is, is this: Act according to a maxim which can . . . be valid as a universal law."[21]

Duty or consequences? Which theory gives the best account of morality? There are many, many theories and approaches to ethics that combine, modify, and even claim to overthrow these basic approaches, but no one theory predominates. For example, the late John Rawls, the most influential political philosopher from the late twentieth century (he died in 2007), developed his own version of deontology: contractualism.[22] How, he asked, would we, as rational actors/citizens, organize ourselves as a society, if we did not know in advance where we would end up in that society (top or bottom)? What principles would we follow? Rawls argues that rational agents would abide certain rules of "fairness": for example, that basic rights, such as freedom of choice and equal opportunity, are more important than ensuring the "good life." For Rawls, inequalities would be tolerated if those with the least benefitted the most. This could be a defence of inequality rather than prioritizing justice, as some critics have claimed,[23] but I think it is not, and we will return to it in the chapter on justice.

Interestingly, one prominent modern philosopher, the British philosopher, Derek Parfit, has argued, at some level of abstraction and also at some considerable length, that while the perspectives of utilitarianism and deontology differ, they are ultimately concerned with the same end, the search for a "single true morality."[24] His arguments have not settled the issue but are helpful for those of us who see advantages in combining both types of ethical theorizing. The ethics decision procedure adopted in this book and described in Chapter 1 incorporates the perspectives of deontology and consequentialism. Neither theory will suffice on its own; both are needed. And both types of theories are quite compatible with the idea of "mid-level" principles serving as guides to action for moral agents.

The following well-known, mid-level principles of ethics form the backbone of the ethics decision procedure that will be used in this book: (1) the autonomy principle (acting on the basis of respect due persons: what does this patient need and want?); (2) the beneficence and the non-maleficence principles (acting in the patient's best interests: what can be done to avoid harm and provide help to this patient?); and (3) the justice principle (acting on fairness: to what resources may this patient lay claim?).

The autonomy principle is largely a deontological principle; the beneficence principle is consequentialist; the justice principle contains aspects of both (the basic notion of justice as fairness could be considered deontological, whereas distributive justice could be given a utilitarian cast). The toolbox approach to ethics is admittedly eclectic, but it does depend on one common commitment: the "respect for humans" (or "respect for human dignity") principle that is required in everything that we, as healthcare providers, do.[25]

Other ethical perspectives

This approach to doing ethics is not meant to imply that other perspectives are not possible or useful. I will return to and at times utilize these other views throughout the book, but will briefly mention some of them here.

Virtue theory looks at the motivations and intentions of actors: a good action is what a virtuous agent would do. This theory relies, ultimately, on the moral intuitions of persons and is a reminder as to what ethics is all about. There is an emphasis on the type of person making the decision: *Am I the kind of person I want to be in taking such an action? What kind of person am I in taking this action?*[26] Virtues obviously cannot be ignored in clinical ethics; they are attitudes and behaviours—such as honesty, loyalty, fair-mindedness—that motivate us to do the right thing, can be recommended to others, and are a hedge against "breaking bad." The prime virtue this book recommends to practitioners is *prudence*, taking due care and exhibiting due diligence in one's deliberations and actions. *Altruism*, putting the interests of others before one's own, would come a close second. Prudence leads to (or derives from) the principle of non-maleficence whereas altruism is connected with beneficence and justice.

Narrative ethics focuses its attention on making coherent sense of the stories behind the lives of our patients, "Illness itself unfolds as a narrative."[27] Understanding the patient's story should be the goal in any good clinical encounter, but eliciting such stories requires time, compassion, and having a "receptive ear."[28] Narrative ethics enriches, rather than replaces, a principle-based approach to clinical ethics. However, narrative ethics in treating the patient's story as a text to be interpreted is less interested in applying ethical rules than it is in understanding the patient's story *from the inside*: what is life really like for the patient, the family, the practitioner? The goal is to find the hidden treasure, the moral heart, that will help a story make sense. "I can only answer the question 'What am I to do?' if I can answer the prior question 'Of what stories do I find myself a part?' "[29]

Feminist bioethics is not one approach but is a complexity of many strands that include cultural critiques and studies of inequalities between the sexes. One core theme in feminism is the emphasis on an "ethics of care" over the use of abstract ethical principles, such as rights-based individualism. Feminism reminds us of the importance of relations with others and of social structures that limit the choices that people—especially women and minorities—face.[30] Restrictions on the choice and freedom of women are "advantage-increasing" rules for men ("patriarchal" rules) that discriminate against women. Feminist bioethics also tends to look at less examined topics such as reproductive ethics, disability ethics, women in research, and hierarchies of power in medicine. It is not one theory of ethics but pushes its boundaries into a more inclusive field. It reminds us of the importance of relational ethics, "persons are, inevitably, connected with other persons and with social institutions."[31] There are hidden interests and voices of the disadvantaged and the powerless that feminism tries to render visible.[32]

Casuistry is a long-discredited branch of philosophy reviled for its picayune analysis of ecclesiastical and mundane cases that seemed to justify opposing opinions ("apologies") for the same dilemma; hence, it appeared to use reason to justify any stance. Its close analysis of cases, however, is instructive and has been recently revived by some very able philosophers who argue that by using casuistical reasoning we can find mid-level maxims or a typology of cases that can guide us in similar situations. It eschews higher-order principles and a coherent account of medical morality as it considers these to imply a deductive algorithm that will lead to answers to difficult cases. Casuistry would look at a case where promise-breaking is wrong (e.g., where a father has promised to take his daughter out for her birthday but not turn up because he has decided to go out with friends instead) and then find changed circumstances that might justify the promise-breaking (e.g., if the father was a health professional and was called away for an emergency). What justifies an action is not a rule but local circumstances.[33]

Legalism is another response to ethical dilemmas in medicine but is not so much a theory as a trend. Legalism replaces ethical debate with jurisprudential reasoning (i.e., the opinions of lawyers). When faced with moral dilemmas, practitioners often ask what the law says, mistakenly seeing this as the bottom-line answer.[34] While legal rulings are almost always relevant to what we ought to do (they are part of the professional's moral landscape), following the law too assiduously can lead to purely self-protective behaviour ("What can I do so as not to be sued?"), and to egregiously unethical events. So it was in 2012 when a woman in Ireland, imperiled by her pregnancy, needlessly died, her doctors having been guided by their interpretation of Irish law prohibiting the termination of pregnancy as long as a fetal heartbeat was detected.[35] The clinician exhibiting the virtue of prudence would have asked: which is worse—allowing the mother to die or not following the letter of the law? Physicians are not lawyers or judges. Where a law seems to stand in the way of what obviously should be done to save the patient before you, the clinician ought to follow his or her professional judgment and act to save the patient.

Thus, what the law says should not bring discussion to a halt. Medicine is about doing what is best for a patient "all things considered," whereas the law has a whole range of social interests and concerns to balance. Practically speaking, when a dispute comes to court, the legal resolution *can* seem to have the last word about what to do. Medicine's boundaries are for the profession itself to determine, but "within the framework of . . . law."[36] The law is, however, rarely uniquely determinative. It typically allows for professional discretion as to what to do, especially, for example, if a patient's life is at stake and the clinician is acting in "good faith." Moreover, the social currents the law reflects (and influences) are in constant evolution, as evidenced, for example, by recurring debates throughout the world over abortion, euthanasia, and assisted suicide. The law also changes in part with input from professional ethics.

So, where a clinician disagrees with existing law, taking a judge through one's considered ethical opinion can help the court see how "the reasonable standard of professional care" (such as that regarding end-of-life care or truthtelling by clinicians) is changing.

This is not a source book on the law and so cannot be comprehensive. Nevertheless, I have tried to focus on the important legal cases—largely Canadian, but also some from American and British law, with which the clinician needs to be familiar. Whether a judgment cited is the right guide in any particular case will depend upon the reader's considered moral judgment.

Professional Ethics

There is not one medical morality for doctors and different ones for everyone else. Ethics is for everyone—professional, patient, and public alike. This does not mean that each has the same duties, but the *professional's* duties ought to reflect society's expectations of medicine. The good clinician is one who is predisposed to act in morally defensible ways and act out of the virtues of trustworthiness, altruism, prudence, humility, and compassion. Society must understand and endorse what healthcare professionals do, and strive to do, in carrying out their healing mandate, otherwise the trust between healers and patients may be lost and the whole healthcare enterprise is threatened. The Hippocratic oath saw trust as possible only if the doctor kept his professional training a secret—as perhaps befitted a tradition that had few truly helpful interventions.

Today, trust in medicine requires informational transparency and patient involvement. More than ever, trust and truth go together. The old, narrow guild mentality and the monetary self-interest of some modern healthcare professionals are ongoing threats to the public's trust in the profession. So, too, is the laconic view of medicine as a corporate enterprise. This will be discussed more fully in later chapters.

Ethics utilizes the human penchant for regulation to transform and increasingly moralize aspects of social life, such as healthcare. *Ethical rules are, frequently, "advantage-reducing" rules,*[37] particularly well-suited to changing hierarchical or authoritarian systems wherever they exist. They reduce, for example, the free hand, the unregulated practices, the unfair advantages of the more powerful, such as doctors and researchers, and up-regulate the position of the less well-situated, of patients, and the public generally. Rules about consent, confidentiality, truthtelling, and so on, attempt to level out to some degree what is an unlevel playing field. Together, ethics and the new technologies of information transcend the deceptive Hippocratic ethos in their emphasis on patient self-determination.

The international equalizing trend of medical morality has been strengthened by the era of the Internet. Patients are less dependent on doctors for information and seem to have more choices than ever. Transparency and access to information are keys to informed decision-making and increasingly put power in the hands of patients.[38] The idea of the physician as captain of the ship must give way to the notion of the patient as the driver of the system. This is not the end of professionalism, as some have claimed.[39] Healthcare is *not* a zero sum game: we all gain when patients and professionals partner together in the activity of improving healthcare; it's a win-win proposition. Barring some world-wide conflagration and environmental or economic collapse (unfortunately, always possible[40]), the ongoing process of moralization of healthcare, and of the social world more generally, makes it less and less likely that medicine can serve evil purposes such as Nazism or Stalinism again without dissent.

Book outline

The plan of the book is as follows. Chapter 1 sets out a way to approach and manage ethical problems in medicine typically encountered when conflicting responsibilities must be balanced, and it serves as a useful summary for the book as a whole. Chapter 2 examines a crucial principle of contemporary medicine, patient autonomy. Because this principle engenders duties regarding confidentiality and disclosure, these are presented next in Chapters 3 and 4. Chapter 5 looks at informed consent, while Chapter 6 considers the ethical problems involved in incapacity and substitute decision-making. Chapter 7 examines another fundamental principle of medicine, beneficence. Chapter 8 discusses the new professionalism and the issue of medical error—when medicine goes astray. Chapter 9 examines justice, a less familiar principle for many but one recognized by Hippocrates and now of increasing concern in everyday healthcare practice. Chapter 10 looks at new life issues and the new reproductive technology. Chapter 11 concerns the care of the dying and assisted death. Chapter 12 looks at the influence of culture and genetic knowledge on ethics and at ethical issues in medical research. The Conclusion contains suggestions for further reading.

Throughout this book I provide cases followed by a focused discussion of each. Many of the cases are taken from real-life dilemmas in clinical practice but details altered to protect privacy. None of this case discussion should in any way be taken as legal advice. Nor should my opinions be taken as the "right answers." In the ethical problems of real life, as in medicine generally, decisions are fraught with uncertainty and even the seemingly best choice may have reasonable alternatives. I encourage you to develop your own opinions in each of the cases; you will also have the opportunity to apply these in the new material presented at the end of each chapter.

By the end of this book you should be able to analyze and manage ethical problems in medicine in a reasonable way. Although there can be no guarantees that you will have done, or will have been able to do, the best thing in responding to an ethical problem, you should be satisfied that you have tried to solve the problem in a comprehensive and careful fashion. Medicine is a challenging job. Trainees and mentors can suffer under the weight of information and decision-making.[41] Better and more satisfying experiences with learning and practising medicine are possible if the advantages of ethical, patient-based decision-making are utilized: decision-making can be shared, responsibilities a little lightened, humility practised, and perfectionism eased up on.

Many healthcare professionals view their future, and their patients' futures, with dismay, feeling that theirs is a profession under siege.[42, 43, 44] Patients and families, too, are restive and critical, and know all is not right with healthcare. Dickens' book title, *Hard Times*, seems apt for our times: *hard times are here and also lie ahead*. Nonetheless, hard times can be catalysts for development and improvement.[45] In any times, an emphasis on the key ethical principles and values, such as trust and mutual respect, enhances the relationships between practitioner, patient, and other healthcare workers, and makes for a more satisfying practice.[46]

Studies suggest that healthcare professionals experience less burn-out and cynicism if they remain in touch with the meaning and significance of what they do.[47] Medical trainees find benefit from ethics awareness as well.[48] The "joys and challenges" of medical work can prevail over its discouragements if practitioners can "re-moralize" their practice. They can do so by making connections with patients, by recognizing them as unique persons with always fascinating stories, and by remembering the opportunities we have to make remarkable and unforgettable differences in their lives.[49] Ethical sensitivity can help patients and clinicians alike by enabling them to recognize and strive for best possible outcomes not only in good times but also in hard times: when resources are scarce, practices criticized, and outcomes uncertain. Assiduous attention to ethical concerns can help those involved do their best to do what seems right and feel confident they have done so. This enriches us all. Hard times, perhaps, but also exciting times when we are able to combine science with humanism to renew medicine, "the greatest benefit to mankind."[50]

Ethics Matters
Doing Ethically Sound Medicine

The mental and moral, like the muscular powers, are improved only by being used.

John Stuart Mill, 1859[1]

The foundations of moral motivations are not the procedural rules on a kind of discourse, but the feelings to which we can rise. As Confucius saw long ago, benevolence or concern for humanity is the indispensable root of it all.

Simon Blackburn, 2001[2]

I. Ethical Reasoning and Principles in Medicine

As healthcare professionals, we frequently encounter ethical dilemmas in our work with patients—situations where we have to make a decision about what to do when there are conflicting options. Although we want to do the right thing, just what that is may not be obvious. How do we assess what is right? Is it right for the patient? For his or her family? For ourselves? For co-workers, our profession, or society?

In this chapter we will be introduced not only to the basic principles of medical ethics, but also to an analytic tool to help effectively manage moral problems in healthcare. The best way to *learn* medical ethics is to consider cases and how healthcare professionals should respond to them. The best way to *do* medical ethics is, of course, to apply what you learn to the real world of medicine and patients. You will have to do *that* on your own time.

We begin with a case familiar to clinicians and patients. We will then consider two other cases that illustrate troubling ethical situations and end with a deeper exploration of a more challenging case.

CASE 1.1 TO PRESCRIBE OR NOT TO PRESCRIBE

You are a young primary care practitioner in the downtown core of a large city. You see a new patient, a 32-year-old factory worker, Mr M, who has been unwell for 24 hours with a runny nose, aching muscles, a dry cough, and hoarseness. Apart from some tender muscles, his physical examination is normal; indeed, he barely seems ill. You say, "We can get to the moon, but we cannot cure the common cold. It will get better on its own."

Unconvinced, Mr M requests an antibiotic because he "always got one from the clinic down the road." He then, rather loudly, voices concern that you do not really have the experience or skills to make the proper diagnosis. "I felt so under the weather today that I couldn't go to work! How do you know I don't have one of those new superbugs I heard about? One of my buddies at work picked something up. He went to see his doctor who said it was nothing and the next thing you know he's almost dead in the ICU."

Is there an ethical issue here? Should you do what the patient requests or what you, the professional, think is appropriate?

DISCUSSION OF CASE 1.1

There is a conflict here between what you, a trained health professional, believe is the right treatment for the patient and what the patient wants or believes he needs. The choice seems to be either to prescribe the antibiotics or not to do so.

In this case there are some pros for prescribing antibiotics:

- the healthcare practitioner may be mistaken about the nature of the patient's illness;
- the patient may benefit because of a placebo effect;
- they can be prescribed quickly, and the patient will not go away disappointed.

However, there are many cons to prescribing unnecessary antibiotics:

- they drain away scarce medical resources;
- they may cause side effects;
- they may encourage resistant organisms to grow;
- they perpetuate the idea of a quick cure for every illness.

Although patients have the right to voice their wishes for treatment, such preferences should not always be granted. As a general rule, practitioners should provide only the care likely to help their patients. Granted, the line between helpful and useless care may not always be clear (and can be quite contentious, as we will see in future chapters), but the overuse of drugs, especially antibiotics, is well known. As well, each time clinicians give in to inappropriate demands for tests or treatment, their ethical fibre is weakened, making it less likely they will act properly in other situations and "hold the line."

Rather than a blanket refusal, you should take some time to talk with Mr M. Perhaps he felt your response to his request was dismissive of his concerns. Inquire about his expectations, find out more about his background, and spend a little time explaining the reasoning behind your reluctance to prescribe the antibiotic. Although time is at a premium in modern-day healthcare practices, time spent listening to the patient can be time well spent. If Mr M remains unconvinced, you *might* propose a compromise: offer to call his pharmacy in a day or two with a prescription if he is not improving. However, sometimes even *this* degree of compromise is inappropriate, given the contemporary concerns over antibiotics.[3] Indeed, if it is clear that antibiotics are not going to help, it is better and more professional just to say no.

Principles

Principles are fundamental elements of a moral system and refer to ideas or beliefs that come first or are primary considerations. "Doing right" can mean many things: following the proper rules, treating others fairly, acting out of good intentions, or seeing that the "good" is done or achieved. Patients are due care that will fulfill the basic goals of medicine to alleviate suffering or prevent illness and premature death. This task can be captured as the moral obligation of healthcare professionals to act according to the principle of beneficence. But in modern healthcare there is an equally compelling and, at times, *more* compelling obligation: to be guided by the principle of respect for persons and for personal autonomy. This means providing care that patients will find beneficial according to their *own* values and beliefs, care that also helps to empower them and maximize their opportunities for "self-actualization." This is what "patient-centred" care should be about.

Conflict resolution

The principles of beneficence and autonomy may be congruent or may appear to conflict. Trouble lies ahead for the clinician and patient if such principles or conflicts go unrecognized and are not properly addressed. The first step is to recognize and acknowledge that there *is* an issue, often rooted in an apparent disagreement, or "dis-ease," between clinician and patient. The skilled practitioner is sensitive to such issues, and tries to resolve the conflict in an open and principled, professional way.

One aspect of Case 1.1, for example, is the patient's criticism of the clinician's expertise. It is important not to ignore this, as an adversarial relationship has already been set up that may hinder good patient care. The patient may view the clinician as dismissive and uncaring, which does not augur well for a "therapeutic alliance." Rather than openly addressing the patient's criticism, the practitioner might be tempted to write the patient off as difficult and demanding, and ignore legitimate concerns.

Beyond principles

Adhering to ethical principles will not resolve every real-world dilemma. The modern philosopher Frankfurt argues there are other concerns—familial, cultural, or religious—that an individual may consider more important than ethical considerations in making a decision.[4] Moral agents may, for example, be swayed from doing the right thing by lack of fortitude, fear or intimidation, discriminatory attitudes, or local mores (not mutually exclusive facts).

The tension of ethics versus "non-moral" factors applies particularly to healthcare trainees in subordinate positions who may be uncertain of their rights.[5] In hospitals, power and prestige traditionally seemed to often hold sway over sense and reason.[6] That is, one did things, right or wrong, because of "doctors' orders" and feared for one's professional survival if they weren't followed. Doctors were at the top of the heap (and specialists on top of generalists), other health professionals next, and patients usually last. (Or at least that was the perception anyway; sometimes fear or intimidation, like the power of the wizard in the Wizard of Oz, is in the mind of the beholder.[7]) This hierarchy continues to some degree today (and more in some places than others). Physician assistants and nurses may be asked to undertake tasks or perform procedures they consider wrong.[8] Likewise, junior medical trainees may still be subject to intimidation. For example, a survey conducted by University of Toronto medical students revealed that about half their class had experienced or witnessed ethical misbehaviour, such as being asked to perform pelvic examinations on anesthetized patients just prior to surgery.[9] Such infractions are common and not unique to one country or one medical school.[10]

A hidden curriculum

That hierarchically-induced unethical practices still exist in many places is a measure of the degree to which various institutions such as medicine remain "under-moralized." Something is wrong—in rigid hierarchies, there is a power imbalance with too little ethical regulation—and health-care could do better. More ethics awareness could help even out an uneven terrain. Under-moralized practices in education create what has been called the "informal" or "hidden" curriculum that can escape scrutiny. This can dominate teaching and care at a clinical level and override abstract classroom lessons about ethics. Ethical principles do not always come first.

Here is one such case.

CASE 1.2 A RISKY TEACHING TOOL

A fourth-year medical student on a two-week elective in anesthesia is observing a patient being intubated in preparation for surgery. Suddenly, the staff anesthetist removes the patient's endotracheal tube, asking the student to show him how he would re-intubate the patient. Not surprisingly, the student cannot do so and the staff person must eventually do the re-intubation himself. The student feels embarrassed about his failure and does not mention the episode to anyone until much later.

What should the student have done at the time?

DISCUSSION OF CASE 1.2

This situation is unacceptable for many reasons. The student is unprepared and the patient's well-being is endangered.[11] As well, such action is an assault upon the patient, unless the patient had given prior consent to this teaching lesson. The student feels overwhelmed and unable to see past his own embarrassment to do anything about it: is the staff physician simply mistaken about the trainee's capacities? Or is he in the habit of challenging novice learners? Such pedagogic practices are liabilities, whether or not this particular patient suffers some tangible adverse outcome related to the failed intubation. The not-so-hidden message is that it's acceptable to treat patients in this fashion.

Although intimidated, the student could tell the supervisor how difficult the situation is for him (this may not be a realistic option, however—a clinician who teaches in this way is not likely to let a trainee question his pedagogic technique!). Failing an adequate response from the staff physician, there should be another hospital or university resource for the student to access, such as a student advocacy office, where concerns are taken seriously.

There is no easy way to overcome such roadblocks to acting ethically in practice. If you are the one encountering them, you should not ignore your feelings of outrage, disappointment, and sadness. You could start by seeking support from your peers. Then, if the ethical infraction is serious, consider having a second, perhaps more tactful, conversation with other clinicians, sympathetic teachers, or members of the healthcare institution's administration. It is critical to act and to raise your concerns in some venue; it is only by the voiced opinions of many people that institutions and unethical routines change. This is the value of virtue (and the "danger" of critical thinking): it can call into question the established order of healthcare.

The institutions of medicine *are* changing. Hitherto, there were few, if any resources to address ethical infractions within institutions. There are now complaints processes, patient advocates, patient safety offices, bioethics departments, and so on—all of which can lend sympathetic ears to disenchanted staff and learners, as well as to patients and families. Many medical schools also now have, or should have, resources to help trainees, troubled by the medical hierarchy, to raise issues with less fear of reprisal.

The role of virtues

It can be challenging for moral agents to know when to defy versus when to go along with unethical practices. Virtues play an important role in this discriminating ability. These are the character traits and attitudes that incline people to recognize and to do the right thing. Virtues such as honesty, trustworthiness, reliability, and the capacity for empathy are some of the traits of the "good clinician." Other virtues include fortitude, courage, prudence, and altruism. Deeds that abide by or arise from virtues are typically considered good actions. Indeed, it is hard to see how one would denote a performance or practice as right or good if the person involved is motivated by the opposite of virtue—vice—with characteristics such as dishonesty, avarice, or prejudice. What is unique about virtues is that they are those personal characteristics we would generally promote or encourage in others.[12]

From where do virtues come? In the classical philosophy of Aristotle, one came to know the "good" by *doing* good deeds. The virtuous agent is not born with virtues but provided "by nature" with the capacity to receive them and then to act on them. The more one practises doing right, the more likely one will learn how to act properly. Through practice, each person in particular circumstances should be able to properly judge for him or herself what to do. "Moral virtue . . . is formed by habit, *ethos* . . . Whether one habit or another habit is inculcated in us from an early age makes all the difference."[13] This seems true indeed; environmental factors in early childhood no doubt have a profound influence on one's moral development and "doing right" can be habituated.

But "doing right" and achieving good ends cannot rest with an acquired sense of what is right and wrong alone. It may tell you it's wrong to steal your mother's jewelry but not whether it is wrong to do so if your life depends on it. In complicated and novel situations you may need some rules and regulations to guide you. This is one role for "practical wisdom" or "prudence." Knowing when and how to follow the rules, as well as when and how one may bend or break them, requires some knowledge of ethics and the law.

Ethical values *should* outweigh other considerations in most instances. Indeed, today, institutions are increasingly aware of their moral mandate. Universities, hospitals, regulatory colleges, and so on, are there to ensure that clinicians and trainees act on *professional* moral concerns and not on less appropriate values, such as naked self-interest, or on vices such as dishonesty, disrespectfulness, or greed.

The role of law

Following laws and regulations seems the suitable route to choose by many. Yet the law often does not address, let alone provide a resolution of, difficult moral issues. Established legal precedent—the kind of law that healthcare professionals like to know—may come many years after a moral issue arises, too late to help the practising clinician. It is problematic to accept the law uncritically, as a gold standard for ethically exemplary practice, because the law can itself be immoral and unjust.[14]

A healthcare professional's critique of law should derive from the intrinsic values of medicine. Laws that may interfere with offering proper care to patients, for example, are ethically questionable. For instance, the requirement in many countries to report illegal immigrants (who then may be subject to summary deportation, even if critically ill) should be called into question by healthcare professionals.[15]

How openly a healthcare professional should defy such laws or practices depends on the social context and the fortitude of the practitioner. Where the consequence might be imprisonment, open opposition obviously may not be a wise option. Practitioners might better pursue safer routes of defiance such as advocating to have the law changed or seeking support from the international community.

This issue regarding the limits of the law says something important about ethics. Doing right, thinking critically, is not always the path of least resistance. Following moral rules and acting virtuously may require some degree of risk and hazarding self-sacrifice. In challenging the under-moralized aspects of society, you are allowed to pick the battles you are capable of winning and want to win.

Are healthcare professionals special?

In 1967, Dr Reg Perkin, one of the founders of the College of Family Physicians of Canada, instructed senior level medical students that, throughout their careers as physicians, they will have their ethics continu-ally examined—by their patients, their peers, and society. He went on to say

> Physicians are . . . recognized as being in a class set apart . . . The practice of medicine asks more morally of the practitioner than the community as a whole asks of its members . . . The professional . . . is expected to go the second mile [for his or her patient].[16]

These wise words still ring true today. His words, however, pertain not just to doctors but also to the members of any regulated healthcare profession. Moral courage, altruism, and trustworthiness are virtues that all healthcare professionals should try to exhibit. Whether physicians or any other healthcare practitioners have a special obligation to counter society's ills is an open question. Some days it is hard enough just to do your job. Going the extra mile for one's patients may be far enough.

II. Three Ethical Principles and Questions

How can you prepare yourself, as a healthcare professional, to provide good care? Let's start with where ethics begins in medicine: the connec-tions between people. Medical care is especially all about connections—about lending a helping hand to those in need. It's about the relations among physicians, allied healthcare providers, patients, and families. There are people in need and we want to help them. To do so we need to understand as well as we can, no matter where we work, the stories that lie behind a patient's presentation.

Narrative-based medicine is a helpful adjunct in this task by empha-sizing the depth of, and the meaning to be found in, these complex stories (see Box 1.1.). Ethical perspectives can, in turn, help us put these stories into an order that makes sense, from which we can learn lessons for the future, and that can be applied to other cases. In this chapter we look at a "decision procedure," or better an ethics "work-up," applicable to ethically challenging cases that we may encounter in our day-to-day work.

BOX 1.1

Some strategies for narrative medicine are[17]

- ask patients, "What would you like me to know about you?";
- don't interrupt;
- elicit patients' views of their condition;
- ask patients about the impact of the illness on their lives;
- don't forget to assess patient distress and suffering;
- examine your assumptions and stereotypes about patients and their culture;
- see patient noncompliance as a hidden story.

Central to the ethics work-up are the ethical duties of healthcare professionals to provide beneficial care and show respect for patients. These responsibilities are always relevant to medical practice—the "*prima facie*" duties—and are meant to be followed unless there is some stronger reason not to do so. Certain authors have analyzed these duties as deriving from the key moral principles of medical practice. It is their analyses I use in this book.[18] The principle-based analysis has its limitations, as it can fail to capture the complexity and nuances of real-life cases.[19] Nevertheless, it is a very helpful way to become familiar with the core ethical responsibilities of healthcare practitioners generally as well as the ethical expectations of the public.

The ethical principles fundamental to healthcare are well-known: autonomy, beneficence, and justice. (In later chapters we will discuss each principle in greater detail.) In the beginning, in considering what should be done, the practitioner or trainee needs to ask and address three simple questions corresponding to those principles (see Box 1.2). This is the beginning of practical wisdom.

BOX 1.2

The core ethical questions are

1. What are the patient's wishes and values? (Autonomy)
2. What can be done for the patient and what are the harms and benefits? (Beneficence)
3. Is the patient being treated fairly and can his or her needs be satisfied? (Justice)

These questions lead to three basic duties that are almost always relevant to every healthcare practitioner's everyday clinical practice. We should

- listen to patients and respect their wishes and values;
- seek to prevent harm to patients and serve their interests; and
- strive to ensure patients get treatment they are "fairly" due.

The last two duties are recognized in the traditional Hippocratic Oath.[20] What is new in modern medicine is the importance attached to the patient's perspective.

The principle of autonomy

The medical encounter often begins with a simple question, "What can I do for you today?" or "How can I help you?" These questions immediately put the clinician at the service of the patient. What are the patient's concerns, wishes, and values? Consider, for example, the competent patient's wishes for treatment. So long as these are informed wishes that do not contravene any other important moral principles, the patient's wishes should guide his or her treatment. While the "patient's agenda" sets the tone for a meeting, it does not always "rule the roost." Patient-based medicine is a collaborative enterprise. A good clinician will listen but also question the patient to be able to understand the issues as the patient sees them. This is more challenging if the patient is incapable. Others—the clinician in collaboration with a patient "proxy" or, better termed, a "substitute decision-maker"—will usually be called upon to help make decisions as the patient would have. This can be a treacherous road to take, with many pitfalls waiting for the unwary. We will discuss these issues throughout this book.

The principle of beneficence

Having (at least initially) established the patient's main concerns, the skillful clinician will carefully attend to his or her professional "agenda." The appropriate dialogue with the patient begins by initiating a conversation and a set of focused questions in order to better establish what troubles the patient. Problems can arise when healthcare professionals make assumptions about what their patients believe, value, or should do, or what resources, financial and social, patients have at their disposal. They need to know *what life is like* for their patients, what it means to step into their shoes.[21] This can only happen by conversation, listening, examination, and careful observation.

The principle of justice

This principle includes that of fairness: is a person receiving his or her fair share of scarce resources? A patient's wishes and concerns are rarely considered in isolation from the needs of others: will other persons, such as the family, other patients, or professional staff, be unduly burdened by the treatment chosen? The job of the clinician is to try to access appropriate, not inordinate, care for patients and to attempt to give priority of focus to the needs of those patients, all the while not ignoring the impact of the recommendations on the interests of others—not an easy task. There is always a social background for our medical recommendations.

Non-maleficence: "Above all, do no harm"

I have not made non-maleficence a fundamental principle. This is the Hippocratic principle of *primum non nocere* ("above all, do no harm"), the oldest and seemingly least controversial moral rule in medicine. For our purposes this principle can be included in the principle of beneficence. Other things being equal, the wise practitioner would, of course, recommend the intervention that would result in no possibility of harm to the patient.[22]

Unfortunately, truly non-maleficent interventions are rare in medicine. Even simple interventions, such as taking a venous blood sample or discussing a diagnosis with a patient, involve some small risk of harm, even if done well. While many healthcare professionals refer to the non-maleficence principle, it rarely serves as a guiding principle for medical practice. Otherwise, some fear, "therapeutic nihilism" (the view that *all* medical treatment is worse than the disease) may ensue.[23] Skepticism about medical interventions can be appropriate, as much of what we practitioners do is not helpful or can actually harm patients. At times a wait-and-see attitude, rather than intervening with risky or uncertain measures, is the better route to take. (See Chapter 5 on the "zero option.")

Think of "do no harm" as an ideal to be incorporated into the principle of beneficence. The best choice is the option where the benefits outweigh the harm. Although there are evil clinicians about (such as the now deceased Harold Shipman in the UK who killed several hundred patients in the late twentieth century before being arrested), most clinicians do not go to work with the conscious intent to harm their patients.[24] They can act maleficently, however, as a result of ignorance, incompetence, dishonesty, mental illness, or, when faced with the "reality" of rationing (see Chapter 9 on justice), lack of fortitude. They can also do harm to patients by being overly aggressive with unproven therapies.[25]

Patient-centred harm and benefit

In general, harm and benefit cannot be purely objective notions. They must be defined with some input from the patient and tailored to that patient's situation. What might be a great harm to one patient could be relatively no harm at all to another. Lack of awareness of a patient's values is one factor that can lead practitioners to inadvertently act in a maleficent manner (see Chapter 7 on beneficence).

CASE 1.3 DESPERATE HOPES

A 46-year-old man, Mr H, dying of multiple myeloma, has fought the disease every step of the way with a remarkable determination to live. He has undergone every known treatment—bone marrow transplantations, experimental therapies, naturopathic remedies. Mr H is now thin and wasted and on dialysis. The disease has, it seems, finally reached its terminal stages, and he has but a few weeks to live. He recognizes he is dying but refuses to agree to a "palliative care only" order. For him this would mean giving up. He wants any extra moment of life that aggressive interventions might give him. His treating team wants to transfer him to a palliative care facility which could better serve his many needs. The patient refuses this.

Mr H seems to be asking his caregivers to break the *primum non nocere* rule: he is asking them to do something that will almost certainly cause him more harm than good.

Is this ever acceptable?

DISCUSSION OF CASE 1.3

Desperate situations can lead to desperate hopes, and this is probably one of them. If we strictly followed the non-maleficence principle, we might not agree to the dying man's request to continue to receive aggressive care. On balance, however, it is Mr H's life and his death. On his scale of values it would be better to try likely futile gestures than none at all. The clinician needs to understand how Mr H views his circumstances. He may believe that accepting palliative care means others will give up on him. He would have to be reassured otherwise by deed and attitude of those looking after him that this would not be so.

Empathic communication, such as the questions and comments given below, can enable care providers to understand the story behind the patient's perspective and help address the impasse.

- What do you understand about your situation now?
- What are you hoping for?

- How do you want things to be when you die?
- Tell me how you feel about all of this.
- It sounds like you are worried we will give up on you. We won't and we will do everything we can to help you in your illness.[26]

This conversation tries to close the gap between patient and care providers by acknowledging the patient's perspective and assuring him he will not be abandoned. The right response to this patient is the exercise of compassion[27]—"to suffer with" the patient—to not abandon him or show him indifference, but to try to see what life is like for him, at his life's end, and hope that "going the extra mile" for this patient may help loosen his fixation on technology.

III. "Resolving" Ethical Dilemmas

Various formal approaches to "resolving" ethical dilemmas were developed some time ago by, among others, Lo, Thomasma, Siegler, and McCullough.[28] All have used some variety of the "ethics principles" approach and presumed an organized approach to understanding an ethical dilemma in medicine is helpful to its appropriate resolution. Thomasma deemed such an organized approach an "ethics work-up" to make it seem familiar to medical students used to "working up" the causes of a patient presenting with, for example, new onset heart failure or fever of unknown origin.

The importance of circumstances

In ethical matters, as in other matters, the right people must be involved for good decision-making. It is not surprising to find great variance in this. The people involved, the circumstances of the case, and the milieu will often help to determine the "right thing" to do. Doing right for a particular patient will mean being aware of such circumstances as

- institutional regulations;
- local laws;
- the attitudes of your fellow healthcare professionals;
- your emotions; and
- your cultural background and that of the patient and his or her "significant others."

This cultural factor may seem overwhelming in some circumstances (See Chapter 12 on cross-cultural care). Issues such as race, class, gender, income, and education—of the healthcare practitioner and the patient and the similarities or gaps between the two—have an obvious impact on the care that may be requested and that can be provided.[29] Factor in the cultural norms and practices in the communities where practitioners and their patients reside and you have fertile grounds for seemingly insoluble problems. Ethics cannot treat patients as abstract entities but must be able to recognize their distinctness and individuality. We are "diversely diverse," as the economist Amartya Sen has written.[30]

Importantly, as ethics may risk very real sacrifices and may involve hard choices, whatever solution is proposed, one should try to consider what the opinion of a disinterested or hypothetical decision-maker would be. Most importantly, ask yourself: "Is this what a ('reasonably') good person would do?" If you cannot in good faith answer this (admittedly, somewhat vague) question, it suggests you may not be ready to address or resolve the dilemma.

Really hard choices are not always about ethics

The decision procedure here outlined is not a moral algorithm that will churn out right answers to any dilemma like a sausage-making machine. As well, not all dilemmas are *ethical* dilemmas; many difficult decisions concern matters of living—so-called "existential" dilemmas. The most heartbreaking example I can think of is in the movie *Sophie's Choice*, based on the book by William Styron, in which a mother is forced to decide which one of her two children she must give up to the Nazis and certain death.[31]

There is nothing that Philosophy can do that could ever make such a choice right in any way. This situation really has nothing to do with ethics as there are no reasons that could ever justify forcing a parent to make such a decision in the first place and no good moral reasons to choose among the alternatives Sophie faced. The feelings of distress and guilt accompanying this type of dilemma are inescapable. In the aftermath one could only listen to, exhibit compassion towards, and bear witness with the person in despair.

IV. "Doing Right": A Decision-Making Procedure for Clinical Ethics

The procedure for analyzing and addressing ethical problems in the care of patients (clinical ethics) has eight steps (see Box 1.3). Keep in mind that case resolutions do not always follow every step. In some instances it will be obvious how to proceed after a few moments' reflection because one ethical principle or the context may suggest the best way to proceed. The full procedure is most helpful for deciding difficult cases or when you wish to ensure that your decision is backed up by careful reflection.

Step 1. Recognize that a case raises an important ethical problem.

Ethical problems arise, as suggested earlier, when there is a seeming conflict of values or ethical principles leading to different paths of action. For example, the relatives of an elderly woman with dementia wish to have her placed in a nursing home, something she refuses to consider (safety versus autonomy); a patient does not want his sexual partner to know he carries the hepatitis B virus (confidentiality vs non-maleficence); a 15-year-old girl, 16 weeks pregnant, is resisting the abortion her parents insist she have (autonomy versus beneficence). In all these cases, clinicians must make a difficult decision about what to do or to recommend. Remember, however, *it is the patient who has the problem*. We are there to help patients worry through the problem and the possible choices—not necessarily solve it for them, but to help them solve it.

It is important to be as knowledgeable as possible about the situation. You should know the most relevant aspects of the patient's life story and family context, his or her medical condition, the working diagnosis, and the various treatment options as well as their associated burdens and benefits. A true ethics consultation for a case will usually not rest content with the kind of "thin" case studies used (due to space limitations) in this book. The devil, they say, often lies in the details, but sometimes in the details is the angel, the best solution to the case.

Step 2. What is the problem that has to be solved?

State what you take to be the central problem. This is often the most important step. Should the woman with dementia be institutionalized without her consent? Should the partner of the hepatitis patient be informed of his partner's condition? Should parents have a say in their daughter's decision?

Always be clear on what needs to be resolved. Seemingly intractable ethical problems can arise when the participants are not asking the same question. For example, a family resists for some time the transfer of their cognitively impaired father to another ward. Consultation reveals the problem is not that the family wants something inappropriate; the problem is a disagreement among the siblings. What they need is help as a family in resolving their differences. When this is achieved, a solution to the ward problem is found. Sometimes an ethical dilemma turns out to be a communication problem or a cultural factor or an issue for Psychiatry. Once the problem is precisely identified, you will be better able to decide what resources you'll need to resolve it.

Step 3. Determine reasonable alternative courses of action.

Asking what is the right thing to do for the patient presupposes there are alternative procedures—usually two or three—for this patient. The list of options need not be exhaustive, but clear alternatives should be given. They may be quite simple: for example, either the woman with dementia should be placed or not; the partner should be told or not; the parents should have a say in their daughter's decision or not. The final resolution of the case will probably be one of these options or some compromise among them.

Step 4. Consider each option in relation to the three fundamental ethical principles.

This is a critical and difficult step. The ethical healthcare practitioner or trainee is expected to utilize and consider the three fundamental ethical principles of autonomy, beneficence, and justice. Knowing just how to interpret the principles in light of circumstances and the agents involved can be problematic. What to do when the principles seemingly conflict is another, and not infrequent, problem. Broadly speaking, the patient's wishes come first, but the acceptability of these wishes will sometimes depend upon the medically possible and culturally plausible options. You obviously need not agree to fulfill a patient's wishes if they are illegal, immoral (even if locally accepted), or unusually burdensome to others. For example, for the woman with dementia who refuses to leave her home, you will want to weigh the significance of her wish against its effect on her well-being and the safety of others. Does she pose a risk serious enough to outweigh her wish? What if she is a smoker—in bed? What if she is prone to leaving the stove on? Or wanders in the snow shoeless?

Step 5. Consider who should be involved and other circumstances.

You will want to ensure, insofar as this is possible, the right people—other healthcare providers, clinicians—are brought into the patient's circle of care and consulted. If the patient is not capable or is doing something potentially harmful and acting out of character you should attempt to contact the patient's family or substitute decision-maker. You may also need to involve others, such as a public guardian or a local sage or healer, who may have been appointed or may be expected to "look after" an incapable person in their community.

You should also consider other circumstances, such as institutional policies, professional guidelines, cultural norms, and personal or emotional factors. In deciding what to do for the woman with dementia, for example, you will have to take into account specific factors such as legislation that might allow an incapable person to be removed from her home. You may also wish to reflect on practical matters such as how strenuously the patient would resist being "placed" without her consent.

Step 6. Decide on a resolution to the problem.

You must take a stand as to what you think is the right course of action. Try to follow your best guess as to the right thing to do, all things considered. Your conclusion may be disputed, so you should be able to justify your choice as the best one. Be flexible—if the evidence changes, be prepared to change.

Step 7. Consider your position critically.

Before and after the decision, keep an open mind and consider what could be done differently. The reflective practitioner will ask: *under what circumstances would I/we advocate a different course of action*? It may help to formulate one's position as a general "maxim" or principle. For example, if you decide the woman with dementia should be allowed to stay at home, you might generalize this into a statement such as: persons with dementia may stay at home providing they are not putting others in danger. The next step would be to consider the limits of such a principle. What if the impaired person refused any help or monitoring of his or her condition? What if she didn't smoke but had weak legs, which could result in a high risk of falling down the stairs? What if the society has no home-support resources for patients with dementia?

At the end of the day, ask yourself: will you be able to sleep soundly given your decision? Would you be comfortable if your decision were to be made public? Will your colleagues stand behind you? If they will not step forward to support you, this may be telling you something you should not ignore. If you or others feel ill at ease with the decision, carefully reconsider the main features of the case. Take into account the cultural or ethnic factors that may result in differing views. Where no option seems right, compromises may have to be made.

Also, consider what *your* role would be in achieving what you take to be the right choice. Do not be pushed by abstract ethical principles to do something your conscience or emotions tell you is wrong. Emotions can be a helpful corrective to reason.[32] One's conscience, emotional reaction, and, yes, intuition in relation to a case can provide reasonable brakes on action. They can represent your deepest values, identity, and integrity as a professional. For example, you can in good conscience refuse to go along with a practice, such as abortion, that you find morally objectionable (but in consideration of concern for the patient, you may have some obligation to refer the patient to another doctor—see Chapter 10 on abortion).[33] Not all moral disagreements can be readily settled. In the end, people in disagreement have to learn to work with one another or agree to disagree.

Step 8. Do the right thing!

This step should go without saying but there are many roadblocks to acting ethically in practice. Doing the right thing may be difficult because of conflicting loyalties, cultural differences, survival needs, and extreme circumstances like war and natural disasters. Professional ethics may seem a slim reed to grasp onto in extreme situations. Those who do cleave to the moral route in such circumstances may fare better in the long run than those who shuck their ethics, as if it were a mere moral carapace, for the "easy" thing to do. Although the right thing is not always easy to do, attempting to do it allows you to develop your "moral muscles," as Mill wrote.[34] Learning ethics by doing was Aristotle's view: the virtuous person learns to be "good" by habitually doing or, at least, trying to do the right thing, and in so doing developing "moral dispositions."[35]

BOX 1.3

The ethics decision-making procedure

1. The case: express simply but with pertinent facts and circumstances.
2. What is the dilemma? What decision needs to be made?
3. What are the alternatives?
4. How do the key considerations apply?

- (a) Autonomy: what are the patient's wishes and values?
- Consider the patient's capable wishes, beliefs, goals, hopes, and fears. If incapable, look to a substitute decision-maker.
- (b) Beneficence: what can be done for the patient?
- Consider the benefits and burdens of the various alternatives from the perspective of the clinician, the patient, and possibly the family, and the probable result of each one.
- (c) Justice: is the patient receiving what is fair?
- Consider the patient's fundamental right to his or her fair share of medical resources as well as the interests and claims of the family, other patients, and healthcare staff.

---

5. Consider involving others and consider context: are there other situational factors that are important? Consider others who ought to be involved. Be familiar with cultural and local practices, institutional policies and guidelines, professional norms, and legal precedents.
6. Propose a resolution: weigh these factors for each alternative; then say what you would do or recommend. Consider, in the circumstances, what your role would be—what would a "good person" do?
7. Consider your choice critically: when would you be prepared to alter it? Consider the opinions of your peers, your conscience, and emotional reactions. Know your resources. Formulate your choice as a general maxim and how far it might extend, suggest cases where it wouldn't apply, decide if you—and others—are comfortable with the choice made. If not, reconsider key considerations and consider consultations with specialists in ethics, law, or in the local culture.
8. Do the right thing—"all things considered."

A note on the cases

In this book I use many clinical vignettes to illustrate typical ethical problems in medicine. My discussion tends to be brief and pragmatic, using the ethics decision-making procedure as a template only. This procedure is assumed in many of the discussions; I do not pause to make each step explicit. A more in-depth analysis by the reader of each case is encouraged.

V. Applying the Ethics Decision-Making Procedure

Now, let's consider the use of the decision-making procedure in a complicated, controversial and very sad real-life case with which I was involved many years ago.

CASE 1.4 TO FEED OR NOT TO FEED?

Ms E, a 22-year-old woman ill since age 14 with severe anorexia nervosa, an illness of self-starvation, was brought into the emergency room in cardiovascular collapse. She was extremely emaciated, weighing less than 60 lbs., and virtually unresponsive. After receiving a bolus of intravenous glucose, she perked up just long enough to pull out her intravenous line.

Ms E had been admitted numerous times in her starved state and had spent most of her previous eight years in hospital. She had been considered one of the most "difficult" patients by specialty units of various tertiary care hospitals. All corrective therapy had failed. Drug therapy using antipsychotics and antidepressants was unsuccessful. Different psychotherapeutic approaches over many years—including cognitive-behavioral, family therapy, and even "paradoxical" therapy (admitting to the patient that she is going to die and hoping she will struggle against this pessimistic message)—had also been unsuccessful. On previous admissions she had nutritional rehabilitation, including force-feeding which required restraints and caused major disruptions on the ward. She had expressed a wish to die but not consistently so. She had recently told her family doctor that she wished her suffering would soon end and at that time requested no forced feedings in the future. She thought she was always overweight and did not believe her food refusals endangered her life. The various tertiary care hospitals refused her readmission because of her previous extreme resistance and disruptiveness.

The clinicians involved in her care considered the option of providing her nutrition through a gastrostomy tube (a tube inserted directly into her stomach through a small incision in the abdominal wall). This would have entailed a surgical procedure and putting her in physical restraints. "Forced feeding" would be considered a form of torture in other circumstances[36] so why would it be an acceptable form of treatment here?

What should have been done on this admission?

DISCUSSION OF CASE 1.4

1. The case
The first step is to acknowledge an ethical dilemma exists here. Sometimes we become so focused on what we are doing in medicine that we fail to question—wait a minute—what are we doing here? Are we sure about this? Should we be doing something different? Once these questions are raised, the ethical moment has been recognized. The care providers for this patient felt it was their duty to feed her but were troubled by the *consequences*—for the patient primarily, but for everyone else as well.

2. The problem
This case contains a number of problems, but the central one is whether the patient should be force-fed or not. The standard of care

for such patients is nutritional rehabilitation and weight restoration. Patients who do not respond require "higher levels of care"[37] including involuntary hospitalization and feeding by any means possible. Does the standard of care, however, require you to do so again and again with a protesting patient?[38] When might not feeding a starving patient ever be appropriate? How important are the interests of others when it comes to readmitting her?

3. The alternatives

Obviously, the central immediate problem of severe starvation and imminent vascular collapse posed the question of emergency fluid resuscitation and then pursuing the option of more aggressive force-feeding. What was the status of her recent wish not to be force-fed? Or her action of pulling out her intravenous line? Were these simply the products of a mind unbalanced by delusions (firm, fixed beliefs unamenable to criticism or evidence) and starvation? What if she had been resuscitated long enough to be conscious again? Would her wishes have been considered any more reliable? Not rehydrating her and not re-feeding at this critical point would result in her death.

4. Applying the principles

As rehydrating/feeding and not rehydrating/not feeding her are two sides of the same coin, let us consider the problem from the "not feeding" side. What are the pros and cons of not feeding her?

Autonomy

PRO: Not force-feeding was what the patient had previously requested, so this option accorded with her wishes.[39] For some people these days, anorexia is not so much an illness as a "life-style" choice.[40] This view is popular among some with the disorder and others who are resistant to the idea of psychiatric illness altogether.[41]

CON: While it appeared that this patient seemed to understand, when not in a starved state, what she was doing and the risks she was taking, it can be argued that this understanding was not competent and therefore not authentically autonomous (and therefore quite distinguishable from that of a person on a hunger strike for political reasons). Following her wishes would result in her death by starvation, an outcome she had not consistently or clearly requested. Perhaps her request for her suffering to be over was a wish for healing and not for death—it may have been a cry for more help, not less. Her failure to truly appreciate the consequences of self-starvation and prior refusal of all forms of nutritional rehabilitation, as is the case for many anorexic patients, made her views incapable and therefore unreliable.[42]

Beneficence

PRO: The benefits of not rehydrating/not force-feeding the patient included not prolonging her suffering and not having to restrain her to maintain the nutritional therapy. There was also an implicit recognition that Ms E was terminally ill and could not be rescued—it might, therefore, have been a "mercy" to let her go.

CON: The most important harm in not feeding her was obvious: the patient would die. This patient was delusional about her weight and engaging in self-destructive behaviour as a result. Although suicide and attempted suicide are not crimes in most jurisdictions, healthcare professionals are generally obliged to intervene when patients under their care place themselves at risk of death in the context of a mental illness.

Justice

PRO: The patient's care *per se* was not expensive but the demands on others were high. The family and healthcare staff felt burdened by her care. Letting her go would have relieved them of the emotional burdens of looking after her. As well, if treatment were truly futile, then resources would have been "wasted" in trying to keep someone alive who was doomed to die.

CON: As she was the patient, the focus of care must be on her, not others. She deserved her fair share of medical resources. One standard for this would be what treatment would other patients in her situation have received from a "reasonably competent practitioner"? Starving anorexic patients receive nutritional treatment, including force-feeding, if need be. A lack of resources was not an issue; thus, this intervention ("the standard of care") was due to her unless there were strong countervailing reasons.

5. Context

Contextual factors included the possible negative emotional reaction of staff to a difficult, "unlikable" and so, in their eyes, "untreatable" patient, not an ethical rationale at all. There were fears of legal liability, such as negligence, if the patient were allowed to die. Courts have generally ruled against forced feeding but that has usually been in the context of competent refusals of food, such as by prisoners who go on hunger strikes.[43]

6. One resolution

Autonomy triumphs—usually. On the other hand, when autonomy is thwarted by illness, we, as care providers, must try to "rescue" patients in harm's way (see Chapter 7 on the "rule of rescue" and its limits). It would seem to have been in the patient's best interests to rehydrate her on an emergency basis and subsequently offer nutritional therapy, as well as providing all other appropriate care for her, because she would otherwise die, something she had not consistently verbalized as her wish (although her body language spoke otherwise). This may have added burdens onto the staff and her family, but it is not clear that such burdens were intolerable. Their emotional reactions may indicate that the limits to their tolerance were being reached, however. Finally, while there is no legal duty to force-feed starving patients, there is an obligation to rescue incapable patients who are in imminent peril.[44] Weighing these factors together supports the position that this patient should have been resuscitated by fluids and food.

The options as to how this might best be done should be discussed with the appropriate substitute decision-maker, because the patient is currently incapable. If and when she ever seems to regain capacity over nutritional matters, the patient needs a careful assessment of the ability to authentically make a "food and fluids" decision. If she is found capable of making such a decision, her most authentic wishes ought to be explored: does she want to be saved again should the need arise even if she insists the opposite (a "Ulysses" contract) or is she suffering so much that she does not wish resuscitation (a "reverse Ulysses" contract)? (In the ancient myth of Ulysses, the Sirens were sea nymphs whose singing could reveal the way home to lost sailors but could also cause mariners to throw themselves into the ocean. Ulysses ordered his crew to stuff their ears with wax and to bind him to the mast of his ship and not release him, no matter what he said, until they passed safely by the Sirens' island. Indeed, as they sailed by, the Sirens' song was so sweet and attractive that Ulysses struggled to loosen his ropes, begging his men to release him. They ignored him and bound him even tighter until they were able to safely pass by. In a "reverse Ulysses" contract the sailor would ask *not* to be saved from the Sirens entreaties, and, so, presumably, be allowed to go to his doom.) It may seem odd, but if she ever *could* be found capable of making such a decision, her wishes would have to be respected in such circumstances. It is, however, unlikely she would be found so capable because patients with such severe anorexia are almost always delusional about sustenance.

7. Critical considerations

This position could be generalized into a principle such as "Incapable patients in danger of dying from self-starvation should receive non-voluntary nutritional rehabilitation." When might this be unacceptable? It would certainly seem so when the patient has a *competently* expressed wish not to be so fed. It would also be unacceptable when it is clear that further feeding can no longer benefit the patient. In other words, if the patient is going to die anyway, further feedings would be futile and should be withheld.[45] This might be the case if the patient had, for example, a terminal illness such as advanced cancer or advanced dementia. One need not give treatment that cannot achieve any reasonable medical goal. It may well be that the patient has already reached this near-death stage in this case. Although not suffering from a recognized terminal illness, it may be that she is so emaciated and so intractable in her belief that she is overweight that she cannot be rescued. The duty to rescue should be a proportionate one and not an excuse to torture the dying with extravagant therapy.[46] The care providers in the ER might win today's skirmish, were they to re-feed her, but the war is being lost.

8. Action required

The healthcare professionals should have proceeded to provide Ms E whatever rehydration and nutritional support was required, at least until a further assessment could have been done.

FOLLOW-UP TO CASE 1.4

This patient was, in fact, not resuscitated. After meeting with her family and obtaining consultations in hospital with the departments of Psychiatry and Internal Medicine, and the hospital ethics committee, her physicians deemed her terminally ill and, on grounds of compassion, did not rehydrate or force-feed her. She died shortly after being admitted.[47]

Of some concern is the possibility that the decision to limit care in this case was due to an unexplored animosity of the healthcare providers toward a seemingly hopeless and demanding patient. Did they give up too soon because she seemed incurable and imposed such a burden on others? Some hold that *no* patient with anorexia should be considered hopeless but this may be overly optimistic.[48] Would a better physician in a better institution have done better? Or would she have simply suffered more? Needless to say, such cases are very troubling for all concerned.

My own views have evolved in the years since I was involved in the care of this patient. I try to guard against negative reactions to patients that might lead to under-treatment while not ignoring the emotions invested in a patient that can lead to over-treatment. Emotions have an important role to play in healthcare: they cause us to *care* about what we do, as reason alone may not. Feelings, such as empathy, root us to what matters to us and to what we care about. Ethics is never just an intellectual enterprise.

Arguing for the importance of feeling and sentiment to moral judgment, the Scottish philosopher of the enlightenment, David Hume, wrote several centuries ago, "*Morality, therefore, is more properly felt than judged of.*"[49] I'm not sure that feelings are *more* important than judgments but they are not to be ignored. A "good person" marries emotion with reason. This is where one's personal psychology and virtues necessarily enter; virtues inform our intuitions about doing right. The virtue of prudence can stay the hand of an anxious clinician; the virtue of altruism can encourage a timid soul to expend extra effort for a patient. Feelings of benevolence—caring about our patients and a concern for humanity—ground and extend our ethical judgments. They allow our ethical "sympathies" to extend "beyond ourselves," indeed, to a "great distance," something even Hume's more limited view of reason in ethics avowed.[50]

Case 1.4 demonstrates how difficult the resolution of ethical dilemmas can be in the real world of everyday medicine. Facts are uncertain, wishes hard to ascertain, truth elusive, and authentic choice tenuous. Nevertheless, we should not cease seeking for a sense of the "truth" in our deliberations, that is, for "better" resolutions.[51]

Conclusion

Ethics is a complex and sometimes confusing field. In this chapter I have presented an approach to sorting out and addressing ethical dilemmas in medicine—a kind of ethics toolbox. It is a method of analysis to introduce some consistency in how healthcare professionals should view and manage moral questions in medicine. Future chapters will examine in more detail the ethical principles that form the foundation for the acceptable professional practice of modern medicine.

Cases for Discussion

CASE 1: SILENT WITNESS

You are in your first year of training in a healthcare profession. Recently learning about the dangers of suntanning, you have taken to cautioning your friends about melanoma, the most serious form of skin cancer. You've seen pictures of some pretty nasty looking lesions in your Dermatology atlas. One hot summer's day, as you are standing in a crowded bus going to school, you happen to notice a small but ominous-looking lesion on the posterior shoulder of a fellow passenger wearing a halter top. You have never seen her before.

Questions For Discussion

1. Is this an ethical dilemma? If so, how would you analyze the situation using the "ethics decision procedure"?
2. Would you say anything to her? If so, what? Under what circumstances would you *not* say something?
3. How do you think the public and the medical community view what should be done in these situations?

CASE 2: A FAMILY AFFAIR

You are a nurse practitioner working on the oncology service. On one of the wards is Mr O, a 72-year-old male admitted with nausea and ataxia. While in hospital he had several brief seizures and is now on phenytoin. An enhanced MRI revealed a thin coating of tumour wrapped around his brainstem: he has leptomeningeal carcinomatosis. This is an uncommon but very lethal condition that is virtually untreatable. Time to death after diagnosis is usually weeks to a few months.

Mr O does not know the diagnosis but his family does—they had an acquaintance in the MRI suite who tipped them off. The large and supportive family has formed a protective cordon about Mr O.

His wife, herself a doctor from another country, pleads with you not to tell Mr O what you know. "I know the prognosis for my husband is terrible. We have all come to accept that. Now we only want to be able to take him home and let him die there in peace," she says with tears in her eyes, "It would be cruel and do him no good to be told his exact diagnosis. We have told him he has a seizure disorder from a brain abnormality, that it cannot be fixed, and left it at that. In our country the patient is only told good news; anything else would only make him feel worse. We accept that it is the family's responsibility to look after the patient. You can't do anything for him, we will do everything for him."

Questions For Discussion

1. What are the ethical conflicts here? On which dilemma would you focus, if you were the healthcare practitioner in this case?
2. Discuss the issue of culture in deciding what to do in this case.

2 The Almost Revolution
Autonomy and Patient-Based Care

Autonomy, the liberty to live after one's own law.
Henry Cockerham, 1623[1]

Every human being of adult years and sound mind has a right to determine what shall be done with his own body.
Justice Cardozo, 1914[2]

The idea that individual patients should have the freedom to make choices about their lives and healthcare has *almost* revolutionized medicine over the past 50 years. In significant portions of the world, even in places not considered "democratic," the notion of "patient autonomy" has irreversibly changed how clinicians, patients, and the public think about acceptable medical care.

Eager for a stronger voice in social matters generally, citizens around the world are pressing for more liberty to make choices without fear or intimidation. They also expect healthcare, as with other hierarchical structures, to mirror these changes. Choice is an essential ingredient of modern medicine: effective care means patients can choose, if they so wish, among truly different options. Thus, in modern medicine, the right thing to do requires incorporating patient values and wishes into medical decision-making. The question is not *whether*, but *how* best to do so. Unfortunately, the sad reality throughout the world is of "massive inequalities in the opportunities different people have" to access known effective medical care.[3]

I. The Autonomy Principle

CASE 2.1 THE PATIENT'S AGENDA

Mr P, a 49-year-old overweight smoker, has poorly controlled hypertension and mildly elevated serum lipids. He also has a family history of heart disease: his father died at 52 of a massive myocardial infarction. You have worked a year with this patient as his family physician trying to get him to change, but to no avail. Weight loss is followed by weight gain, exercise by non-exercise, periods of abstinence from smoking followed by chain-smoking. (The patient quips, paraphrasing Mark Twain, "It's easy to quit smoking, I've done it hundreds of times!") His blood pressure today is 190/110.

Despite being cautioned about the threats to his health, he refuses for the umpteenth time to take any medications. "Doc," Mr P states, "I gotta do this on my own! I swear, see me in six months, I'll be a new man."

Should you threaten to terminate the therapeutic relationship if the patient continues in his self-destructive ways? Should you try to browbeat him with the cudgel of evidence? Should you sound the panic alarm?

DISCUSSION OF AND FOLLOW-UP TO CASE 2.1

This type of "non-compliant" patient can make health professionals contemplate changing careers! It's patient autonomy versus beneficence, right? The patient is an adult, possesses decision-making capacity, but exercises it in a seemingly self-destructive way. It would be easy to say he's mature, he's autonomous, let him be, or, alternatively, to see his decision-making as the product of some mental malady. One author, commenting on this sort of patient, writes: "The physician should do more than consider whether there is something wrong with the patient; the physician should ask what might be wrong with the doctor–patient communication."[4] Clinical care relying solely on a simple "logic of choice" ("it's all up to you, the patient, to decide . . .") seems anemic compared to the complexity of the "logic of care" (how clinicians and patients negotiate compromise) required for optimized patient outcomes.[5]

Indeed, communication is a root issue for many "non-compliant" patients. Rather than acting out of alarm or abandoning the patient, the clinician needs to better understand his fears and concerns (see Box 2.1).

As it turns out, the patient is worried about side effects from medication. Two years ago, his previous doctor had put him on pills causing erectile problems and swollen ankles, making him feel like an old man, he says. He stopped them and never went back to the doctor. He is in a new relationship now and wants nothing to do with pills that might interfere with his sex life.

Once these issues are addressed, the patient is willing to work at lifestyle changes and to try some alternative medications. Recognition and management of the ethical dilemma, by incorporating the patient's wishes (autonomy) with best-evidence care (beneficence), resolves the problem. While simple, there is something important in this kind of reasoning: it does not rely on the autonomy principle or the beneficence principle alone. Rather, the physician strives to do the right thing by taking into account the patient's preferences and experiences but does not forget the professional responsibilities of minimizing harm and maximizing a "good outcome." Just what a good outcome is will depend on the patient's perspective.

Patient-based interviewing

Patient-based medicine starts with attempting to understand patient needs and wants in the context of the patient's life. Patient-based interviewing creates an atmosphere of trust whereby the patient feels respected and heard—it is an essential step in establishing rapport between the healthcare professional and the patient (see Box 2.1).

BOX 2.1

The following are some guidelines for patient-based interviewing. After introducing yourself, try to

- be at eye level by sitting on the edge of the patient's bed or a chair;[6]
- put patients at ease with a touch or a handshake, if appropriate;
- avoid medical jargon and be sensitive to patient cues of fear, anxiety, and the like;
- allow the patient to finish his or her initial monologue;[7]
- facilitate communication by active listening: nodding, echoing, saying "hmm-hmm";
- elicit the patient's agenda: "What else?" "What other concerns do you have?";[8]
- prioritize if there are many issues: "You have a lot of concerns, what were you most hoping we could do today?";
- review with the patient: "What I hear you saying is . . ." "Is it all right if we focus on your main concern . . .";
- not prematurely reassure—first, hear the whole story. Pause and ask, "Let me see if I have this right . . ." Or, "Sounds like . . .";[9]
- be transparent: consider sharing your notes or your computer screen with the patient;[10] present the patient's story to your mentor in the patient's presence.

Patient-based care

Patient-based interviewing leads to "patient-based care" which is intimately bound up with the ethical notions of patient autonomy and respect for persons. Health professionals and their institutions are obliged to put patients' views and interests at the foundation of appropriate healthcare.

Respecting patients also implies an allegiance to a patient-based notion of benefit—benefit as seen and experienced by the patient. It does not entail a model of medicine as a business enterprise where the patient is a "client" or a "consumer" of bits of healthcare; neither "buyer beware," nor "the client-is-always-right" has any place in healthcare. Partly because power and information tend to flow *away* from the patient, it is an uneven playing field favouring the healthcare professional. The ethical practitioner must work at levelling out that field. Respect due persons, as a principle, applies to "capable" patients with the wherewithal to express their wishes as well as to those who, due to a defect in decision-making, are "incapable." (See Chapter 6 for the notions of capacity and competence.) Regarding *capable* persons, autonomy means two things:

1. having the right to decide what they want when it comes to healthcare; and
2. having the right to be treated in respectful ways by healthcare professionals.

Expressing these notions as "rights" implies that healthcare professionals have corresponding duties towards patients. Indeed, they do, but more is involved—if clinicians are to help patients live their lives as they desire (and they should do so, if the aims are reasonable ones), then this means not only respecting but also, at times, helping to promote and actualize the choices and values of capable patients.

Regarding *incapable* persons, autonomy requires the following:

1. showing fidelity to patients' prior capable views; and
2. treating those patients as individuals with inherent worth and dignity.

Among other things, the commitment to incapable individuals means attempting to restore or support their autonomy and help them actualize their capacities as much as possible. This is a social and political task, not just a medical one, as adequate resources are required to support and assist those living with disabilities or deprivations.

The meaning of autonomy

Autonomy is derived from the Greek "*autos*" meaning "self" and "*nomos*" meaning "rule" or "law." *Autonomous* patients are those capable of exercising deliberate and meaningful choices, choices consistent with their own values—making their own laws.[11] They are persons with the cognitive and emotional "competence" or "capacity" (in this book, I will not distinguish between these two terms) to make decisions for themselves. (This has obvious implications for decision-making that will be explored in Chapter 5 on consent.)

The opposite in a binary model are heteronomous patients who cannot, or will not, make decisions for themselves. Literally, they are subject to the laws of others. They may exhibit "decidophobia," an inability to compare alternatives and make decisions "with one's eyes open."[12] This may be because of familial, cultural, or social factors that encourage an inordinate (or appropriate or acceptable) dependence on others.[13] Heteronomy may also result from a lack of certain mental capacities, for example, as in a newborn or a comatose or severely demented patient or to a seeming "lack of will," as in depressive or compulsive disorders. It may also relate to aptitude and interest and can fluctuate with time or conditions. For example, although a person with deafness may be quite capable of communication, living in a non-signing community can make comprehension of his or her wishes difficult and has traditionally resulted in much prejudice against members of the Deaf culture.

The concept of a binary opposition of autonomy versus heteronomy will not suffice. The proper exercise of autonomy requires the right social conditions. Autonomy does not imply one must make all decisions by oneself.[14] An autonomous individual—capable, rational, well-informed—can relinquish or "waive" the right to make his or her own decisions in favour of a spouse, family unit, community, or the like. Alternatively, he or she can "share" the decision with, or relinquish it to, the healthcare professional, various others, or indeed, a whole community (be it secular, political, religious, fundamentalist[15]). Sharing our concerns with those to whom we are the closest can help us consider alternatives in a more well-rounded way and strengthen us as integral, rooted persons. This does not have to diminish our autonomy.

Autonomy as used in this book simply means being true to one's self. How one experiences and achieves this has much to do with one's family, the local culture, and mores. But there is a deep well of thought here. The seventeenth-century French Enlightenment philosopher and mathematician René Descartes' argument that the only statement of which one can be absolutely certain is *cogito ergo sum* ("I think, therefore I am") was a remarkably novel and radical departure from the punishing conformist attitude of the time.[16] Just think how radical Descartes' dangerous idea still is: only the individual can (and must) decide what is right and true; everything else—family, society, religion, god—is uncertain.[17] Once the self is recognized as the fount of decision-making and the locus of certitude, other ideas naturally flow from that—ideas about independence of thought and action, idiosyncrasy of interpretation, the right to be "wrong" and not be sanctioned for this, and so on.

Autonomy as the patient's preference

Autonomy as a principle makes the patient's own priorities and aspirations the focal point, although never the sole objective, of medical care. A healthcare practitioner ought not, in general, substitute his or her wishes and preferences for those of the patient, even if what the physician wants seems more likely to promote the patient's best interests. A successful medical encounter depends on the practitioner understanding and working with the patient's unique wishes, perceptions, and beliefs. (This leads to the notion of "concordance" to be explored in Chapter 5.)

CASE 2.2 PATIENT KNOWS BEST?

A patient, Ms N, had undergone menopause at age 54 in the mid-1990s. At the time she had significant menopausal symptoms (flushing) but was otherwise healthy. Her mother had died in her early sixties of heart disease. Her primary care physician, following well-established "evidence-based" guidelines at the time that recommended estrogen replacement therapy (ERT) to both alleviate menopausal symptoms and to lessen the risk of heart disease, suggested she start ERT soon. This, Ms N adamantly refused to do, believing that menopause was a natural process and should not be "medicalized."

How should a practitioner evaluate a patient's refusal of evidence-based "best care"?

DISCUSSION OF CASE 2.2

From an evidence-based point of view, this patient's refusal of therapy at that time might have seemed less than optimal because the benefits of ERT seemed the gospel truth. As it turned out the patient was quite prescient: the evidence from the 1990s *was* seriously flawed. Later research suggested that ERT increased cardiovascular risks as well as the risk of breast cancer. Obviously, Ms N was not irrational (far from it); she simply had different beliefs from her clinician. She preferred her symptoms and the risks of future problems (such as osteoporosis) to taking any hormonal therapy. Thus, abiding by the patient's choice was the right thing to do.

Despite "evidence" and guidelines, the right of patients to refuse recommended therapy—especially informed refusals such as this— ought to be respected and other avenues should be pursued to help them achieve the medical outcomes they have chosen (for example, to alleviate their symptoms and reduce the risks to their health). Healthcare professionals may overrate the success of new and approved treatments while patients, generally more risk-averse than clinicians, may be more skeptical of the latest medical fashion. The principle of patient autonomy entails respect for patients' decisions even if thought to be "sub-optimal." Clinicians are expected to provide patients with information and guidance needed to empower them to make authentic choices, approaching this task with the appropriate caution and humility.

Patient-centred care

Clinicians should approach wellness and illness from the patient's point of view as a whole—what is life like for him or her?[18] "Narrative medicine" encourages an enriched history-taking in order to give deeper meaning to the clinical encounter.[19] Similarly, the "phenomenological" approach to illness, so common in post-modernism, based on the work of continental philosophers such as Edmund Husserl, tries to capture medicine from the inside out, as it were, by emphasizing its subjective and experiential dimensions.

These views can be a powerful impetus for moral introspection by the healer ("How do *I* feel about what I am doing? Could *I* be wrong and the patient right?") and are further steps towards true patient-oriented medicine. They make for a deeper foundation for shared decision-making by attempting to break down barriers to understanding between doctor and patient. They also remind us that the patient's experience should be considered the fulcrum of treatment and the doctor's "objectivist" perspective is more limited in scope, the opposite of what is usually thought.[20]

There is, by the way, no better impetus to appreciating the value of autonomy, and how "they" can become "us", than when a clinician becomes a patient.[21] The experience of severe illness can be devastating to patients in ways often not appreciated by healthcare professionals. Oliver Sacks described his own experience as a patient with a severe limb injury. "What seemed, at first, to be no more than a local peripheral breakdown [in my leg] now showed itself in a different, and quite terrible, light . . . *not just a lesion in my muscle but as a lesion in me.*[22] The nadir in his hospital experience came when he realized his clinicians saw him as no more than a leg injury and, so, could not truly help him get well.

Although patients do not always have full insight into their conditions—and thus cannot have a full say over their care—they have experiences that must be elicited and acknowledged. Good clinical care does not consider the patient with serious illness simply as an object to be cured but involves recognition of his or her worth and experience as a human in crisis.

II. The Case of Mrs Malette and Dr Shulman

The legal system sometimes prods medicine to change. According to the following well-known Ontario court case, a patient's deeply held views should be respected and not considered *on their own* as irrational, irrelevant, or untenable, even if they put the person in harm's way.

In 1979 Mrs Malette, a 57-year-old woman, was brought, comatose, to the ER.[23] Involved in a severe motor vehicle accident in which her husband was killed, she appeared to be bleeding to death from a head injury. Dr Shulman, the Emergency Room physician, believed a blood transfusion had to be given to save her life. However, Mrs Malette had a signed card in her wallet, albeit neither dated nor witnessed, stating she was a Jehovah's Witness and would never want to receive blood products. Despite being aware of this card, Dr Shulman ordered a blood transfusion. He felt he had little choice, as he was uncertain about her true beliefs and there were dire consequences of not treating her. In my mind this was a reasonable calculation to make (see Box 2.2).

> **BOX 2.2**
>
> Where a patient currently cannot express his or her wishes, the patient's previously expressed (capable) wishes, whether written or verbal, regarding therapy should be followed.

Reasonableness and beyond

A later court settlement found that the transfusion, although it had saved Mrs Malette's life, had been given against her known wishes. Dr Shulman was found guilty of battery and ordered to pay $20,000 in monetary damages. In commenting on religious refusal, the court reasoned that

> if the objection [to treatment] is on a religious basis, this does not permit the scrutiny of "reasonableness" which is "a transitory standard dependent on the norms of the day." If the patient's

objection has its basis in religion, it is more apt to crystallize in life-threatening situations.[24]

The crucial finding of this judgment is that Dr Shulman's care was substandard because it ignored the prior expressed wishes of Mrs Malette. A higher Ontario Court of Appeal later upheld the earlier judgment: "A doctor is not free to disregard a patient's advance instructions any more than he would be free to disregard instructions given at the time of the emergency."[25]

So, while medicine's goals are to ameliorate suffering and prevent premature death (the beneficence principle), in general, these cannot be achieved at the expense of the patient's preferences (the autonomy principle). For some patients, being saved by treatment that violates their fundamental values is an experience worse than death. Courts countenance this when the decision to refuse care reflects what a person wants, even if such preferences are far from mainstream thought: "If [the doctor] knows that the patient has refused to consent to the proposed procedure, he is not empowered to overrule the patient's decision for her even though he, and most others, may think hers a foolish or unreasonable decision."[26]

The court's remark regarding this case, however, was off target. It is not that Dr Shulman ignored the patient's wishes; he seemed genuinely uncertain as to what they were. It is difficult for doctors to evaluate how good the evidence of a patient's prior wishes must be to require abiding by that individual's apparent refusal of emergency treatment. Should Mrs Malette's wishes have been respected, and she be allowed to die, even though her signed card was neither dated nor witnessed?[27]

Dr Shulman's position was thus an unenviable one. Where the basis of treatment refusal is unclear and the patient will die without treatment, one should, in general, treat that patient until the wishes are clarified. In the court's view, however, if patients leave home with a vaguely worded living will refusing treatment, then they take upon themselves the risk that they will not get that treatment.

Bottom line: clinicians ignore even uncertain evidence of a patient's wishes at their peril. (It must be said, however, that while Canadian courts have been fairly consistent in recognizing the primacy of patients' wishes, the same consistency cannot be said for US or UK courts.)[28]

In another case, concerned with mentally ill patients who refuse antipsychotic treatment, the court wrote that the best-interests standard (the patient's "well-being" from the medical perspective) cannot be used to overrule a patient's wish to refuse treatment (see Box 2.3). If that were allowed, it would violate "the basic tenets of our legal system" and not be in accordance with the "principles of fundamental justice."[29] The law assumes competence until proven otherwise; although the patient may now be mad, bad, or just plain ill, it is the patient's prior expressed preferences that must guide care.

BOX 2.3

"The patient's right to forego treatment, in the absence of some overriding societal interest, is paramount to the doctor's obligation to provide medical care. This right must be honoured, even though the treatment may be beneficial or necessary to preserve the patient's life or health, and regardless of how ill-advised the patient's decision may appear to others."[30]

III. Choices: The Good, the Bad, and the Ugly

1. The good: the right to choose

Patients, by the principle of autonomy, have a right to make choices about the kind of healthcare they receive. The right to a second opinion is an important corollary, as is the right to information. Patients, too, can choose to have or forego tests or surgeries. They can choose what kind of dialysis to go on or choose not to go on it at all (and risk imminent death). They can ask to see the best surgeon for brain or heart surgery—provided they are willing to wait in Canada or to pay big bucks in the US. Patients can ask for almost anything. Whether they will get it depends on the urgency of their problem, where they live, the alternatives, and whether they can afford to wait—in short, it depends on availability and the standard of care (see Chapter 9 on justice).

Reasonable choices by patients are nonetheless resisted by some physicians who still find refuge in paternalism.

CASE 2.3 LIGATION LITIGATION

A 24-year-old unmarried woman is pregnant for the second time with a Caesarian section already scheduled. Well on in her second trimester, she requests to have her "tubes tied" at the time of the delivery. This, the obstetrician refuses to do, citing her young age and unmarried status. "How do I know you won't change your mind in a few years?"

Is the obstetrician acting properly here?

DISCUSSION OF CASE 2.3

This is an all too common doctor-knows-best scenario. The obstetrician has his reasons but, from the autonomy perspective, these are insufficient to support his refusal to perform a tubal ligation on this patient. If she understands and appreciates the proposed procedure, this should suffice. Of course, he can give her information about it and send her away to think about it, but ultimately the choice is hers to make. (Informed choice should be a *process* of communication anyway, not a one-time event.) Patients may regret any procedure they undergo; the best the clinician can do is hope they truly comprehend the likely outcomes (such as, in this case, the irreversibility of the ligation). This professional reluctance to grant a competent patient's request for surgical sterilization may be a holdover from certain religious objections to non-therapeutic sterilization and may be hard to eradicate. Even if the obstetrician had some moral qualms about ligating an unmarried woman, he at a minimum should, from this perspective, refer her to an appropriate colleague.

This is an area, though, where the doctor's peers would probably act similarly. "Experienced, wise gynecologists," it has been argued, will routinely turn down a woman younger than 25 years old asking for tubal ligation.[31] In this view, women have other, very effective and safe, non-surgical methods of birth control. It is also not infrequent for women and men to enter a new relationship several years later and want their irreversible sterilization reversed. Physicians following a young person's wishes fear litigation from a regretted tubal ligation. But while ligation is a litigation-prone procedure, this is usually on account of an unwanted pregnancy from negligent ligation and not because the gynecologist has coerced the woman into it.

Surgeons are understandably reluctant to perform any irreversible procedure on patients if they might be too young to truly appreciate the implications of their request: for example, it is prudent to deny a teenager access to purely cosmetic surgery or most permanent tattooing. There may be some room here for a limited paternalism. Clinicians should make sure to distinguish a defensible community standard from their own personal distaste for a procedure.

Interestingly, young men would have similar difficulty getting a vasectomy, so the problem is not simply one of sexism and is not discipline-specific.

2. The "bad": the right to foolish choices

Autonomy and the freedom to exercise choice mean, among other things, the freedom to make "bad choices," ones that may cause harm. Citizens in our society have the liberty to engage in risk-prone activities (such as drinking alcohol, eating junk food, and smoking), so long as such activities do not harm others. There is an old adage that the right to swing your fist ends where my nose begins. The moral difficulty for clinicians is in knowing how to handle patients' more controversial wishes.

> **BOX 2.4**
>
> "Any accounting for how well we are succeeding in providing care must above all consider the patient's preferred outcomes."[32]

CASE 2.4 DON'T TOUCH MY ARM!

A 64-year-old woman about to undergo elective surgery for a prolapsed bladder told the anesthetist before the operation, "Whatever you do, don't touch my left arm. You'll have nothing but trouble there." The anesthetist accepted this cryptic prohibition without seeking any clarification. Soon after the operation began, he lost intravenous access in her right arm. Ignoring her previous request, he started a new IV in her left arm. The operation was completed without incident.

   Unfortunately, post-operatively the IV in the patient's left arm went interstitial and a toxic fluid leaked into the surrounding arm tissue, resulting in a significant injury to the arm. At trial, no evidence was presented of any medical reason for the left arm not to have been touched. On the other hand, no evidence was offered supporting the necessity of starting an IV in that arm. The patient successfully sued the doctor for assault (non-consensual touching).[33]

Was this an appropriate judgment?

DISCUSSION OF CASE 2.4

It would seem so because the doctor had ignored the patient's prior stated wish. Patients have a right to idiosyncratic beliefs—even if they pose some risk of harm to themselves. In this case, the arm injury was entirely fortuitous—the patient had no foreknowledge that harm would ensue if the doctor touched her left arm. Nevertheless, her instructions were explicit and appeared to have been accepted by the anesthetist. He should have sought IV access anywhere else but the left arm.

Of course, it would have been quite appropriate to question this patient before surgery about her cryptic request. What were the goals that were important for her? If she persisted in her prohibition and he felt this to be unsafe, he could have declined to act as her anesthetist (much as a surgeon would refuse to operate with one hand tied behind her back). *If a patient's request is inherently unsafe and abiding by it skirts negligence or unprofessional conduct, the healthcare professional has no duty to acquiesce to it.* In fact, he or she ought not to comply with it. However, waiting until the patient is asleep under anesthetic is not the best time to question a patient's prior wish.

The principle of autonomy allows patients to set their own goals and define their own ways of living (and dying). While some will be straightforward, others will seem unusual and perhaps eccentric. Unless seriously deranged, these choices should be explored, but not necessarily overruled, by clinicians. Seemingly competent and autonomous patients can choose irrationally by

- thinking about the immediate future and ignoring long-term risks;
- thinking that nothing bad will happen to them;
- acting on unreasonable fears that make them avoid necessary treatment;
- exhibiting extremely eccentric beliefs; or
- adhering to unusual ways of interpreting information.[34]

None of these reasons are sufficient on their own to overrule a patient's wishes. They do suggest that something may be amiss with the patient's cognitive state and act as red flags for the ethical and prudent clinician to probe those patient beliefs more thoroughly. Some "irrational" choices made by patients are true expressions of deeply held convictions, whereas others are products of their defence mechanisms, such as denial, in the face of difficult life events.

3. The "ugly": self-destructive wishes

Abiding by the autonomy principle can cause some healthcare professionals to feel like handmaidens to less than optimal goals of their patients, ones that can border on the self-destructive. This may be something quite different from what they expected when they entered their training program: is their job not to improve and save lives, rather than imperil or end them? Although some patients' goals are clearly illegitimate and must be resisted, others are less clearly so—especially where they arise from illness.

CASE 2.5 TRANQUILLIZER TRAP

An 84-year-old woman, Ms B, has a history of coronary disease. She requests her usual prescription of triazolam, a short-acting benzodiazepine she has taken for years for insomnia. Despite repeated efforts on your part to wean her from this drug, Ms B insists on taking it. Her fervent wish is for a good night's sleep. And, oh yes, she has tried "everything" already to help her sleep. "Only *this* little pill works."

Should the drug be prescribed yet again?

DISCUSSION OF CASE 2.5

Elderly people are notoriously overmedicated. This patient risks falling and confusion secondary to her use of a benzodiazepine, problems not infrequent in her age group.[35] Many long-time users of hypnotics and anxiolytics are not readily weaned from them ("But, doctor, I can't sleep a wink without them . . ."). They can hang on to their drugs as tenaciously as if their lives depended on them ("You'll pry them from my dead hands . . .").[36]

You must balance the task of getting Ms B to agree to reduce these risks (which such patients typically downplay) by coming off such medication against the risk of becoming embroiled in a power struggle. You should try, once more, to remind her of the risks of hypnotics and discuss alternatives with her. In doing so you might have satisfied the beneficence principle—and perhaps also the autonomy principle if the patient's use of hypnotics compromises her independence.

This could be one more battle you are unlikely to win. If you decide to continue prescribing the medication, you should do so prudently: prescribe limited quantities each time; have a discussion about associated risks on a regular basis; document these discussions, making it clear that the patient is making an informed choice; and continue efforts to wean her off. Of course, it goes without saying that patients such as Ms B should be carefully and regularly monitored for the development of such adverse effects and a more forceful discussion undertaken if such symptoms do emerge. On a practical level, the patient could go to another doctor to request the benzodiazepine if you refuse her request. At least you can monitor her use of the medication if you continue to be the one prescribing it.

The modern allegiance to patient autonomy should not be an excuse for not caring for and thereby abandoning a patient. It is the clinician's job—his or her fiduciary responsibility—to explore the choices a patient makes, to invade that person's privacy (with his or her consent, of course) to make sure the patient is not cast off in his or her autonomous shell. The tale of Diogenes, an ancient Greek philosopher who lived in less than pristine conditions in a barrel, is instructive here. In modern parlance, "Diogenes syndrome" has come to refer to those usually antisocial individuals who fail at self-care and live alone in squalor and neglect. Although they typically refuse help, there is also a prevailing reluctance by society to intervene because of the respect for autonomy.

With such a situation in mind, many argue that allowing mentally compromised patients the "right" to their self-harming actions says more about our negative attitudes towards mental and physical impairments and the limits of caring in our society than it does about patient autonomy. Similarly, biased attitudes towards, for example, the mentally ill, the elderly, and those with neurological illnesses in many societies may lead to the under-investigation and under-treatment of their other concurrent conditions.[37]

Cases in which seemingly "autonomous wishes" lead to patient harm may involve the healthcare professional in a more central way.

CASE 2.6 A MAN SHOULD DIE AT HOME!

A spry but frail 94-year-old man, Mr Y, long widowed and living alone, has a history of serious heart failure. Finding himself yet again in a coronary care unit, facing death, he begs to be released ("There is no fate worse than this! A man should not die in a hospital!" he cries out to the Home Care nurse who has lately become his *de facto* primary care provider). The specialists feel he cannot manage at home and argue he will be back in their Emergency Room within the week. Mr Y simply wants to be at home. He argues he is quite prepared to die since, outliving his family and friends, he sees no further possibility of a happy life. His stated goal is to die at home in peace. In his culture, he tells the nurse, no one dies in hospital, alone. Instead, people at the end-of-life are cared for at home by their families. For Mr Y, being part of a wider network of kith and kin is more important than preserving autonomy. Mr Y is clearly not troubled about dying; he is only troubled about having no family on whom to rely.

Should the health professionals aid him in his wish to die at home?

DISCUSSION OF AND FOLLOW-UP TO CASE 2.6

There seem to be very few options in this case. Mr Y is quite alone and feels he has come to the end of his days. If found incapable, he could be confined to hospital and treated against his will. This would seem undignified. Eventually, he is deemed capable of making the decision about where to live and so is released to his home despite the risk of death and of re-admission. His community nurse who, arguably, knows him better than anyone else, agrees letting Mr Y go home is the right thing to do.

After Mr Y is discharged to his apartment, he stops eating and taking his medications, dying several weeks later. The patient's nurse, who helped get him home and was with him when he passed away, feels some complicity in his death. Had she done "everything" to help the patient live? Or did she too quickly comply with his wishes because he was a "sad old guy"? In the end, although troubled by his death, she feels it was her duty to be the patient's advocate ensuring that his doctors heard his plea and respected his rights. Her dedication to the patient is remarkable in these days when care can seem callously anonymous.

On the other hand, it could be argued that this patient was in fact depressed. That he stopped eating upon discharge may indicate he wanted to kill himself. Was this patient carefully assessed for the presence of a treatable depression? Older patients are notoriously under-investigated for depression and suicide risk.[38] Was the nurse projecting her own feelings of hopelessness onto the patient?

In this case, however, the patient's actions seemed very consistent with his culture of origin's views about the acceptability of a "natural death." For Mr Y the enemy was not death but being kept alive (and perhaps dying) on machines in a hospital.

Costs to the professional

Sometimes the right thing to do is to allow avoidable harm to come to a patient, especially when that harm is foreseen by the patient and is less important to him or her than other, more central, goals and aspirations which may themselves be culturally based. This would seem to go against the basic philosophy of the healthcare professions, but it is important to remember that harm and benefit must be defined with patient input. Unfortunately, if helping a patient results in injury or death, the healthcare professional can be left with difficult feelings of guilt and regret; this is part of the hidden costs of respecting the values and choices that patients have and make.

The careful clinician will make sure a patient's decision to forego care, or to embark on a course that will lead to his or her death, is not influenced by modifiable or "reversible" factors, such as despair or loneliness. If such factors are involved, the practitioner should address these as best as possible before going along with a patient who wishes to die or puts him or herself in harm's way (see Chapter 11 on end-of-life decisions).

IV. Reduced Autonomy

Various factors, such as critical illness,[39] deprivation, social isolation, and substance abuse, can create a state of vulnerability in patients. Attention must be paid to these factors as they create roadblocks to the simple exercise of self-determination.

CASE 2.7 A HYPNOTIC REQUEST

Ms B, the 84-year-old patient in Case 2.5, refuses alternative means of sedation. The following year she suffers a myocardial infarction for which she is hospitalized for three weeks. Her illness is complicated by congestive heart failure and arrhythmias. Upon discharge she once again requests triazolam.

Examination reveals an elderly woman in no acute distress but with subtle changes in her mental processes; Ms B seems more confused than before her myocardial infarction. You discover she has been using higher daily doses of triazolam to cope with feelings of anxiety and panic over her diminished stamina. Worried that her overuse of triazolam might be contributing to her mental state, you decide to involve, with the patient's reluctant co-operation, a community geriatric team to help her cope better with her losses and end her dependence on the drug.

Is this an acceptable encroachment on patient liberty?

DISCUSSION OF CASE 2.7

You have judiciously balanced Ms B's wishes with the need to protect her health. Her use of a hypnotic is now excessive and threatening to undermine what autonomy she has left. Her increased physical and mental frailty make you uncomfortable with simply acceding to her wishes. A physician failing to find her drug use problematic would not be living up to professional standards. One of these is to protect patients from themselves. Does this smack of paternalism? It may, but is legitimately exercised here because the patient's autonomy is being compromised by her illness and her drug use.

In such circumstances it is difficult to decide how far to respect a patient's expressed goals. Are they authentic expressions of the patient's self, or do they derive from someone who is suffering and under siege by illness or incapacity? Patients can appear competent but be impaired for more subtle reasons having to do with their illnesses (see Case 7.4 "Not Like Himself").

Patient waiver revisited

Although some patients wish to maintain control as long as they are able, others are only too happy to have someone look after them in a protective, paternalistic fashion. A former editor of the *New England Journal of Medicine* in the 1970s, Franz Ingelfinger, argued that for a treatment to succeed, the patient needs a clinician who will take charge and in whom the patient can believe.[40] His views revealed his own personal need for someone to direct his care when he was ill with an incurable cancer. This hardly seems an ethically worrisome paternalism. His or her autonomy already impaired by illness, a patient may waive the right to make decisions in favour of someone else. Such wishes should be respected. (If the illness or situation changes, of course, it would be proper to discuss with the patient the possibility of resuming control.)

CASE 2.8 A WISH NOT TO HEAR

You are a visiting nurse seeing a new patient, Mr K, a 78-year-old widower, for a post-operative home visit. He claims to feel fine following recent surgery for what he claims was only a "stomach ulcer." Mr K indicates he has a tube to drain bile from his liver. You are perplexed, as a tube is usually only put in to relieve an obstruction, not to treat a simple ulcer. The patient cannot explain this. Later, inspection of his hospital chart and his family doctor's referring note reveals Mr K had been told on at least two occasions that he had inoperable pancreatic cancer.

What should you do?

DISCUSSION OF CASE 2.8

You should see Mr K again to get a better understanding of his personality. It appears he is denying the true nature of his illness. Should you try, once more, to beat down his defenses? If I had satisfied myself that this attempt had been made before, I would not. (A significant number of patients with cancer deny their illness despite clear evidence to the contrary.)[41]

Instead, I would ask him: are you the type of person who likes to know everything about his illness, or would you prefer only your clinicians to know? If he answers yes to the latter, I would let him be. Patients have a right to their defences and the right to expect us to look after them. Such needs should not be run over roughshod by a simple-minded allegiance to the principle of autonomy.

The limits of autonomy?

Some patients' wishes defy easy resolution. When a patient refuses appropriate, basic nursing care, what is to be done? Is this the end result of patient autonomy as we know it?

CASE 2.9 THIS LADY'S NOT FOR TURNING

Ms W is a 56-year-old inpatient with a long history of disabling and destructive rheumatoid arthritis. Her hands and feet are cruelly contracted. Despite numerous surgeries she is unable to bear weight; even sitting is painful. She is admitted to hospital for yet another attempt at corrective surgery. Unfortunately, during this hospitalization she develops C. difficile colitis and, later on, large sacral pressure sores. Now Ms W is refusing to be turned. After several weeks of intense but fruitless negotiation, the hospital ethicist is asked by the treating team to see her.

Ms W seems bright and alert but sad. Confined to bed for almost a year, she has managed with live-in help at home but hates her life: restricted, inactive, and isolated. Why, the ethicist asks, are you refusing care for your pressure ulcers? Ms W complains bitterly about the care on the ward. At first they hardly turned her at all. Now that her condition is so bad, she whispers, they seem to blame her for the problem and turn her more roughly, without attending to the pain this causes her. She seems to understand the gravity of her state and admits her situation is far from ideal.

With this the ethicist has to agree: Ms W has large necrotic pressure ulcers on her sacrum and buttocks. Moreover, the odour from them is noticeable as soon as you arrive on the ward and is almost unbearable. *Horribile dictu*, the ethicist also notices small black flies flitting about the patient.

"Could," the team asks the ethicist, "Ms W be turned despite her wishes not to be?"

DISCUSSION OF CASE 2.9

One can analyze this case using the ethics decision procedure. An ethical dilemma does indeed seem to be present: is it ever acceptable for a patient to refuse basic nursing care, such as sacral ulcer care? There seem to be at least two alternatives to action: one should provide that care without patient consent or one should abide by the patient's firm refusal of care and not do so. One can then analyze the pros and cons of each alternative in terms of the basic principles: providing care would seem contrary to the patient's autonomy but not doing so would, it seems, conflict with beneficence. But would it? From the patient's point of view, she would prefer the hazards of not being treated than being in agony with treatment.

Is Ms W being treated "justly"? Basic care is a right, but she is not obliged to accept it. There is also the issue as to whether her refusal of care has an unfair impact on others. Her refusal of care is draining for the whole ward. She is literally rotting in her bed "with her rights on." As far as context goes, there is no precedent in the hospital for such a refusal. No policies seem applicable but failing to provide basic nursing care seems a grave offense to the nursing staff especially. The patient has no significant others to be called upon.

What is to be done with a patient who refuses basic, dignified care?

CONCLUSION OF CASE 2.9

The odiferous nature of Ms W's untreated ulcers hits one on the nose like a clenched fist. Or so it seems to the ethicist. This case, the ethicist writes in the patient's chart, has gone on far too long: staff are alienated from the patient; nurses and trainees fail to turn up when expected; and even the attending surgeon has not been around for days. A difficult situation has literally festered. This case warrants a "root cause analysis" (keep asking why until one gets a satisfactory understanding of the situation). This seeks not blame but understanding as to how an unwanted state of affairs has occurred and what can be done to prevent its recurrence. Discussion with staff should ensue to examine their own attitudes to a "hateful patient."[42] The team should determine how Ms W might be treated more humanely, for example, by treatment under anaesthesia. Psychiatry and Palliative Care could also be consulted for other appropriate options. However, autonomy has its limits, [43] as this case illustrates. There is only so far a patient in an institution, where the welfare of other patients is at stake, can refuse care. Ms W has to be treated. Her right to refuse is limited where it threatens to undermine the welfare of other patients.

Ms W's perspective is that she is experiencing her care as torture. She is not really refusing care, only excessively painful care. As even the lightest touch provokes a pain response from her, the resolution of the issue would require some concerted efforts and imagination in order to treat her humanely. At the end of the day this case isn't really about the limits of autonomy but rather about the limits of beneficence and how far the team is from understanding the patient's experience of illness. But the flies definitely have to go. It is simply undignified.[44]

BOX 2.5

Limits to autonomy include
- requests for illegal or unprofessional care (see Chapter 8);
- patient incapacity (see Chapter 6);
- limited resources (see Chapter 9);
- social welfare/public health: control of contagious disease, violent persons, terrorism, and the protection of the public generally (see Chapter 3).

Conclusion

How patients exercise their autonomy may not be straightforward. Their goals and wishes may require at the same time both respect and exploration. Clinicians should use their skills to decide what they feel is appropriate, not only in the light of the patient's hopes, fears, and values but also what best evidence supports. In the proper application of clinical judgment, practitioners should not only know when to respect a patient's wishes and to help them to achieve their goals, but also when it is advisable not to do so (for example, when and how to protect the vulnerable and the ill from serious harm). Where the evidence is uncertain, clinicians must acknowledge this and learn how to share it with patients.[45]

When patient and doctor clash, whose view should prevail? The answer is often neither view on its own. Instead, the participants ought to try principled negotiation; common ground should be sought through mutual understanding and respect.[46] By examining one's own feelings and the patient's feelings, expectations, worries, and, because of illness, changed functioning in the world, the self-reflective clinician will be better able to devise a treatment plan that combines the patient's goals with the physician's obligations. This finding of a common ground by dialogue tries to avoid unnecessary power struggles and simplistic kow-towing to the patient's expectations. Shared decision-making is the right way to go.

In Chapters 6 and 7, we will return to the clinician's duty of beneficence and care for non-autonomous patients. The next three chapters will deal with other implications of the principle of autonomy for the practice of medicine.

Cases for Discussion

CASE 1: "I'M NOT DONE YET"

An 81-year-old male with very advanced metastatic prostate cancer is at home, willing to try anything that might extend his life. "I'm not ready to die," he tells his doctor. He had found online that an injectible substance, P-41X, although expensive, could reverse advanced cancer. "Don't give up on me, Doc, I'm not done yet." Having felt obliged to give two previous injections of this substance to the patient, his doctor has concluded from his own review of the evidence that there is little to support its use. He also knows this patient wants to hear only "good news." "If I wanted to be depressed, I'd read the front page of the newspaper," he has said.

QUESTIONS FOR DISCUSSION

1. Would you go along with his request? Discuss this using an ethical analysis.
2. When would you not go along with a request from a patient?
3. What if he was pursuing this option in place of an effective treatment?

CASE 2: INTERESTING CASE

"Interesting case in bed two!" barks the clinician to the medical trainee. "Go get a history from her." The student wanders into the patient's room, not knowing what to expect. Ms U is 56 years old, but is frail and seems much older than her stated age. Her history is complex and not easily pigeonholed. In several weeks she had gone from a state of generally good health to being unable to walk, dress, or feed herself. Despite countless investigations, no diagnosis has been made. The student feels out of her depth. Ms U's answers do not clarify the situation so the student begins to chat with her about how all this has affected her and her husband. She responds she no longer feels like a human being, but as an interesting curio, a "guinea-pig."

At Grand Rounds a few days later, Ms U is presented by one of the ward doctors. He expresses his own perplexity as to the patient's diagnosis. "Whatever it is, her future is not rosy," he states matter-of-factly, "I don't know what's wrong with her, but the patient will likely die soon."

"Why doesn't she know this?" the student asks, "Why are you still doing so many scans which are causing her so much anxiety? Maybe she should be referred for palliative care." The attending dismisses this and responds they can't "give up" on her until they have come up with a diagnosis and are sure she is terminally ill.[47]

Questions For Discussion

1. What is the central problem here?
2. Can you formulate a response using the ethics work-up?
3. Keeping in mind you are a trainee, how would you best manage this situation?

3 No Man an Island
Confidentiality and Trust

Thou art the only one to whom I dare confide my Folly.
George Lyttelton, 1744[1]

Achilles: Of this my privacy, I have strong reasons.
Ulysses: But against your privacy, the reasons are more potent and heroic.
William Shakespeare, c. 1602[2]

Deciding on the right thing to do in medicine can be a complicated task, rarely accomplished by simply adhering to one particular moral principle or duty. Nowhere is this more obvious than in the conflicting professional responsibilities concerning the management of patients' private information. Healthcare professionals are expected and, indeed, required to respect the confidential nature of patient information and protect it from inappropriate disclosure. In certain circumstances, however, circumscribed and outlined in law and ethics, privacy expectations cannot be met for reasons of public safety and private welfare.

I. Rights of Privacy, Confidential Duties

CASE 3.1 DON'T TELL!

You are a fertility specialist seeing Ms R, a 34-year-old woman, for the first time. She and her partner have been trying unsuccessfully for the last five years to have their first child. After spending time talking to the couple, you ask Ms R to disrobe in the next room so you can conduct your physical examination. As you enter the room, she appears nervous and hesitant. Finally, she says to you, "I have to be really honest with you, I had an abortion when I was 19 and then again when I was 25. I never told my partner, please don't tell him now."

This information is important in your work-up of her infertility.

What do you say to her?

Privacy, confidentiality, and trust

The right to privacy is a fundamental tenet of liberal democracies. The values of autonomy, liberty, and dignity—all versions of the "respect for persons" principle—underpin the concept of privacy.[3] At the end of the nineteenth century two American Supreme Court justices defined privacy as "the right to be left alone."[4] In other words, privacy is the right to be free from intrusion or interference.

BOX 3.1

The right of privacy is constitutionally embedded in many countries, and belongs to the individual. The right to prevent disclosure of sensitive information can be invoked to prevent the government and some others from gaining access to personal health information or to hold them legally responsible if they access/disclose the information improperly.

Protection of informational privacy can be justified on duty-based and utilitarian grounds. "The confiding of information to the physician for medical purposes gives rise to an expectation that the patient's interest in and control of the information will continue."[5] This is more than a mere "expectation" on the patient's part, however. The right of the patient to have control over his or her own information is a kind of "promise" made by clinicians and the healthcare system in general to patients. Kant would say that promises, once made, ("irrespective-of-consequences") are to be kept.

This duty has been expected of physicians long before modern law. Hippocrates said that whatever one heard in the course of medical practice must never be "spread abroad."[6] The special relationship between doctors and patients has been referred to as a "fiduciary" relationship, and is protected in common law.[7] Clinicians ignore promises they make at their and their patients' peril.

BOX 3.2

The duty of confidentiality is imposed on those who have access to or possess sensitive information of a "private" nature. The duty of confidentiality protects an individual's/patient's right to privacy regarding his or her personal information.

Individuals should be able to define how far others may access their private space, both physical and informational. In healthcare, this translates into the patient's right to control how personal healthcare information is communicated to others.

There is a "consequentialist" ("dependent-on-outcomes") perspective on the right to privacy as well. As breaching privacythreatens the trust on which healthcare depends, this in turn may lead to negative outcomes such as avoidance of care by patients and disciplinary proceedings against healthcare professionals.

But healthcare professionals cannot do an adequate job if they are unable to appropriately "invade" a patient's physical and mental privacy. This is both a great allowance and a hefty responsibility. Good medical practice would be difficult if patients felt vulnerable in sharing information about their private lives with healthcare professionals. In the very first meeting, patients come prepared to confide tremendously personal aspects of themselves—their "follies," perhaps. Such information, at times intimate and secret, is disclosed on the assumption it will not be shared with others.[8]

Confidentiality refers to the duty of healthcare professionals to respect patient wishes regarding their private information. The courts have defined it as "the obligations of individuals and institutions to use information under their control appropriately once it has been disclosed to them. One observes rules of confidentiality out of respect for, and to protect and preserve, the privacy of others."[9] This is a standing legal obligation for all healthcare professionals.[10]

BOX 3.3

"Certain duties arise from the special relationship of trust and confidence [between doctor and patient]. These include the duties of the doctor to act with utmost good faith and loyalty, to hold information received from or about a patient in confidence, and to make proper disclosure of information to a patient ... When a patient releases personal information in the context of the doctor–patient relationship, he or she does so with the legitimate expectation that these duties will be respected."[11]

The judicial and ethical recognition of privacy is not universal, of course. Some countries devalue privacy and routinely access and misuse the medical records and other personal information of their citizens. In China, for example, privacy has been considered to be of "instrumental," not intrinsic, value.[12] We should be concerned about a purely instrumentalist view of privacy—that privacy is respected only insofar as it serves other ends—of the state, one's family, the health of the community (views widely held throughout the Western world as well). Privacy has an intrinsic value too; it is required for a robust sense of one's self. Thus, it is most morally defensible to balance a state's or an institution's (sometimes legitimate) interest in certain information and an individual's interests in protecting some (or much) personal information from public scrutiny. In this chapter we will explore the tension faced by healthcare professionals in attempting to maintain this delicate balance.

DISCUSSION OF CASE 3.1

Ms R's request to keep her past hidden from her husband is quite reasonable. She simply needs to be told that whatever she discloses in private to any health professional in the clinic will be kept that way.

Although medical confidentiality is protected by professional regulations and standards, doctor–patient communications are not "privileged" *per se* in Canada except in Quebec under the Civil Code. (Privilege means, traditionally, the right to withhold information gained within the context of a "special relationship"—such as that between doctor–patient or therapist–patient or attorney–client.)[13] This means doctors must disclose information about a patient if properly requested to do so by the courts. Legal advice around just what is required to be disclosed in court should be sought. For example, a "subpoena" is not in itself a licence to breach patient confidentiality by releasing any and all private information to lawyers and others but simply a command to attend court.[14] However, as one commentator has observed, despite "lofty" court language espousing medical confidentiality, *none* of the most important precedent cases before the Supreme Court of Canada actually find in favour of confidentiality.[15] That may be so, but there are still many other legal and regulatory protections for privacy.

> **BOX 3.4**
>
> The rule of privilege can prevent the person who owes a duty of confidentiality (arising from the special nature of the relationship) from disclosing it to others without patient consent.[16]

Informational protection for psychiatry?

More protection has traditionally been given to psychiatrist–patient communications. presumably on account of the more private matters that are discussed and the ill consequences that can accrue to a patient if his or her psychiatric history is revealed to others.[17] A trusting therapeutic relationship is essential for effective psychiatric care, especially for those who already may be struggling with trust issues due to traumatic life experiences. The Canadian Psychiatric Association's 2000 position paper on confidentiality and privacy in Psychiatry states, "Without confidentiality there can be no trust; without trust there can be no therapy."[18] Nonetheless, psychiatrists and other mental health professionals are permitted and can be compelled to give evidence in court anywhere in Canada. The "interests of justice" (as in *Smith v. Jones*, to be discussed later in the chapter) may at times quite legitimately outweigh the benefits of privacy despite the therapeutic relationship.

Trade secrets

Patients who find truths about themselves hard to handle or difficult to disclose to others may look to the healthcare provider to engage in "deception." This can put healthcare providers in the difficult position of having to weigh a patient's requests for privacy against the duty to protect that patient from harm.

BOX 3.5

"We cannot avoid secrets, disconcerting or otherwise. They come to us unsolicited and by surprise, and, once heard, they change forever the way we feel about a patient . . ."[19]

CASE 3.2 SELF SECRETS

You are the primary care provider for Ms T, a 45-year-old woman admitted with syncope and a possible seizure disorder. This is her second such admission. During a similar hospitalization three months ago, a complete neurological work-up, including a brain scan, failed to reveal a cause for these symptoms. The attending physician on this admission orders the same tests to be repeated.

Informed of the admission, you come to visit Ms T in the hospital. You are extremely worried. Two days previously, the patient had come to see you and had confided the real cause of her last admission was a beating, one of many she had suffered at the hands of her abusive husband. Ms T had never disclosed this to anyone before and asked you to keep the matter a secret. In their culture, she explained, men are allowed to beat their wives for actions such as going out without the husband's approval. Ms T does not disagree with this cultural allowance. She does not even regard this as "abuse"—it's "just how things are." It's what she learned growing up. You are sure that the husband's actions are again the cause for her admission. After reviewing the admission notes, you realize this has not been considered by the attending physician.

Should you reveal the patient's secret to her admitting doctor? Suppose the patient resists help to deal with the violence she experiences at home. Is that a matter for the healthcare team?

DISCUSSION OF AND FOLLOW-UP TO CASE 3.2

Spousal abuse is underreported and often not suspected by healthcare professionals.[20] Cultural factors and norms can play a role in its occurrence. This does not make it acceptable as just another cultural custom. There are important screening questions to identify domestic violence that the clinician should initiate in private (e.g., does your partner ever physically hurt you? Insult or talk down to you? Threaten you with harm? Scream or curse at you? How often does this happen?).[21]

It is remarkable Ms T has been able to confide this much to you. (If she does not share a common language with you, this is where reliance on a professional interpreter, as opposed to a family member such as the husband, is critical.) Abused women commonly resist help even when the problem is identified; this reluctance to seek help must be of concern to healthcare professionals. But, unless a patient is in "imminent" or serious danger,[22] you cannot breach her confidentiality until she is ready to have her secret revealed. In most jurisdictions, a patient's consent for medical information to be shared among members of the "circle of care" (those healthcare professionals and entities such as pharmacies, laboratories, and hospitals providing or assisting in providing healthcare to a specific patient) is implied. However, this patient's explicit refusal of such information-sharing must be respected. Premature disclosure could undermine the patient's confidence in you and make it harder for her to ask for the help she needs. Although Ms T may be given unnecessary medical tests if you do not reveal her secret, this is not a strong enough reason to override the duty of confidentiality.

The greater worry would be the consequences of Ms T returning to her husband. You should try to explain how all involved in her care must respect her privacy. You could also try to ensure her physical safety by referring her to culturally sensitive services and shelters. The unacceptable cultural mores that tolerate domestic violence need to be addressed as well.

In the end, Ms T is persuaded that she can safely disclose the true cause of her injuries to the admitting medical team and seeks help for her troubled home situation.

Not an arm of the law

The duty of confidentiality prevents healthcare professionals from becoming a simple part of the administration of justice—a reminder once again that the health professional's main allegiance is usually to the patient, not to third parties. The police, for example, may ask a clinician to perform a blood test on or release the toxicology report of a patient suspected of impaired driving. Unless the patient has given consent or the police have a valid warrant, the clinician should not breach confidentiality and comply with such requests.[23]

Charges of sexual assault

One area where medical information is more protected is in the case of sexual assault charges. The fear of having one's personal, psychiatric, and medical information laid bare in a courtroom has made many victims of sexual assault wary of laying charges. Bill C-46 of the Canadian *Criminal Code* (amended in 1996) is aimed at encouraging the reporting of such crimes by restricting access to medical, counselling, therapeutic, and other personal records of complainants in sexual offence prosecutions.[24] Psychiatrists and other healthcare professionals are protected from having to release information from an alleged victim's medical records *unless* the accused can come up with compelling reasons for this. This prevents "fishing expeditions" by defense lawyers looking for some reason to cast aspersions on the trustworthiness or credibility of the plaintiff.

All applications by an accused for access to such records must go through two stages: (1) the accused must establish that the records contain information likely to be relevant to an issue at trial or to the competence of a witness to testify, and (2) the trial judge must deem this a legitimate request and only then will review the records in private and decide if they are indeed relevant. This complicated process of review is why doctors should not simply hand over their records when asked to do so.[25]

II. Professional Regulations

Regulated health professionals may be found guilty of professional misconduct, with resultant disciplinary proceedings, should they, without appropriate rationale, disclose private information about a patient without the patient's permission or unless required by law. For example, the *Regulated Health Professions Act*, covering all regulated healthcare professionals in Ontario, states that professional misconduct includes "giving information concerning a patient's condition or any professional services performed for a patient to any person other than the patient without the consent of the patient unless required to do so by law."[26]

Despite this, breaches of confidentiality happen all the time: patients are discussed in the halls and even in hospital elevators within earshot of visitors,[27] filing cabinets are left unlocked overnight, patient information is faxed to a wrong number, a hospital healthcare team doing ward rounds talks to a patient about his medical issues in full hearing range of the roommate on the other side of the curtain.[28] Most hospitals have training and information for practitioners to remind them of their responsibilities and how to avoid inadvertent breaches of confidentiality. This is especially important as large numbers of people—from residents, healthcare trainees, and other healthcare professionals to data clerks and hospital administration employees—may have access to confidential information in a patient's chart. But such access by many people can still allow patients to have an interest in maintaining some element of privacy. By analogy, as a wise judge in 1814 stated, "Though the defendant might not object to a small window looking into his yard, a larger one might be very inconvenient to him, disturbing his privacy and enabling people to come through to trespass upon his property."[29]

In the antediluvian days before privacy became a big issue, a well-known physician and newspaper columnist was found guilty of professional misconduct after disclosing personal medical information about a woman (named in the article!) in his column. This confidential material, obtained from her record, contained information of which even she was unaware. Because she was not his patient, the doctor claimed he owed her no duty of confidentiality. Not surprisingly, the court was unimpressed by this argument.[30] It is hard to imagine a healthcare professional taking such liberties with patient information these days. Such cavalier attitudes to patient identifying information should be, and largely are, gone from healthcare—gone for good now, like cigarettes, from the clinic, in a puff of smoke. (Unless you are celebrity patient in which case, it seems, almost anything goes.)

The fog of war, however, can still obscure things.

CASE 3.3 A CASUALTY OF WAR

Dr Kevin Patterson, a Canadian surgeon-novelist who had recently finished a tour of duty as a physician in Afghanistan, decided to write a story about the death of a Canadian soldier he treated. The article, describing in explicit and gruesome detail the soldier's final hours, was published in a widely circulated American magazine. The soldier was identified by name. The magazine contacted the soldier's mother in Nova Scotia to alert her of the article's impending publication.[31]

Did the physician breach confidentiality in publishing this article?

DISCUSSION OF CASE 3.3

The duty of confidentiality *should* persist after a patient's death. Deceased persons and their families may have an interest in the preserving the privacy of the deceased. The length of time which must elapse before personal information can be *legally* released without prior patient or family consent varies from place to place; in some countries there may be no posthumous protection, in others, such as Canada, more than a century must elapse. According to the magazine, the soldier's mother did not object to publication of the story and, in fact, several family members expressed gratitude for Dr Patterson's heroic efforts to save their loved one. However, the Department of National Defence viewed this as an illegitimate breach of confidentiality for which he could face court martial and possible jail time. Family members later agreed the article had caused much distress. Although the surgeon had the best of intentions—to honour the death of the soldier and to enable others to understand the ongoing sacrifices made by the troops—the level of individual detail was unnecessary and had a negative impact on other family members and friends of the deceased. Dr Patterson was ultimately exonerated by the Dept of National Defense. But he *was* found guilty, by his provincial governing body for physicians, of professional misconduct for breaching patient confidentiality. The penalties imposed included a formal written reprimand, a fine of $5000, and an agreement to donate $7,000 to charity. Dr Patterson assured the governing body that "in any future writings based on medical scenarios, or in any future works of journalism or fiction" he "will not include any information that could identify patients."[32]

Thus, while it may be that patients or their families rarely recover damages through the courts from a medical professional for breaching of their confidentiality,[33] others may still be prepared to judge a healthcare professional's disregard for protecting patient data.

The respect due persons does not end with the death of the person. Just as we treat his or her physical remains in a respectful and dignified way, so should we treat his or her "informational remains." This is just common decency.

Privacy laws

The advent of health information privacy laws in many jurisdictions is a response to widespread concerns over the loss of privacy in social life generally. In Canada since 2004, the floor to protection of privacy is set by PIPEDA (*Personal Information Protection and Electronic Documents Act*), a national act that sets the standard for the use, collection, and disclosure of personal information. Provinces must substantially meet, or may exceed, these standards in their own legislation (such as in Ontario, PHIPA, *Personal Health Information Protection Act*). In the US similar federal legislation exists under HIPPA (*Health Insurance Portability and Accountability Act*), which governs personal electronic data. These legislative initiatives now exist in many countries so medical professionals need to be familiar with applicable laws in their jurisdictions.

Taking information privacy seriously and trying to ensure consistency of access to and control over information—acknowledging the "intrinsic" value of privacy—is an example of the moralization of social life and how ethical regulation is "advantage-reducing." Privacy laws beef up personal information security so that identifiable patient information is not accessed and becomes vulnerable to misuse by insurance firms, pharmaceutical companies, or the government. Secure information practices help ensure healthcare professionals do not become "long arms" of the law or long limbs of any other outside parties.

Express and implied consent

Where collected data uniquely identifies a person, its use and disclosure requires patient consent—basically, the patient must know who can access that data and for what purposes. Such consent may be either express (or explicit) or implied (or implicit). Express consent is consent given either verbally or in writing. Implied consent, on the other hand, is permission implied by a patient's action or inaction. For example, permission to share information when a patient is transferred from one facility to another is implied.

Many fear an overemphasis on privacy will be bad for patients and bad for research. They argue this might inhibit healthcare professionals from disclosing needed information to other clinicians in the patient's "circle of care"[34] and might make research too unwieldy. These arguments are not without merit. It is quite possible, however, for laws to be crafted that allow for reasonable access to patient information and that do not impair high quality research.[35]

In fact, in most jurisdictions these days, those in the patient's circle of care may share information amongst themselves for the purposes of care without express consent, as it is assumed the patient would want all his or her healthcare providers to have this information (patients may still forbid sharing of personal medical information within the circle of care if that is their wish). In certain cases, where the information is anonymized, medical researchers may access patient charts for retrospective ("past looking") research without any type of patient consent,[36] if they follow a suitable approved research plan, or if they are a member of a "designated entity."[37]

When it comes to serious illness, most people who are suffering will not sit fretting about gaps in data protection. However, others—such as youth or marginalized persons—may avoid appropriate medical care (such as a young teen seeking contraceptives) if they perceive that medical practitioners are not sufficiently sensitive to their privacy concerns.

Medical practitioners should (1) be aware of pertinent laws or regulations in the jurisdictions in which they practise and (2) avoid careless ways in which sensitive patient information might be revealed.[38]

CASE 3.4 A RISKY RECORD

A 31-year-old patient, Ms N, is transferring her care to a new physician. A request is made to her former doctor's office to send a copy of her file to the new physician. Her former physician releases the patient's entire file except for some of the consultants' letters. She cannot do so, she says, because the letters were the property of other physicians. Some of the consultants' letters are stamped "Confidential. Not to be released without permission." Most importantly, she is reluctant to release one from a psychiatrist noting that Ms N has a "borderline personality" disorder and likely to be a "challenging patient."

Is the physician correct in holding back part of the patient's chart?

The medical record

In North America, in general, the information in a medical chart "belongs" to the patient. Although the *physical* record belongs to the recording professional or his or her institution, the *contents* of the record belong to the patient. It is ultimately the patient who controls what information may be disclosed and to whom it may be disclosed. Patients may permit their personal health information to be released, such as to a lawyer for a medico-legal report or an insurance company or to other physicians.

Because the chart belongs to the patient, its contents can be read by the patient. Patients can access their record, they can ask to "correct" it, they can close off part of it, or indeed all of it, from scrutiny. Sensitive personal information, such as that found in a psychiatric record, may be protected in a "lock[ed] box." Access to such information is very restricted and only allowed for identifiable individuals and only with good reason, such as if the contents are thought necessary to save a patient's life.

DISCUSSION OF CASE 3.4

If a doctor is very worried about the impact on the patient or on others of releasing portions of the record, he or she may withhold that information. It is an exception to the disclosure rule that should rarely be needed. In this case it seems unlikely that the conclusion that Ms N is "challenging" and has a borderline personality disorder would fit the bill. Her doctor might wish to consult with Ms N's psychiatrist. If there still is genuine concern about the letter's impact, denying access *may* be ethically acceptable. This denial may, in turn, be subject to court challenge by the patient.

The right of patients to access their medical records does suggest clinicians must be careful about their documentation. Objective descriptions are preferrable to terminology which could be interpreted as derogatory. The question to consider when entering anything into a patient's record is, would you feel comfortable having the patient read what you have written?

It is worth noting that the "confidential-not-to-be-released" stamp does not apply to the patient, but to third parties such as insurance companies. Consent to copy and release her entire record is implied in this case as the receiving physician is considered part of the patient's circle of care.

BOX 3.6

- The content of the medical record belongs to the patient; the physical record is the property of the "health custodian"—doctor or institution—and is held for the benefit of the patient.
- Patients may have access to their records in all but a small number of cases and may cordon off all or part of it from the scrutiny of others by a virtual "lock box."
- Access and control by the patient of the chart, or parts of it, may be denied if this might compromise the safety of the patient or third parties. The burden of proving this danger is on the practitioner so claiming.
- Denial of access or control may be subject to legal challenge.

While the law aims to strengthen privacy and confidentiality, it must at the same time specify when they may legitimately be breached. When the welfare of other individuals and the public is threatened, individual privacy rights may be eclipsed.[39]

III. Limits To Confidentiality

Respecting privacy and maintaining confidentiality are important responsibilities of a healthcare professional—but not the sole responsibilities. "[T]here may be cases in which reasons connected with the safety of individuals or of the public, physical or moral, would be sufficiently cogent to supersede or qualify the obligations *prima facie* imposed by the confidential relation."[40] *Confidentiality in medicine is a duty whose exercise must be concerned with its consequences for others and for the administration of justice.*

Mandatory disclosure

In most jurisdictions today, there are a number of circumstances in which it is mandatory to divulge a patient's private medical information (see Box 3.7).

BOX 3.7

The following is a region-dependent and not exhaustive list of circumstances requiring mandatory disclosure:

1. Communicable disease
2. Child abuse and neglect
3. Vulnerable adults
4. Driving safety
5. Flying, train, and marine safety
6. Fitness to work
7. Gunshot wounds
8. "Management of the healthcare system"
9. Certain criminal activities

---

1. Communicable disease
All North American jurisdictions require notification in cases of contagious, communicable, and virulent diseases. For example, in Ontario, healthcare practitioners need only form an "*opinion* that the person is or may be infected with an agent of a reportable disease [and] shall as soon as possible . . . report thereof to the medical officer of health." This kind of phrasing is found in most public health regulations.[41]

2. Child abuse and neglect

In almost all jurisdictions, medical practitioners are required to report any information about the *possible* mistreatment or neglect of children. Again, the threshold for reporting is having an *opinion*, based on "reasonable grounds," that the abuse is taking place. Children may be in need of protection because of neglect, failure to provide proper medical treatment, emotional, physical or sexual abuse, and so on. Reporting suspected child abuse or neglect does not require the consent of the suspected abuser.[42]

3. Vulnerable adults

Laws to protect vulnerable adults, including the elderly, are not as consistent or available as for children.[43] At the present time, for example, there are few mandates for healthcare professionals to report elder abuse and neglect. In some jurisdictions, there is mandatory reporting of abuse of the elderly or "serious incidents" in long-term care institutions.[44] For community-dwelling elderly, there is little requirement in cases of suspected neglect, physical, financial, or emotional abuse. Even if there are no "elder specific" laws, however, practitioners need to be aware that many current laws (such as Guardianship laws) can be applied to protect the rights and interests of vulnerable adults (See Chapter 6).[45]

4. Driving safety

In the Ontario case of *Toms v. Foster*, a car driven by a 73-year-old man struck a motorcycle, seriously injuring the two riders.[46] Before the accident, despite knowing for two years that the man was suffering from weakness of the legs and diminished agility due to cervical spondylosis that could affect his ability to drive safely, his family doctor and neurologist failed to report this to the Registrar of Motor Vehicles. Although the physicians argued that reporting was a matter of discretion, the court concluded that there are no such exceptions. In this case, the plaintiff was awarded $616,000 with 20 per cent liability assessed against the GP, and 10 per cent liability against the neurologist.

In some jurisdictions such as the UK, reporting one's concerns about driving safety is allowed but not mandated.[47] In other areas, as in Australia,[48] it is up to the individual to self-report. In most jurisdictions, as long as physicians report in good faith, they are typically protected from legal liability. Where there is mandatory reporting, the physician reports the name of the patient (and a statement that he or she suffers from a medical condition making vehicle operation potentially unsafe) to the transport authority, which may then suspend the person's licence, pending an investigation.[49] While you do not require patients' consent to report them, it is respectful to inform them you are going to do so.

Physicians typically do not relish this responsibility and frequently shirk it.[50] Reporting patients can create great distress as driving may be one of their last vestiges of autonomy. Warnings to potentially unfit drivers may reduce the risk of road trauma but may also compromise the doctor–patient relationship. Nevertheless, the principle of autonomy does not involve the right to run over others.

How weak must someone's legs be, how tardy his or her reflexes, to impair his or her driving? Despite the court's view in the *Toms v. Foster* case above that reporting is not a matter of "discretion," physicians must use discretion every day in reporting—is three drinks a day sufficient to impair driving? Five? What about the use of sedatives? Antidepressants? Is driving safe in very early dementia? When to report and when not to report can be difficult to determine. Guidelines have been provided and should be known to all doctors.[51] Nonetheless, there are still many questions around the proper assessment of driving ability. Ongoing research may result in the development of tools to better assess driving risk.[52]

5. Flying, train, and marine safety

Physicians and optometrists are similarly required by the federal *Aeronautics Act* to report pilots and air traffic controllers if they have conditions that might affect flight safety.[53] Similarly, the *Railway Safety Act* requires them to report individuals in positions critical to railway safety who may be unable to perform their duties.[54] Merchant seamen may also be required to undergo medical examinations with mandatory submission of a report by the examining physician.[55]

6. Fitness to work

A physician may be asked to report on the "fitness" of one of his or her patients for employment purposes (e.g., after a prolonged illness). In doing so, the physician needs to be aware of the requirements of the patient's work and may simply state whether or not the patient is "fit" for work. The doctor does not have to identify the specific medical conditions of the patient and ought not to do so without the patient's consent. More complicated relations arise where a physician acts as a "third party" examiner. For example, an insurance company may request an independent medical examination of one of their clients. In Canada the Canadian Medical Protective Association reminds its members (most physicians in Canada) that employees who undergo "fitness-to-work" assessments are owed a duty of confidentiality, even if the assessment reveals that the employee has impaired functional capacities.[56]

Whether or not you are that person's own physician, as regards the examination and the report, the client is owed duties of consent and confidentiality. Among other things, the patient must be told the purposes of the examination and to whom the report will be made, as well as any consequences that might follow, such as benefit eligibility, and who bears the costs of the process. Generally, the patient's consent must be obtained; this consent may be terminated at any time.

Although patients may attempt to put limits on what can be disclosed, the third party physician, who must be accurate in the submitted report, may be unable to submit a complete report and is obliged to note this incompleteness. Even if the examination is done for third party purposes, suspicious or unanticipated findings with consequences for the patient's welfare must be disclosed to the patient and, with his or her consent, to that person's doctor.[57]

It is not always clear what to do with a patient who refuses to permit disclosure to the employer of a condition that might constitute a grave danger to others at work. In cases of serious and foreseeable harm to others, especially if imminent, a patient's refusal to consent to the release of pertinent information should not prevent appropriate disclosure by the physician.

7. Gunshot wounds

Ontario's *Mandatory Gunshot Wound Reporting Act* of 2005 requires public hospitals to report gunshot wounds of patients who present at their facilities. Saskatchewan, Manitoba, and Nova Scotia have extended this obligation to mandate reporting of both gunshot wounds and stab wounds, similar to legislation in many US states. Ontario's Act allows police to act as soon as possible to prevent further violence, injury, or death. Any facility identified by the Act must (1) make a verbal report to local police authorities if someone is being treated for a gunshot wound; (2) provide that person's name, if known; and (3) give the name and location of the facility. The report must be made as soon as practically possible without interfering with the person's treatment or disrupting the regular activities of the facility.[58]

There is no obligation to keep the patient at the facility until the police come. Releasing to the police any information other than that mandated by the Act would be considered a breach of confidentiality. For example, it is not required to disclose what the patient said about how the gunshot wound occurred. It is important to note that this Act does not mandate physicians to report gunshot wounds; only the facility must do so which then can designate the most responsible person to make this report. This duty to report has generated some concern that people so injured may not seek treatment. In fact, experience with other mandatory reporting laws have not shown fall-off in medical attendance of those affected by the laws.[59, 60]

8. *"Management of the healthcare system"*

Physicians must disclose births, stillbirths, and deaths they attend or of which they are aware. Certain deaths—ones that are unexpected, suspicious, or occur in unusual circumstances—require prompt reports to medico-legal death investigators, such as the coroner or the local medical examiner (see Box 3.8).[61] Death certificates must be accurate; properly filling them out takes some training.[62] Healthcare fraud, loss or theft of narcotics, and termination of the employment of a healthcare professional for reasons of incompetence or incapacity must also be disclosed to the proper authorities.

BOX 3.8

Medico-legal death investigators' cases are deaths

- resulting from violence, negligence, malpractice;
- by "unfair means" ("suspicious deaths");
- related to parturition and childbirth;
- which are sudden and unexpected;
- from illness not treated by a legally qualified medical practitioner;
- from any cause other than disease; and
- under circumstances that may require investigation.

---

9. *Certain criminal activities*

It is sometimes asked, is there a duty to report *past* crimes committed by a patient? The answer must be, "it depends." Doctors, in general, have no duty to disclose crimes their patients may have committed.[63] New legislation in many jurisdictions requires practitioners of medicine—and indeed other members of the public generally—to report those who may be involved with terrorism. In this regard, the *Patriot Act* in the US allows authorities by a secret court order to seize patients' medical records without a warrant and forbids the physician from telling anyone such records have been seized.[64] No such equivalent legislation applies in Canada.

It is a different matter if the concern is about future serious crimes, however.

Smith v. Jones

A precedent to breach the duty of confidentiality was set in Canada in *Smith v. Jones,* a case which went to the Supreme Court of Canada. A psychiatrist was retained by a defence lawyer to examine his client who had been charged with aggravated assault of a prostitute.[65] The lawyer indicated to the accused that anything he said during the consultation would be privileged.

During the interview with the psychiatrist, the accused described in some detail his plan to kidnap, rape, and kill prostitutes in the future. The psychiatrist informed the defence lawyer he believed the accused was dangerous and likely to commit future offences unless he received sufficient treatment. The accused subsequently entered a plea of guilty to the assault charge.

Discovering his concerns about the client's past and future dangerousness would not be addressed in the sentencing hearing, the psychiatrist subsequently commenced action for declaration that he would be allowed to disclose his concerns in the interests of public safety. The trial judge ruled the psychiatrist should be mandated to breach confidentiality; when the case was subsequently brought up to the Court of Appeal, it was agreed disclosure was warranted in this case. The threat was clear, serious, imminent, and directed against an identifiable group of persons. It then went to the Supreme Court of Canada which recognized and allowed a public safety exception to the "privileged" relationship between solicitor and clinic that would normally prevent evidence from defence counsel from being used against the defendant.

Forty years ago a jurist sagely observed: "No patient has the moral right to convince his psychiatrist that he is going to commit a crime and then expect him to do nothing because of the principle of confidentiality."[66] Clearly, a judgment of proportionality must be made here: minor crime is one thing, murder another.

IV. To Warn and to Protect

In cases of patients who are a current or future danger to *others*, there is now a widely recognized legal concept of "duty to warn" others which eclipses privacy. (In Chapter 7, section III, we will look at breaching privacy to protect patients from *themselves*, that is, the issue of suicide.) The US has a fairly clear judicial precedent set by the *Tarasoff* case. In 1969, a university psychologist was told by his patient, Mr Poddar, that he intended to kill a former girlfriend, Tatiana Tarasoff. Concerned, the psychologist and his supervising psychiatrist asked the campus police to detain Mr Poddar, but he was released when he appeared rational and promised to stay away from Ms Tarasoff. Two months later, Mr Poddar, who did not return for therapy, murdered Ms Tarasoff. Because no one had warned the victim of her peril the California Supreme Court found the two parties most responsible for this to be the psychologist and university. They were considered negligent in failing to do so.[67]

The court weighed the importance of protecting Mr Poddar's privacy but concluded that this must take second place to "the public interest in safety from violent assault. The protective privilege ends where the public peril begins." According to this ruling, where there is a real hazard to an individual or the community and no other way of relieving this hazard, the patient–therapist confidentiality rule must yield to the interests of safety.

In another US ruling on *Tarasoff* ("*Tarasoff II*"), the court reaffirmed its view that medical professionals ought to err on the side of public safety when it comes to dangerous patients, despite the possible negative implications for privacy: "The risk that unnecessary warnings may be given is a reasonable price to pay for the lives of possible victims that may be saved."[68] *Tarasoff II* emphasized the duty not only to warn but to protect possible victims. Since *Tarasoff*, virtually every US jurisdiction that has ruled on the issue has found a Tarasoff-like duty to warn and/or protect.[69]

BOX 3.9

A clinician has a duty to protect under the following circumstances:

- the clinician has a duty of care towards a patient who has made a serious threat of harm;
- an identifiable person(s) is (are) in danger of grave harm from that patient;
- that harm may be ameliorated or alleviated by an intervention; and
- there is a special relationship of care between the person(s) in danger and the physician.[70]

Although Ms Tarasoff was not the therapists' patient, the court felt she was owed a duty of care because of their relationship with Mr Poddar. There need not be a direct relationship of care between the endangered person and the clinician in order to find a duty to protect. The dangerousness of the clinician's direct client engenders duties to take due care and prevent harm to members of the public that could, predictably, be expected to occur were not proper precautions taken (see Box 3.10). A clinician, for example, who does not attempt to confine or seek to restrain (by involving the police) a homicidal mentally ill patient could be liable for failing to provide due care if the patient should harm another person[71]— even if that victim were unknown to the clinician.

Hospitals and healthcare professionals, similarly, have a duty to protect the public and third parties from harm that might be caused by their mentally ill patients if not "appropriately supervised and controlled . . . The psychiatrist's duty to protect will depend on such factors as the particular risk posed by the patient, the predictability of future behavior giving rise to the risk, and the ability to identify the person or class exposed to the risk."[72]

> **BOX 3.10**
>
> Ways for clinicians to fulfill their duty to protect include the following:
>
> - warn the intended victim and/or the relevant authorities, such as the police; *and*
> - carefully supervise the patient by:
>   - hospitalizing the patient voluntarily; or
>   - seeking involuntary commitment of the patient.[73]

Not universal

The limits to confidentiality outlined here may seem morally reasonable but are not universal. Some jurisdictions seem to forbid a weighing of the consequences of non-disclosure and simply make it a duty almost without exception to respect patient confidences. For example, Europe is vague as regards any "duty to warn." The UK has permitted non-consensual disclosure where there is an identifiable target group. Germany recognizes such disclosure might be justified in an "emergency" threat to life, as a "defence of necessity."

France has no legislative allowance for breaching confidentiality except in "emergencies" when the doctor might have to defend himself—although it is not clear from whom or to whom the breach should be made.[74] Physicians there can be imprisoned if found guilty under the criminal code for violating patient confidentiality—even in circumstances where the patient consents or where the public might be protected from harm. In one case, a physician treated and made his report on a young girl who had been the victim of a sexual assault. When it came to trial, however, he refused to give testimony, despite authorization by the girl's parents, citing the "absolute" nature of medical confidentiality.[75]

Even in France this may be changing, however. In late 2012 it was reported that a French psychiatrist was sentenced to prison after failing to recognize and report the public danger posed by one of his patients who had gone on to murder someone.[76]

A sea change in opinion in Canada came about at least in part due to the murder trial of Colin McGregor, convicted in 1993 of the first-degree murder of his estranged wife, Patricia Allen, an Ottawa lawyer. Six weeks earlier, Mr McGregor had informed his physician he planned to murder his wife. His doctor took no action to warn Ms Allen, following the Code of Ethics of the Canadian Medical Association at that time.

A consensus panel, in part funded by the Estate of Ms Allen, made recommendations in 1998 regarding the duty to warn for the medical profession (see Box 3.11).

> **BOX 3.11**
>
> "A duty to inform [arises] when a patient reveals that he or she intends to do serious harm to another person or persons and it is more likely than not that the threat will be carried out . . . Taking all the circumstances into account, physicians will want to consider very carefully whether they should report threats and will, if there is any doubt, err on the side of informing the police because of the potential seriousness of the consequences in the event that they decide not to inform."[77]

In cases where the patient's secret concerns only himself or herself, the patient is generally owed the duty of confidentiality. If the healthcare professional feels the patient is wrong to keep a matter secret, he or she should try to persuade the patient to change his or her mind. The clinician has to abide by the patient's wishes, ill-advised though they may be, until he or she is ready to change. The only exception to this might be if the patient is (a) suicidal or (b) in imminent danger of serious harm to life or limb, such as returning to a house where the abusive husband has threatened to shoot her. In this case, it should become a police matter before it becomes a coroner's matter.

Professional reporting

Until now, we have focused on the different circumstances under which health professionals may or must breach confidentiality. Health professionals may also be expected to disclose private information about the risks that they themselves, other physicians, or other health professionals may pose to the public.

Fitness to practise medicine
It behooves healthcare professionals with a condition that might affect the safety of their patients and that may worsen over time to be knowledgeable about it, to be vigilant in monitoring it, to seek care from appropriate medical practitioners, and to accept recommendations regarding care and treatment. Professionals who carry diseases such as Hepatitis B or HIV—ones that are transmissible, serious, and might impair the ability to practise safely—are required in some jurisdictions to inform their regulatory organizations, which may then require medical monitoring and set limits on their practice.

The same rules of self-disclosure to medical licensing authorities would apply to any health professional with a condition—depression, early cognitive impairment, psychosis—that may have an impact on their fitness to practise. Many jurisdictions now require self-disclosure of potential or past impairments for purposes of public protection. Such disclosure would be expected at times of licensure enrolment and/or at renewal. However, this must be balanced against the professional's right to privacy.[78] Professional associations should be interested only in a clinician's *current* conditions that are active or might deteriorate in a way that might cause harm to patients. Regulatory authorities typically offer confidential help for impaired professionals. *Healthcare professionals are not obliged to disclose their own health status to their patients unless required to do so by regulatory authorities.*

Physicians in Canada are permitted and, indeed, encouraged, to report to the appropriate local authorities colleagues whom they suspect to be unfit to practise because of illness or addiction. After several rather horrendous cases,[79] the United Kingdom has enacted far-reaching legislation making it mandatory to report unfit healthcare professionals while protecting the "whistle-blowers."[80] Whatever the legal status of such reporting, there would seem to be strong professional reasons to report colleagues who are a danger to others. Traditionally, healthcare professionals have been reluctant to discuss the mistakes of others or to "blow the whistle" on an incapacitated colleague. This may be out of misguided loyalty or fear of repercussions for themselves.[81]

Some jurisdictions besides the UK have legislation in place to protect whistle-blowers. Even when a colleague's mistakes are serious, reporting such conduct will not necessarily be easy or find peer support. A profession can close ranks against a member who makes waves. Though whistle-blowing can protect the public from harm, many whistle-blowers have done so at considerable personal risk.

BOX 3.12

Guidelines for whistle-blowing are as follows:[82]

- the wrongdoing ought to be grave;
- the disclosure must be made in good faith and when ordinary channels of complaint fail;
- the disclosure should have support from others and be prepared for "going viral"; and
- there should be clear and full documentation of one's concerns.

V. The Digital Age

The medical profession as a whole has been slow to adapt to the digital revolution.[83] Although in its infant stages, this revolution promises to fundamentally alter and improve how we learn and practise medicine.[84] The new technologies of information can at times be daunting but they can help prevent medical error by making some tasks of medicine—such as keeping up good medical records, sending consultations, reviewing tests, and applying guidelines—less time-consuming, less onerous, and more efficient. Modern information technologies also pose challenges to privacy and confidentiality.

CASE 3.5 THE POSE THAT PAUSES

You enjoy trawling the Internet and come upon a site that links persons in the community with health professionals. One part of this site is devoted to graduate-level trainees and newly minted health practitioners acting as mentors—providing hints and insights into medical culture—to younger would-be medical students. A physician assistant (PA) posts a number of pictures of himself establishing a central venous line in a patient. In one photo he holds a syringe at a man's neck with a caption, "When you can't start a line in a junkie's arm, go for the neck."[85]

As it happens, you recognize the PA—what, if anything, should you do?

DISCUSSION OF CASE 3.5

It's obvious something very wrong has happened here. The professionalism of the physician assistant has been tarnished and this in turn tarnishes the reputation of medicine. He should not even have to be told this. Cavalier use of medical information invites cynicism and mistrust of healthcare professionals generally. The only dilemma is a practical one: to whom would you talk first: the PA whom you don't really know or your program director?

What is appropriate in the digital age? May a health practitioner accept a friend request from a patient on a social media site? Is it acceptable to Google a patient? May a practitioner post personal information about him or herself online, by blogging or on social media sites? Is it appropriate as a healthcare professional to join an online discussion group devoted to a disease he or she treats? What are the limits to treating/communicating with a patient by email?

The answers to almost all of these questions are tentative and "under review." Ready and timely communication between provider and patient may be facilitated by digital media—especially for patients housebound or at a great distance. Friendship requests may be quite benign as long as they do not intrude on the proper processes of care. (No queue jumping by friends allowed!) Searching for a patient may be informative and helpful; it can also be voyeuristic—and sometimes no different than reading about a well-known patient in the news. Practitioners may reveal information about themselves but should be cautious in doing so when it comes to personal information and only do so to exhibit empathic communication and trust in the profession generally. Practitioners need to be wary about sites that may compromise on promises about privacy. Joining an online discussion group may be a great way to educate and encourage patients; it obviously should not be used as a lure to attract patients to one's practice. Communications with patients by email can be convenient and easy, but messages must be retained or summarized as part of the patient's record. Email messages and online discussion groups are also notoriously not secure. Psychiatrists and other healthcare professionals who engage in psychotherapy, thus, ought to follow especially vigilant stipulations, such as avoiding online relationships with patients. [86]

Many of these concerns were raised by the advent of the telephone and telemedicine.[87] But the gain in information access and permanent data storage as well as the multiplicity of ways in which people can now interact across borders and boundaries, by stealth or by open access, will result in unforeseen and surprising challenges for future healthcare practitioners.

CASE 3.6 TRAINEE TROUBLE

A senior medical trainee finally gets to look after his own patients. He enjoys the responsibilities and is often at the hospital late looking up lab reports and studying the intricacies of his patients' illnesses. A close friend asks if he wouldn't mind looking in on his sister who was admitted recently. The student vaguely knows her and readily offers to help out. He pulls up her chart on the ward computer. To his surprise he finds out she has been admitted following a suicidal drug overdose. The admitting history documents previous attempts at suicide and an impulsive, borderline personality disorder. The student logs off the computer and wonders what he should do with his new-found knowledge.

What should the medical trainee do?

DISCUSSION OF CASE 3.6

The student is now in a bit of a sticky wicket. He will feel pressured by his friend to disclose this information about his sister. On the other hand he will know such information is intensely personal and not to be shared with others. The student has, without the patient's consent, invaded her privacy and has violated the hospital's code of privacy by accessing the chart of a patient not under his care. To make amends he should seek out the appropriate staff person— or perhaps the hospital's privacy officer—and admit the error of his ways. As done with good intentions and followed by appropriate apologies, his actions may not result in disciplinary actions.

Conclusion

Confidentiality is far from a decrepit concept, as has been claimed.[88] It remains a core component of patient autonomy and respect for the person—it still has intrinsic value even if not absolute value. It is defended in many diverse destinations by the regulatory authorities, the courts, and commissioners for privacy. When confidentiality and privacy are casually breached, patients' autonomy and their trust in medicine and authorities generally are undermined. They can feel as violated as if their dwelling were burglarized or intimate promises broken.

In Chapter 4, the subject of another key feature of autonomy (of intrinsic value)—truthtelling—will be considered.

Cases For Discussion

CASE 1: A VIRTUAL PRACTICE

Dr D has recently completed his medical training and is ready to go into independent practice. He and several colleagues are unhappy with being a "doc in a box" with the usual ten-minute-per-patient-visit routine. They decide to set up a "virtual clinic" that will combine the power of modern computing with the ability to interact on-line with sick patients at home. Patients will be able to book appointments on-line and have access to advice by email. Fees will be charged for on-line advice or on-line assessments and be paid through PayPal. Access to the patient's hospital files, research participation, and genetic testing will be incorporated into the patient's EMR.

Question For Discussion

1.   What are the pros and cons for patients and for healthcare professionals of such a virtual clinical arrangement?

CASE 2: IT'S A SMALL WORLD

You are a second-year Dermatology resident attending this week's Grand Rounds being presented by one of your fellow residents. The patient, identified as Ms J, is described as a 23-year-old drug addict who has had multiple sex partners. A photograph of the lesion on her chest area is presented on the screen. To your great surprise, you recognize the tattoo just above the patient's left breast and realize Ms J is one of your younger sister's best friends.

Questions For Discussion

1. As Ms J's name has been anonymized, is there a breach of confidentiality in this case?
2. Using ethical principles, discuss why or why not consent needs to be obtained to use patient information for teaching purposes.

The Power to Heal
Truth and Deception in Clinical Practice

Words which burnt like surgical spirit on an open wound, but which cleansed, as all truth does.

Lawrence Durrell, 1960[1]

Patients have a need for and an interest in medical information independent of issues concerned with consent to medical treatment. This chapter discusses the nature of and complexities associated with truth-telling in healthcare. Disclosure related specifically to consent will be considered in Chapter 5.

I. On Not Telling the Truth

Healthcare professionals regularly make decisions regarding how and how much to tell patients and their families about the patient's medical condition. Although most acknowledge the importance of telling the truth, medicine has long been known for its parsimonious approach to truth-telling. Consider the not very flattering origin of the phrase *doctoring the truth*: "to treat so as to alter the appearance, flavour, or character of, to disguise, falsify, tamper with, adulterate, sophisticate, cook."[2]

CASE 4.1 THE WORRIER

A married, 72-year-old retired construction worker, Mr G, has a history of severe coronary artery disease (CAD), Type 2 diabetes, and recurrent depression. Perpetually in a gloomy state of mind, he worries considerably about his health, fearing he won't make it past 74, the age his father and his father's father died of CAD. One day his family doctor receives a letter from the local hospital informing her Mr G may have had his prostate biopsy done last year with an improperly sterilized re-usable instrument. A patient on whom it had been used just prior to Mr G later died of Creutzfeldt-Jakob disease (CJD).[3] The doctor wonders what, if anything, to say to Mr G. She had read of CJD being transmitted by neurosurgical instruments, but by a prostate biopsy device "the risk must be incredibly low," she thought. She has seen no evidence for this disorder in this patient. She also recalls Mr G reacting almost hysterically when she asked him several years ago about testing for HIV ("What is this? You want to give me another illness to worry about? I'm sick enough already."); it took her an hour to calm him down, but eventually Mr G did the test (which was negative). She reads in the notes from his last full physical that Mr G complained of impotence and was not having intercourse with his wife.

She decides, on grounds of compassion, not to tell him about his possible exposure to CJD.

Was this the right course of action?

The eighteenth-century philosopher Kant viewed lying as *always* wrong—even if necessary, for example, to prevent a would-be killer from tracking down someone you know.[4] Deceiving a would-be murderer, by lying about where your friend is, he [in]famously argued, would be to treat that person as a "means" and not an "end." Most of us would agree that Kant's position is too extreme: putting truth first and saving a life second is the wrong order of priorities. But what if, as in Case 4.1, you simply don't tell the *whole* truth—is that as bad as telling an outright lie? The answer is *sometimes*. It will depend on the consequences of the withholding of information. (A deontologist might say not telling the whole truth is as bad as lying if your intent is the same: to deceive.)

The standards and expectations for truthtelling in clinical practice may be quite different than those in everyday life.[5] In the everyday world, tact, lying, and subterfuge are often used to avoid uncomfortable issues or bad outcomes. For example, lying to save face or to maintain someone else's self-image may seem appropriate. Discomfiting outcomes cannot be so easily avoided in medicine. Nevertheless, the "truth" in medicine was, historically, used in the service of therapeutics. Providing information was done if it would encourage "patient compliance" but avoided if it might lead to non-compliance, anxiety, worry, or suffering on the patient's part. The truth is that the truth can sometimes hurt patients. This is not a rationale for non-disclosure in medicine but it does remind us to choose our words carefully.

DISCUSSION OF CASE 4.1

Mr G needs to be told about the letter at some time.[6] One cannot be certain he was not infected. If he is, it has implications for others. Of course care has to be taken as to how and when one should disclose the news and in whose presence (with or without the spouse, for example). One would want to assess his current mental state and his own assessment of his medical status. The right words need to be found as well—"We all know you worry a lot about your health. How have you been coping with these issues lately? I have some news to tell you that shouldn't make you worry but probably will anyway. Are you in any state to receive such news today?"—pausing after each question and allowing the patient time to respond. If the day is right, you might just get away with telling the truth bereft of a tsunami of emotion.

Advanced malignancies, dementia, HIV seropositivity, and neurological conditions such as multiple sclerosis, some of which are still not very amenable to treatment, all have posed challenges for clinicians around how to disclose in a forthright and compassionate way. Patients can likewise avoid unwelcome truths: for example, many of those at risk for Huntington's Chorea decline to be tested for the causative gene—in large part as it is an untreatable, fatal illness.[7]

Consider this: how many of us would really want to know how or when we will die if it were written in the stars or in one's genome? Interestingly, perhaps as we are getting used to the idea of genetic testing, many people say they would get tested for a serious psychiatric disorder, such as schizophrenia—but more likely to say so if there was effective treatment and the test was reliable.[8]

The truth can result in "labelling" patients which then can lead to negative consequences such as excessive worry about the future or the failure to fulfill role expectations such as work attendance and family obligations. For example, one study found that patients who were told they had hypertension exhibited decreased emotional well-being and more frequent absence from work.[9] In another study, giving more information to patients with cancer resulted in higher anxiety levels than those not so informed.[10] Labelling can also result in shunning, discrimination, and exile. (Think of how patients diagnosed with leprosy, AIDS, or schizophrenia were and are treated.) Concerns regarding other very bad outcomes of disclosure—complete loss of hope, premature death, or suicide—are largely anecdotal and require closer study. Insensitive truthtelling by a cold, unempathic clinician can have outcomes as bad as those of deception. The experience can be particularly traumatic for ill-prepared patients in cultures less comfortable with openness about critical illness.[11]

In any case, the news to be told to patients is rarely black or white. Uncertainty about the diagnosis, prognosis, and the potential impact of various therapies makes clinicians wary of a simplistic approach to telling the truth. For this reason, many practitioners feel that ruling out deceptive and paternalistic practices is to forbid use of a needed part of the therapeutic armamentarium, the "therapeutic (white) lie." Some patients, it is said, may "wish to be deceived" or, at least, not be told "everything." In this view, medicine is seen as inherently deceptive and paternalistic. Its success rests as much in art and acting as in science and evidence.

Clinician as drug

The psychiatrist Michael Balint, in his analysis of general practice in the 1950s and 1960s, wrote one of the most profound books on medicine, *The Doctor, His Patient and the Illness*. In it, he examined what lies behind the therapeutic impact that primary care doctors have on their patients. Balint held that the strongest drug in medicine is the "doctor" and his or her "apostolic role," that is, how he or she can guide patients through their illnesses.[12] "There are some people," he writes, "who . . . carry more responsibility than is good for them, especially when ill."[13] The doctor's task is to "educate" the patient, not necessarily about the "truth" of their condition, but as to what is a "reasonable" attitude to take when ill.

There is wisdom in these observations, as "parentalistic" as they may seem. Balint's views as to the complexity and depth of the clinician–patient relationship, the balance that takes place in patients between maturity and dependence, should make one hesitate before revealing everything to patients all at once, in the "fell sweep of a full swoop."[14]

If practitioners must always and only disclose the truth, they may be unable to maintain patient hope, the patient's belief that he or she will get better, in the face of terrible news. Indeed, some patients, against all odds, under the influence of the "less-than-the-full-truth" disclosure, do get better (for a while anyway). One could argue that hope is, by its very nature, unrealistic and lies behind quotidian human attempts to overcome the finite and fragile limits of human existence. (On the other hand, many others do not get better and, due to overly optimistic prognoses and unrealistic hopes, seek and sometimes receive overly aggressive medical treatment.[15])

For their own good

Given all this, it is perhaps not surprising to find how deferential law and social custom used to be to the common practice of "doctoring the truth." Until 40 or 50 years ago, even in Western democratic societies with some sort of commitment to "informed consent," deceptive actions by physicians were commonly sanctioned as acceptable practice.

In a 1954 case, a gynecologist failed to inform a patient of a large needle left accidentally in her perineum following an episiotomy because he thought it might cause her "excessive worry." The judge opined that this failure to disclose was acceptable because it was done for the patient's own good: "I cannot admit any abstract duty to tell patients what is the matter with them . . . it all depends on circumstances . . . the patient's character, health, social position . . ."[16]

"Done for her own good." This is a common refrain we hear from those who would act in deceptive ways. Is it simply a way of justifying mistakes, failures to communicate, and deceptive practices by making them appear beneficent? "You want answers?!" Jack Nicholson exploded in the 1992 movie, *A Few Good Men*, "You can't handle the truth!" While not quite so dramatic in real life, there is a sense of a benevolent protectionism ever present in the medicine of many times and cultures.

Patients, especially when ill, were and are presumed to have difficulty handling the unvarnished truth. It often was, and sometimes still is, the doctor's duty to keep the "whole truth," or even a "partial truth," from them.[17] Some cultures and families believe truthtelling is cruel because it may cause avoidable worry in the ailing or frail patient. This "protective deception" has some credence, especially at times when, and in those places where, medicine could offer little tangible help to patients.

Truthtelling cannot be an absolute or stand-alone duty. There are times when telling the "full truth" must be restrained in proportion to the hazards and pitfalls of doing so and the impact it may have on others. Truthtelling is clearly both an art and a skill requiring years of experience to learn how to do it well. Sometimes, faced with great loss or suffering, one simply is at a loss for words. It is inevitable in training and in practice that to tell the truth will at times be very hard indeed. Here is one role for silence or a measured disclosure by the clinician who takes cues from the patient in terms of how much truth he or she can handle at any one time.

II. The Truthtelling Task

Truthtelling is the attitude and practice of being open and forthright with patients. It is not necessarily about telling the "whole truth," a usually impossible task, but about intending not to mislead or deceive. Information necessary for patients to "make sense" of their medical situation is conveyed. There are so many ways to mislead, it can take clinicians some work and thought to decide how best to present patients with information in unbiased ways.[18]

Deception, by contrast, turns clinicians away from efforts to help patients gain better insight into their conditions. It involves withholding information from, or actively lying to, patients in order to bring about a certain outcome desired by the healthcare provider. Healthcare professionals may deliberately or accidentally engage in deceptive practices with patients for a variety of reasons from the benign (therapeutic) to the malignant (personal gain). The practice of veracity with patients is another example of the "advantage-reducing" role of ethical rules; truthtelling tries to put practitioner and patient on more level ground.

There are many reasons, philosophical and practical, apart from Kant's, to make truthtelling with patients the default position (see Box 4.1).

BOX 4.1

Telling the truth

1. promotes good outcomes;
2. reduces risks of harm to patients;
3. furthers the life choices of patients;
4. shows respect for persons;
5. promotes trust; and
6. reduces litigation.

---

1. Promotes good outcomes

Truthtelling increases patient compliance (concordance) with prescribed medications,[19] reduces morbidity such as pain[20] and anxiety[21] associated with medical interventions, and improves patient comprehension of medical decision-making.[22] Informed patients report more satisfaction with their care and are less apt to change physicians than those not well informed.[23]

2. Reduces risks of harm to patients

Non-disclosure and deceit can harm patients in many ways. For example, if not informed about their medical condition, they may fail to obtain medical attention when they should. (This aspect of disclosure, most intimately associated with consent, will be discussed in greater detail in Chapter 5.) Knowing the level of certainty necessary to trigger disclosure can be difficult. There is no simple answer but, if a serious diagnosis is suspected, there is a professional onus to caution the patient about this as soon as is reasonable. Obviously, as with other factors, there is professional discretion about how much to tell and when.

Clinical uncertainty can be shared with patients.[24] Informing patients about the uncertainties and the range of available treatment options allows them to appreciate the complexities of medicine, to ask questions, to make informed and realistic decisions, to assume responsibility for those decisions, and to be better prepared in case the dire prognosis turns out to be correct.[25] Doubtless some patients find the uncertainty confusing and will need to rely more on the healthcare provider's helping hand in making decisions. It is hard to predict which patients want what information, especially if it makes no difference to the choices before them. Some patients decline prognostic information and play a passive role in the decision-making process.[26]

3. Furthers patients' life choices

CASE 4.2 NOT TO WORRY

In British Columbia in 1986 a woman in the twelfth week of a much-wanted pregnancy contracted chicken pox. Wary of conventional medicine, she hired a midwife for the delivery. The patient and her husband, wanting to keep medical interventions to a minimum, had earlier refused an ultrasound. Her family doctor told the woman the fetus could suffer some abnormalities of limb and skin as a result of the chicken pox but reassured her the risk was small and not a reason for an abortion. The child was carried to term but unfortunately was born with congenital *varicella* syndrome. She has spent much of her life in hospital.

The parents filed a "wrongful life" suit against the doctor (see Chapter 10 for a more detailed discussion of this topic), alleging they would have aborted had they known all the risks to the fetus from exposure to *varicella*. The doctor explained she had not disclosed the serious but unlikely risks (such as cortical atrophy) because she had not wished to worry an expectant mother, especially with reasons that did not, in her mind, justify abortion.

Was the physician right in failing to disclose all the risks?

Failure to provide information that is of central importance to a patient's future means depriving that person of one means by which he or she can live as he or she sees fit. Rather than asking, "Can the patient stand being told?" one should ask: "Can the patient stand not being told?"[27] Certainly, patients should be offered the opportunity to know of medical evils that threaten them. Providing accurate information about an illness that will affect how they will lead their lives in the future allows patients to plan for that future.

Not telling patients some important information about their lives—such as their prognosis—suggests the healthcare professional knows better than they what should be done with this information. Consider how unlikely this is: for this to be so, the professional would have to be familiar with intimate facts concerning the lives of their patients as well as knowing their values and beliefs and how they would apply them.

DISCUSSION OF CASE 4.2

In this case the suit was unsuccessful because the judge was not convinced this couple would have in fact aborted, given the small risk of serious abnormalities and their reluctance to accept conventional medicine. However, the court did find the doctor's explanation negligent as, "without complete candour," she could not "properly assist her patients with such a deep and disturbing decision."[28] It is actually surprising the doctor won this case—the judge used as the standard for disclosure what *this* patient would have wanted to know in order to act. The more common standard is what a "reasonable person" would want to know: a reasonable person, surely, would want to know about potential defects in order to be better prepared for them, not necessarily just to be able to make a decision to abort the fetus.

Although keeping information from patients may be done with good intentions, it is wrong if this results in doctors making intimate decisions for patients—such as an abortion—that should be the patients' to make. This case is also about shared decision-making, which will be discussed in Chapter 5.

4. Shows respect for persons

CASE 4.3 A DARK SECRET

A 20-year-old female student has recently become a patient in your primary care practice. She has been well, other than undergoing surgery as a young teen for what she was told were "diseased reproductive organs." She knows little else about that surgery.

When her medical records are received, there is a letter from her pediatrician stating that "she" is, in fact, genetically a male with Androgen Insensitivity Syndrome. (In this disorder of gonadal dysgenesis, patients usually have an XY karyotype with inguinal testes and a female phenotype. Due to lack of responsiveness to testosterone in utero, male genitalia do not form. The child is often not diagnosed until puberty when such individuals fail to menstruate. The testes are removed during adolescence because of the risk of gonadal cancer.) The patient's family and her physicians had decided not to tell the patient of her "true sex," feeling it would possibly cause great psychological trauma. The letter urges future healthcare providers not to tell her.

You pride yourself on being honest with your patients; you think it is extremely important that patients be as well informed as possible.

What, if anything, should you say to this patient?

Beyond the information needed for decisions about medical treatment, patients have an interest in information concerning who they are as people. Whether patients do anything with medical or "personal health information" is a separate issue. For example, a patient's desire to take an active role in making decisions about treatment "may be less strong than [simply] the need for clear and accurate information."[29]

Patients should, in this view, be told the truth because of the respect due to them as persons; the truth can empower them and encourage authenticity and autonomy. Empowering patients should be recognized as one of the central goals of modern medicine, as important as the amelioration of suffering and the prevention of premature death. Interviews with patients generally support this perspective. For example, in a study done before any treatment for multiple sclerosis existed, patients with the disease felt they had a right to know what was wrong with them. Some were angry about being asked why they wished to know. One said: "Do I have to explain why? Just so that I know."[30]

The principle of respect for persons—encouraging valid choice, promoting patient empowerment, supporting authentic hope—calls for honest disclosure. Doctors who withhold critical information from patients are denying them the opportunity to live and die as they see fit—this practice denies patients an opportunity to cope and hope on their own terms. Hope does not require dishonesty.[31] Very ill patients may want someone to look after and guide them, but this does not necessarily mean a preference for ignorance or deception. Allowing others to make decisions for oneself, to be "taken care of" in the full sense of this phrase, can be consistent with wishing to remain informed about one's condition.

> ### DISCUSSION OF AND FOLLOW-UP TO CASE 4.3
>
> "Testicular feminization syndrome" (or Androgen Insensitivity Syndrome as it is better known today) is a dark secret for some.[32] In the past, the diagnosis was commonly not disclosed to those with this condition. Those who participated in the original treatment of this patient may regret failing to consider how her condition should be revealed to her later in life.
>
> Clearly, we need to know more about the patient: is she the type of person who wishes to be as fully informed as possible? Unless she evinces a clear wish not to know, she should be told. It is, after all, her life. You should seek guidance from skilled counsellors unless you have had experience with other cases. Disclosing this syndrome could be devastating to an unsuspecting patient, and the effect may be compounded if you fail to explain correctly what the condition means. Her sense of herself could be deeply shaken. Sensitive counselling as to the nature of sexuality and gender identity will be vital. You need to investigate what kind of resources are available to help this patient cope in the future.
>
> Interestingly enough, when this patient was told the truth, her longstanding feelings that she was "different" from other women were confirmed. She was relieved to find a physical basis for her feelings. Indeed, she laughed when told about her condition! So much for the expected devastating effects of telling the truth! She did, however, express anger towards her previous doctors and her parents, who had deceived her for so long.

5. Promotes trust

Cabot's 1903 view that physicians should strive to create a "true impression" in the mind of the patient about his or her condition and thereby foster the covenant of trust between physician and patient is consistent with this perspective.[33] This view applies to all healthcare professionals, not just physicians, and nicely contrasts with the centuries-old medical tradition cautioning against veracity with patients.

It is easy to tell one lie but hard to tell only one, Sissela Bok wisely observed in her seminal book, *Lying*. Deceit in medicine is particularly invidious as it undermines the bond of trust between the healthcare provider and patient and produces "corrosive worry" in patients who are deceived.[34] Lies from a health professional, whether done for ill or the best of intentions, can seem particularly shocking when revealed to the public eye; they undermine public faith in medicine. By contrast, proper disclosure to patients saves healthcare providers from entering this labyrinth of lying.

6. Reduces litigation

Failure to be entirely truthful with patients, even if leading to good outcomes (such as sickness amelioration, avoidance of anxiety), can result in healthcare professional domination of decision-making and this can, in turn, provoke patient disappointment, discontent, and litigation. When things don't go well, good communication skills consistent with veracity are even more important as a protective factor against legal actions initiated by patients.[35] (A discussion of disclosure of medical error is to be found in Chapter 8.)

III. Modern Law and the Profession

Not surprisingly, existing jurisprudence relevant to truthtelling varies among countries and is largely focused on negligent disclosure for consent purposes.

Canadian courts have long recognized the physician's obligation to provide information that would be required by a reasonable patient in the plaintiff's position (*Reibl v. Hughes* 1980; see Chapter 5). Australian[36] and most American jurisdictions[37] similarly use this so-called modified-subjective standard while British courts favour more of a "profession-based standard" of disclosure (what a reasonable professional would disclose).[38] Although the latter standard would seem to favour physicians who fail to disclose, "it ain't necessarily so." The profession as a whole is turning in the direction of open disclosure and the UK courts may strike down a profession-based standard of disclosure if it conflicts with good clinical care.

Indeed the profession of medicine, at least in North America, has turned squarely in the direction of openness with patients. The American College of Physicians recommends: "However uncomfortable for the clinician, information that is essential to, and desired by, the patient must be disclosed. How and when to disclose information, and to whom, are important concerns that must be addressed with respect for patient wishes."[39] It adds that the professional duty to be honest with patients requires due care: "Disclosure and the communication of health information should never be a mechanical or perfunctory process. Upsetting news and information should be presented to the patient in a way that minimizes distress."

The British Medical Association notes that the "relationship of trust depends upon 'reciprocal honesty' between patient and doctor" and also encourages the sensitive delivery of bad news.[40] The Canadian Medical Association's Code of Ethics recommends that physicians provide patients with whatever information that, from the patient's perspective, might have a bearing on medical decision-making and communicate that information in a comprehensible way.[41]

IV. The Changing Practice of Medicine

The modern emphasis on truthtelling is reflected in the empirical literature concerning the practice of medicine.

What doctors do

Oken's landmark 1961 survey of 219 physicians in the United States found that 90 per cent would not disclose a diagnosis of cancer to a patient.[42] Attitudes towards disclosure were influenced by personal and emotional factors. Many expressed pessimism and futility about cancer treatment. Others feared their patients would become more depressed or commit suicide, although such fears were based on no actual evidence. Oken's study dates from an era before the advent of informed consent; its findings reflect the era of "medical paternalism," not so long ago, when doctors made decisions for competent patients.

More typical of the attitudes of physicians today were findings published almost 20 years later. A survey of 264 American physicians in 1979 showed that 97 per cent would disclose a diagnosis of cancer.[43] This seems to indicate a complete reversal in the practice of telling patients the truth, at least as far as the diagnosis of cancer goes.

Other studies suggest a less than complete conversion to medical candour. In one US study, physicians who reported that they commonly tell cancer patients the truth said they did so in a way intended to preserve hope and "the will to live," valued notions in US society[44] (and almost anywhere else for that matter). Compared to their North American counterparts, gastroenterologists from southern and eastern Europe are less likely to be candid with patients about serious disease, believing this to be the best way to preserve hope.[45]

Old ways never change completely. A 2009 survey of almost 2,000 US physicians showed that, while the vast majority of physicians endorsed the need for honesty, 10 per cent admitted to having told an adult patient something untrue in the previous year and just over one-half admitted giving a more optimistic prognosis to a patient.[46] The paper did not explore the reasons for the seeming failure to comply with the expectation of honesty.

What patients want

The majority of empirical studies have indicated that patients do want to know the truth. Studies as far back as 1950, reviewed in Oken's 1961 paper, revealed that 80 to 90 per cent of patients wanted to be told if the examination revealed a diagnosis of cancer. Typical of the studies Oken examined was one conducted in 1957 by Samp and Curreri in which 87 per cent of a group of 560 cancer patients and their families felt a patient should be told the truth.[47]

An American survey in 1982 by the President's Commission on Ethical Problems in Medicine revealed that 94 per cent of patients want "to know everything" about their condition, 96 per cent want to know a diagnosis of cancer, and 85 per cent want to know a realistic estimate of their time to live, even if this was less than one year.[48] In a 2006 study 89 per cent of patients with cognitive complaints wanted to be told a diagnosis of Alzheimer's disease[49] and over 80 per cent of patients with amyotrophic lateral sclerosis wanted as much information as possible.[50] Studies of older patients, sometimes thought to be less interested in the truth, have shown that almost 90 per cent want to be told the diagnosis of cancer.[51]

Other studies, not surprisingly, suggest cultural influences upon truthtelling preferences. For example, one study found a greater percentage of Korean-born patients preferred to be given less information than did US-born patients.[52] In Italy, lack of candour about the diagnosis of Alzheimer's disease is common.[53] A greater percentage of patients in Japan as compared with the US (65 per cent versus 22 per cent) would want their families to be told a diagnosis of cancer before being informed themselves, and many more Japanese than US doctors agreed with this (80 per cent versus 6 per cent).[54] As a result, patients with advanced cancer in Japan are often told their prognosis only if their families consent.[55]

Despite such statistics, cultures, societies, and groups within them are not monolithic so it should not be assumed that all members of such share the same attitude to truthtelling and deception. The digital age has helped foster a global public interest in obtaining information and a decline in the more benign reasons ("professional discretion") to withhold it.[56] Countries such as Italy, not known for their frankness, are noticing a change in favour of openness.[57] Religious institutions, boarding schools, businesses, hospitals, and sports groups all have had their reputations tarnished by failing to be transparent and truthful. The democratizing influence of the digital age on authoritarian and closed systems and societies has been, and will continue to be, profound.

V. Truthtelling's Exceptions

Despite modern trends encouraging veracity with patients, there are legitimate "exceptions" to truthtelling in clinical practice (as suggested at the beginning of this chapter). These are not so much exceptions, however, as they are "special circumstances" that require tact and care from the healthcare professional in exercising the duty to tell the truth.

BOX 4.2

"Exceptions" to truthtelling:

1. patient self-image;
2. patient incapacity: dementia;
3. in the case of children;
4. emergencies;
5. therapeutic privilege; and
6. in cases where the news is bad.

---

1. Patient self-image

CASE 4.4 MIRROR, MIRROR ON THE WALL

Mr C is a handsome single male who managed—just—to live through the worst years of the AIDS epidemic. When he had been HIV-positive for six years, it seemed the disease was finally catching up with him. He was losing weight and looked gaunt. On the very day that his doctor thought it might be time to discuss end-of-life issues, Mr C looked at himself in the room's mirror, and happily exclaimed to his doctor, "I look pretty good, don't you think?" The lesions of *molluscum contagiosum* on his face had abated with treatment and he was happy about that. The doctor thought to himself, "You look pretty good all right . . . but only for someone who will likely be dead in a few months." Needless to say, he did not share these thoughts and simply congratulated Mr C for his perseverance.

Later, the patient's doctor reflected on this interaction. "What a coward I am," he thought, "I shouldn't have so readily agreed with him."

Was Mr C's doctor right to be self-critical?

Studies suggest that at least 10 to 20 per cent of all patients do not want to know the details of their condition. For example, some patients with terminal illnesses in previously referenced studies indicated they did not want to know the full truth. Healthcare professionals should be sensitive to such statements or attitudes and try to probe the patient's appreciation of the possible consequences, if any, of not knowing. When such desires are authentic, they should be respected. This is especially true for personal "truths" that have no bearing on care. The less critical for beneficial treatment any information or beliefs that the patient or the clinician may harbour, the less necessary it is for the clinician to "correct" them.

DISCUSSION OF CASE 4.4

Mr C's doctor was self-critical as he felt he missed an opportunity to discuss end-of-life care. But the patient's "self-deception," if you can call it that, was not a road to therapeutic non-compliance. Although the patient was "eagerly anxious" to try new anti-AIDS regimens, he was prone at other times to despondency over the limitations of various treatments for AIDS. "I don't know if I can go on," Mr C would exclaim. "Is it really worth it?" At such times what the patient needed from the clinician was not a pessimistic or overly optimistic response but an exploration of what was so hard for him and a willingness to help him work through it. In fact this patient has done very well since then—with the Highly Active Anti-Retroviral Treatment, he has flourished and rebounded from his clinical nadir.

The doctor and the patient were right, I think, in avoiding the path of pessimism. There was "no harm" done in not challenging his earlier self-perception and much good accomplished in supporting him while new treatments were being developed.

Denial, hope, and optimism may have deleterious effects upon both the patient's and the clinician's "realistic" decisions about treatment but, where that is not an issue, there is no need to take any action other than support and encouragement. We all have our defense mechanisms and ways of coping that may fly in the face of reality but they are still our ways of coping.

2. Patient incapacity: Dementia

CASE 4.5 "I'M SO STUPID"

You are a family physician seeing Ms L, an 88-year-old woman brought by her daughter because of concerns she has become increasingly forgetful and has not been looking after herself properly. Not having seen her for two years, you are shocked at how mentally impaired she seems. She scores poorly on simple testing for cognitive impairment. At one point she begins to cry and says, "What's wrong with me? I'm so stupid!" You stop your interview to console Ms L who quickly settles down, laughing, "Oh, I suppose I'm just getting older. You know, my sister and my mother were just like this."

You feel Ms L almost certainly suffers from either Alzheimer's disease or vascular dementia.

Must you tell her this?

DISCUSSION OF CASE 4.5

Here is where having a longitudinal relationship with the patient helps. There will be ample opportunities in the future to disclose the likely diagnosis if this is what Ms L wants to know and can appreciate. At this time, you may be unsure about what the patient is prepared to hear. It seems appropriate to reserve or delay the "full truth" for another day when you can explore with the patient what she understands about "getting older" and what would best help her cope with her cognitive losses.

If a patient is mentally unable to understand all the information that would under ordinary circumstances be disclosed, the health professional should attempt to tailor such information to the degree that will help the patient appreciate what he or she can—incompetence is rarely total.

3. In the case of children

Special precautions about truthtelling apply to children. Although very young children may be unable to understand their full situation—medically, socially, psychologically—their capacity to grasp complex information increases as they mature.[58] Parents may ask that children not be informed of their condition—such as their genetic heritage or having an untreatable illness—but such requests should not be written in stone. Hard to explain conditions justifying non-disclosure to a young child, such as Androgen Insensitivity Syndrome, may no longer hold as the child matures. Decisions to withhold important information from a child should therefore incorporate a plan for disclosing the information as the child grows older (see Box 4.3).

Failing to be honest with children can have lasting negative psychological consequences for them—such as depression and loss of self-esteem.[59]

Lack of candour with children can also negatively impact their parents as well. In one study, parents able to be forthright about death with their dying child felt such open discussion helped them and their child. Parents unable to be so honest later regretted their reticence and experienced guilt and lasting unhappiness.[60]

> **BOX 4.3**
> Decisions to withhold important information from a child should incorporate a plan for disclosure as the child grows older.

4. Emergencies

When a patient's medical condition is so unstable that telling the truth is considered unsafe or not prudent, it is acceptable to withhold certain information. To be justified, the emergency exception to the truthtelling rule requires that the emotional or physical condition of the patient must be so severely affected at that time so as not to permit safe communication of information. As the condition of the patient may change, the healthcare professional should attempt to revisit the issue of truthtelling when the patient appears more stable, that is, when the emergency abates.

5. Therapeutic privilege

"Therapeutic privilege" is invoked when a health professional decides for a seemingly capable patient that it is in the patient's best interests not to know certain information for purposes of consent to treatment (as in Case 4.1). It should be seen as a variant of the emergency exception to the rule of veracity. (The patient or situation must be so unstable that it is not the time for truthtelling.) Where consent to treatment is not an issue, the law, but not ethics, may be neutral as to whether a clinician has an obligation to share the information with the patient. Ethics would say, even if such information cannot be "used" by the patient (to ameliorate a condition, for example), he or she may still wish to have this, as was noted earlier "just so that I know." Putting a name to a set of symptoms can be comforting to some (and worrying to others), so the symptoms are not seen as an "imaginary" ("all-in-the-head") illness.[61]

6. In cases where the news is bad

It can be difficult to predict what information a patient will find upsetting or how upsetting that information will be. Poor truthtelling practices, even if the information conveyed is accurate, can have devastating consequences for patients.[62] Such disclosure is typically done too hurriedly, in the wrong setting, without appreciation of the patient's circumstances, and without addressing the patient's real needs and fears. Patients need to know, for example, not only a diagnosis, but what it may mean for them and their family, now and in the future.

Studies show that the way in which the information is communicated may be just as important as the information itself.[63] Care must be taken that information is given at the right time and in the right place, a "compassionate milieu." Even if telling the truth does have some negative consequences, this does not in itself warrant non-disclosure (see Box 4.4).

BOX 4.4

"The hurried telling of bad news in a busy clinic with little explanation and no opportunity for the patient to ask questions can result in unnecessary psychological and emotional pain."[64]

It is important to break bad news carefully and compassionately. The news may be brutal for a patient; the telling of it need not be.[65] Good communication skills are essential to truthtelling. Done well, information sharing—which includes conveying "bad news"—will generally improve patient satisfaction and the quality of medical care.[66] In all cases of such sharing, just how and when to discuss the patient's situation, and how much to say at any one time, will vary from one patient to the next.[67] This is the art of truthtelling, relying on the doctor's skills and attitudes to "take the patient into his [or her] confidence"[68] and give a "true impression" of the illness.[69]

Suggestions to clinicians/trainees for sharing information

1. Be well prepared for the session by having a plan for disclosure before the interview. You need to be as informed as possible about the patient's situation and know how to get answers for the patient if unable to answer any questions. You need to know what the patient needs to do next.
2. The sharing of information, whether good or bad, is best done when you and the patient have time for each other. Try not to be or appear rushed.
3. Both parties should be reasonably comfortable; you should sit, not stand. Privacy and a pleasant room are always welcome.
4. Ask if the patient would like anyone else to be present as part of the discussion.

5. If cultural, ethnic, or family barriers to veracity are possible, offer the patient the opportunity to know: "Are you the kind of person who likes to know everything or would you prefer us to speak with someone else?"

6. Straightforwardness in language and lack of prevarication are essential. Try to keep medical terms simple; you must make reasonable efforts to help patients understand the news in their own terms. If translation is required, it may be preferable to use a non-family member, assuming patient autonomy and confidentiality can be assured, as loved ones may sometimes not convey information correctly for their own reasons.

7. You may best prepare a patient for "bad news" by giving a "shot across the bow," a warning that what you are about to disclose is something very difficult (e.g.,"Things have not turned out as well as we'd hoped" or "I have some hard information to share with you . . . ").

8. Patients and professionals give non-verbal cues as to how well each is listening to the other. Patients may express strong emotions; this is to be expected and acknowledged. The late Dr Robert Buckman, author of *How to Break Bad News*, always encouraged practitioners and trainees to identify and try to understand a patient's emotional state before proceeding, and in so doing, engage and empathize with patients at a deeper and more satisfying level.[70] Patients must be able to express their fears and worries and will need to understand how the illness is likely to affect their future.

9. You should be available to schedule follow-up sessions as needed, especially if the information is serious or uncertain.

CASE 4.6 "WHAT'S UP, DOC?"

You are a clinical clerk in your final year of medical school looking after a previously well 66-year-old married male patient, Mr I, admitted recently due to a two-week history of vomiting and dramatic weight loss. Tests done two days ago revealed he has advanced metastatic gastric cancer. The internist responsible for this patient tells you Mr I is unaware he is dying of cancer. "It was the family's wish not to tell him and I went along with it. He doesn't speak much English and the family said in their culture the family is always told first." she says, "He thinks he has a bad infection in his colon, so don't say anything."

One evening, when everyone else has left for the day and you are on call, the patient asks to see you. He tells you he has been gradually feeling worse since admission. "Why am I still vomiting? Is there nothing you can do for me?" His English seems perfectly fine to you. He then adds, "Tell me, Doc, it isn't just an infection, is it?"[71]

How should you respond?

DISCUSSION OF CASE 4.6

Medical trainees are often put in a difficult position by the attending staff if the decision has been made to deceive a patient. Trying to be a good "team player" and not rock the boat may compromise the student's moral integrity.[72] Using the ethics decision procedure makes it easier to decide what to do. The patient is presumed competent unless proven otherwise. Of course we need to know more about the patient and his family. (Sit by the head of his bed, you may be in for a long evening!). What does he know? What does he want to know? What does he suspect? What is his mood? Who are his family members and what are their relationships like? What about the supposed "cultural taboo" against truthtelling? Assuming he is capable and indeed wishes to know "the truth," his wish to be so informed should prevail. (He is not suicidal; there is no evidence the truth will harm him; he is due to the truth as a matter of natural justice; just because others in his culture are reported to not want to know the truth does not mean *he* doesn't want to know.) *How* and *when* to tell him are the practical issues.

You could seek further input from a senior resident or, better still, the attending staff person herself (saying something to her such as, "I was in a difficult situation last night. Mr I confronted me directly about his diagnosis. Help me understand why you went along with the family and what we are going to say to him . . ."). A reasonable answer—one that reflects your humble role—is to say to the patient, truthfully, that you can understand how important the truth is for him, that you are uncertain of what other treatment options exist, but you need first to discuss "what else it might be" with a senior physician. You might gain some time to allow you and your senior staff to finally find a way of breaking the bad news to an already suspicious patient. If he persists in querying you, you should never lie to a patient. Telling him the awful truth is the dignified thing to do. In any case you will also have to figure out how to help his family cope and how to answer the inevitable question from the patient, "Why didn't you tell me earlier?"

Conclusion

There are circumstances justifying non-disclosure of medical information, especially where treatment issues are not at stake. In general, however, modern healthcare professionals have a standing professional recommendation to tell or warn patients about such information that may impact them. Although it can be upsetting to give bad news, clinicians should not feel they always have to protect patients from such news. There are ways of delivering it that can soften the blow. Trust, dignity, prudence, and respect for the patient, all call for care in how "the truth" is revealed to patients and their close ones. The task for healthcare professionals is to combine honesty and respect for patient autonomy with caring and compassion.

In Chapter 5 we will look at healthcare professionals' responsibilities regarding disclosure for the purposes of informed consent.

Cases For Discussion

CASE 1: A "WELL WOMAN" WITH A BLURRY PAST

A 26-year-old accountant, a new patient to your family practice, comes in for a "well-woman" examination. She recounts nothing of significance except for an episode six years ago of weakness in one arm and blurring of vision unaccompanied by headache which disappeared within 24 hours. The patient went to a neurologist who, after conducting several tests, reassured her there was no evidence of stroke and advised her not to worry about the episode. She has indeed thought no more about this. Other than chronic fatigue, the patient seems currently to be symptom-free.

When her medical records arrive, there is a letter from the specialist to the patient's previous doctor stating she likely has multiple sclerosis (MS). The neurologist says it is his custom not to disclose the diagnosis too early as it causes excessive worry. He urges the family physician not to inform the patient.

Questions For Discussion

1. Outline the ethical arguments for or against disclosure of the diagnosis of MS to this patient.
2. What do you say when the patient asks why she wasn't told her diagnosis six years ago?
3. What would your approach to the patient be if she was very anxious?

CASE 2: IS THE TRUTH BAD FOR YOUR HEALTH?

A study of over 6 million Swedish subjects examined the associations between a cancer diagnosis and the immediate risk of suicide or death from cardiovascular causes from 1991 through 2006.[73] As compared with cancer-free persons, the relative risk of suicide among patients receiving a cancer diagnosis was 12.5 during the first week and 3.1 during the first year. The relative risk for cardiovascular death was 5.6 during the first week and 3.3 during the first month. The authors noted that "increased risk was particularly prominent for cancers with a poor prognosis."

Questions For Discussion

1. How would you interpret the results of this study in light of the injunction to be honest with patients?
2. Does this study influence your views on the duty to tell the truth?

The Power to Choose
Due Care and Informed Consent

Over himself, over his own body and mind, the individual is sovereign.
John Stuart Mill, 1859[1]

Respect for the patient's right of self-determination on particular therapy demands a standard [of disclosure] set by law for physicians rather than one which physicians may or may not impose upon themselves.
Canterbury v. Spence, 1972[2]

Informed consent has been called a "sword and shield," a doctrine and a practice by which patients may protect themselves from unwanted interventions and take responsibility for shaping their lives as they see fit.[3] This can also be a shield for the healthcare professional, a protection from litigation. The best defence—and best prevention—against suits alleging failure to obtain consent is to communicate faithfully in a timely and honest way with patients and help them make decisions that best express their genuine wishes. In this chapter we will examine the requirements for consent in greater detail.

The rationale for consent is not primarily a legal one; consent is fundamental to the modern liberal idea of democracy. As the nineteenth-century British philosopher John Stuart Mill wrote in his wonderful essay *On Liberty*: "the only purpose for which power can be rightfully exercised over any member of a civilized society, against his will, is to prevent harm to others. His own good, either physical or moral, is not a sufficient warrant."[4] Consent in healthcare is about free choice, realizing this philosophical ideal in a traditionally hierarchical and paternalistic profession.

CASE 5.1 A SIMPLE PROCESS

You are the primary care clinician for Mr M, a hale but somewhat overweight (BMI = 32) 74-year-old man with a long history of gastrointestinal reflux. His condition has not responded to the usual management so he has sought a surgical opinion, and is scheduled for surgery this week. Mr M is here for his preoperative physical. His abdominal girth is a bit big and he's out of shape, but otherwise nothing seems out of the ordinary. Mr M seems sanguine about the operation. Although you don't question his decision to his face, it strikes you as an excessive intervention for what is a nuisance condition (eructation and reflux).

A week later you get a phone call from his wife telling you your patient had died of a massive myocardial infarction intraoperatively. Mrs M is distraught: "How could you let him go for that operation? I never wanted him to have any type of surgery! And he hadn't even told me about this one, said he was going to his brother's house up north for a few days!" Mr M had not told her about the procedure, not wanting to worry her.

Should you feel any responsibility for Mr M's death?

I. The Essence of Informed Consent

Consent is not always a simple process.

The orthodox opinion on consent in medicine is well known and connected with the principle of autonomy: *no* medical intervention done for *any purpose*—whether diagnostic, investigational, cosmetic, palliative, or therapeutic—*should take place unless the patient has consented to it*. Except in emergencies when consent is presumed (but see below), the healthcare professional providing the service should have a focused discussion with the patient about his or her condition and the treatment alternatives, and then elicit the patient's preferences regarding that treatment.

DISCUSSION OF CASE 5.1

If you were the surgeon for Mr M, you would be directly responsible for the quality of the consent obtained from him. As his primary care clinician you have no direct responsibility for his choice to have surgery or for the consent that authorizes it. Nevertheless, because he is your patient in the long run, it would have been worthwhile exploring with him the dangers of any surgery. Sometimes we are hesitant to explore decisions made by a patient with another practitioner—one may not want to "make waves" or to appear judgmental. But patients often look to their primary care provider, nurse or doctor, for the true "bill of goods."

Mr M, unfortunately, died of an event envisaged neither by you nor the surgeon—an "unanticipated negative outcome of care" or "adverse event" (see Chapter 8). Death had never been mentioned as a possible outcome to him, allowing him to consider the surgery a benign procedure. You had not wanted to disrupt his perception of an operation he had already decided to undergo. You also thought the surgeon was of the "old school," fearing his wrath should Mr M have declined the surgery on account of anything you said. After all, the surgeon was the expert and who were you, the mere primary care provider, to question his judgment? You feel chagrined, however, that you let yourself be intimidated by the medical hierarchy and did not do the "right thing" in reminding Mr M of the well-known nostrum that *anyone* can suffer a catastrophic outcome as a result of any procedure.

Later, when you speak to the surgeon, he tells you he accepted Mr M as a patient as *you* had referred him! Although he thought Mr M wasn't a great surgical risk, he assumed you had assessed him preoperatively. Now you feel really chagrined and together you agree to presume less and communicate more with each other and with families as well in the future.

BOX 5.1

Consent must be:

- specific as to the proposed intervention (or plan of care);
- informed; and
- "freely made" without fraud or under duress.

Consent is not a simple process as patients vary in how much they want to know, need to know, and are able to understand. As well, the potential outcomes of treatment or a plan of care are rarely straightforward, frequently seem complex, and are often unpredictable to patient and provider alike. The risk tables for pre-surgical evaluation, for example, are very good at estimating physiological risks but infrequently incorporate patient preferences and patient-oriented quality of life considerations: there will always be a certain amount of educated guesswork.[5] Clinicians will tailor their disclosure to patients and their significant others depending on circumstances such as urgency, time constraints, and the patient's capacity and situation.

The complexities here can be addressed by remembering what is important when it comes to consent.

II. Ethical Consent

Although there is much legal material relating to consent, which we will soon examine, it is vital to remember its ethical underpinnings. The notion of informed consent is better termed "informed choice," as consent suggests that the patient will go along with the clinician's recommendations. This may not be so, which is why "informed dissent" is just as important a notion. The ideas of consent/dissent/choice are derived from the principle of autonomy which holds that health professionals should not act autocratically. They should respect and enable their patients' views and choices. The legal requirements for consent often tell healthcare professionals the minimum they are required to do, stressing the importance of documentation (which, of course, is important) and legal protection for the healthcare practitioner (important, too). Informed choice can seem an onerous matter if the clinician thinks he or she is duty-bound to explain *every* risk and complication for every procedure or intervention and ensure all this is captured in the patient's chart. But good information sharing with patients will, in many cases, take care of the clinician's legal concerns (see Chapter 4 on truthtelling).

Merely reciting to patients a litany of side effects or possible complications and having them sign a consent form so as to avoid being sued is not the firmest foundation for appropriate patient choice. Patients frequently lack the critical skills required to make accurate risk-to-benefit calculations of medical interventions.[6] They also can have a poor understanding of written consent, believing its primary function to be, as it often is, simply to protect hospitals and doctors.[7] There is an increasing attention to health literacy and materials that may help patients and their families make informed choices—"decision aids." While clinicians may not have a legal duty to ensure patients comprehend the materials and information they provide, they certainly have good reasons for helping patients by simplifying their language and involving translators when needed. (See Chapter 12 for culture and consent.)

Healthcare practitioners at times have a poor understanding of shared decision-making, frequently making decisions for capable patients. One study showed that discussions with patients about risks are often truncated, especially regarding complex interventions, with infrequent assessment of patients' understanding of what is being asked of them.[8] Truly shared decision-making, "concordance," requires new models of sharing complex information and better training of healthcare professionals.[9]

The ethical foundation for consent often calls for clinicians to do something more than what they are legally bound to do. A few unscripted extra minutes with patients, asking them some questions about their lives, can lead to a better understanding of them as individuals. By so doing, clinicians can support their patients in making the decisions that are right for them, as opposed to decisions that simply reflect the professional's recommendations. This conversation can also minimize the risk of unrecognized patient/family expectations.[10]

BOX 5.2

"Performing a professional service without consent, for which consent is required, by law, is an act of professional misconduct."[11]

It should go without saying that any medical intervention requires patient involvement. However, patients vary in their interest in, and current capability for, such involvement in their care. The clinician may be tempted to cut corners around the requirements for informed choice if the patient seems uninterested in being involved in the decision. However, some decisions are weightier than others and require more scrupulous attention to how they are made. Decisions especially calling for the involvement of the patient include those in which:

- there are major differences in the possible outcomes (e.g., death or disability) of different treatments;
- the likelihood of complications is much greater for one treatment than for another;
- the choice of treatment involves trade-offs between near and distant benefits;
- the apparent difference between outcomes seems marginal, but the treatment options are quite distinct;
- a patient is particularly averse to certain risks; and
- a patient attaches special importance to certain outcomes.[12]

Failing to provide adequate information to patients so they may make informed choices can place healthcare professionals at legal risk. *Reibl v. Hughes* was the landmark Canadian case from the 1970s illustrating this.

III. The Doctor Who Didn't: The Case of Mr Reibl v. Dr Hughes

Mr Reibl, a 44-year-old patient with a history of severe migraines, was operated on by Dr Hughes to remove a partial blockage in his left internal carotid artery. As the blockage was asymptomatic, surgery was performed on an elective, not emergency, basis. (This blockage was not even responsible for the patient's migraines, although it might have caused him trouble later.)

Unfortunately, Mr Reibl suffered a stroke as a result of the procedure (a recognized surgical risk) that left him impotent and profoundly paralyzed on his right side. Dr Hughes had not specifically warned the patient of this risk or of the 1 in 7 likelihood of its occurring due to the procedure. The doctor later explained his rule was "never to tell such things" to his patients. Instead, he told Mr Reibl that, in a general way, he would "be better off with the surgery."

Dr Hughes did not obtain consent in the modern way.

After 10 years of litigation, the Supreme Court of Canada found Dr Hughes guilty of negligence, not because of the bad outcome (that was just ill luck), but for failing to ensure true informed consent when he neglected to provide critical information to Mr Reibl. The court decided a reasonable person in Mr Reibl's position would have waited to have the surgery if information about the risk of stroke had been given. This was especially so since the surgery was elective, that is, optional, at least in terms of timing. In addition, because Mr Reibl would have been eligible for a full disability pension in just 18 months, a reasonable person in his position would have delayed surgery until then, in case such a bad outcome did eventuate. Thus, it was the particular circumstances of this patient that made the doctor's omission in disclosure so erroneous. The court wrote:

> [T]he issue of informed consent to treatment is a concomitant of the physician's duty of care. A surgeon's duty to exercise due skill and care in giving his patient reasonable information and advice with respect to the risks specifically attendant on a proposed procedure arises out of the special relationship between them. It is a particular case of the duty which is cast on professional persons in a fiduciary position called upon . . . to give information or advice to a patient.[13]

To avoid negligence, physicians and surgeons must not only be technically proficient but exhibit certain moral skills as well. Their fiduciary, or trust-like, relationship with their patients means they must try to have their interventions serve their patients' wishes and interests. At a minimum this requires truthful and adequate disclosures to patients (see Box 5.3). Dr Hughes abrogated his ethical responsibility by not ensuring Mr Reibl's choice was an accurate and considered reflection of his own views and interests.

BOX 5.3

The lesson: Securing informed consent to treatment is a necessary part of the physician's duty of care.

The rule: Disclose what a reasonable person in the patient's position would want to know.

Unprofessional practice

Unprofessional practice will encompass not just faulty technical skill but also failure to involve patients properly in their own care—for example, failing to inform them of the important side effects of a drug.

CASE 5.2 THE UNDISCLOSED SIDE EFFECT

A 35-year-old female patient with a five-month history of a sore shoulder was treated by her physician with drugs that included an antipsychotic and an antidepressant. The physician had not disclosed to the patient that these were psychotropic medications nor had he told her about possible side effects. Only on discussion with a relative who was a nurse did the patient realize that the drowsiness, weakness, and blurred vision she had experienced could be due to the drugs. The physician was found guilty of failing to maintain the standards of the profession because he had not informed the patient of these potential adverse effects.[14]

DISCUSSION OF CASE 5.2

It can sometimes be difficult to decide what side effects to discuss with patients. Patients often say they want to be informed about "all possible side effects"—an impossible task.[15] In such discussions, the focus should be on the likely adverse effects and the serious, but less common, side effects. In general, the more serious the possible side effects, the more careful the clinician must be in disclosing such information to the patient. If in doubt, it is better to take extra time and inform the patient. Clinicians should also be aware of the different ways of communicating the benefits and harms of drugs— for example, studies have shown that using a succinct percentage format[16] or a simplified "drug facts box" for patients improved patient understanding and resulted in better choices between drugs.[17]

IV. The Essential Elements of Consent: When, Who, What, How?

1. When should consent be obtained?

Now to some details—details that matter a great deal to healthcare providers and patients. Prescribing drugs, ordering tests, giving vaccines, proposing surgery for curative, cosmetic, or palliative purposes, recommending a plan of care—anything done for a medical purpose for or to a patient—requires consent. Consent may be sought for discrete medical interventions or for a "plan of treatment" (e.g., consent for an operation should include an understanding of, and consent to, pre- and post-operative care) as a whole. The more serious the patient's condition or complex the plan of treatment, the more careful the clinician should be in obtaining consent from the patient.

While anything that clinicians do to their patients, such as psychotherapy or prescribing and administering drugs, has potentially serious adverse consequences, it is more common for healthcare professionals who physically "invade" their patients' bodies to be sued for negligent consent. In general, procedures that involve physical "trespass" upon a person's body must meet a higher standard of consent. These would include not only surgical procedures but also any touching of a patient, including the penetration by hand, device, or drug of any orifice of the patient's body. Rectal and vaginal examinations and treatments are particularly intimate and should call for explicit consent.[18] It is also clearly important, where possible, to obtain consent for procedures done while patients are unconscious (such as intimate examinations done under anesthesia).[19]

Practitioners are authorized by their patients to do only the treatment for which the consent was obtained. There is wrong done to a patient who, for example, consents to a hernia repair but has a testicle removed or agrees to a Caesarean section and gets a sterilization as well. If the patient gets something substantially different from what was agreed to, the doctor is liable for charges of trespass or battery. (The doctor who removed the testicle was found not liable because the patient's testicle was diseased and its removal considered an emergency operation necessary to save the patient's life—not something requiring explicit consent. The doctor who sterilized the woman was found liable as tubal ligation was not life-saving.)[20]

2. From whom should consent be obtained?

Consent must be obtained from the person undergoing the treatment unless that person is considered incapable for the purposes of that treatment. (Consent to do with minors will be discussed at greater length in Chapter 7.) Barring evidence to the contrary, patients are *presumed* to be competent, that is, having the mental capacity to give consent to or to refuse the treatment. So, a medical intervention or care plan should take place only if (1) the patient has the appropriate capacity and has given consent or (2) someone else authorized to make decisions on behalf of an incapable patient has consented to it. (See Chapter 6 for a fuller discussion of capacity and substitute decision-makers.)

CASE 5.3 "YOU HAVE NO RIGHT TO TOUCH ME!"

You are a medical trainee doing your rotation in a community health centre. An 80-year-old widow, Ms B, is brought by her son for her annual influenza vaccine. In explaining its risks and benefits, you realize the patient is not following your explanation. An inspection of her chart reveals a five-year history of progressive dementia with a decline in many aspects of daily functioning. A brief examination reveals Ms B to be very confused, having difficulty understanding what is being asked of her. She blankly looks at her son and asks, "Who is that person and what does she want?" The son gives you permission to give his mother the injection, saying she always wanted it in the past. However, normally quiet, she refuses, exclaiming, "What do you want my arm for? You have no right to touch me there!?!"

May you vaccinate the patient?

Whether or not a patient agrees with the proposed intervention, the healthcare professional must assess the patient's mental capacity. This does not have to be a complicated or detailed assessment, unless there are particular reasons to be concerned. Nurse, social worker, occupational therapist, medical trainee, and physician, as well as families or others close to the patient, may all have roles to play in the assessment of a patient's capacity. (Is a patient, for example, acting in or out of character in going along with or refusing care?)

Seek a surrogate

If the patient is found to be incapable, then consent must be obtained from a "substitute decision-maker" or a patient "surrogate." Until recently, the search for the proxy decision-maker in medicine was an informal one (and still is in many parts of the world). However, with the advent of legislation in certain jurisdictions, especially concerning advance directives and substitute decision-making, this process has become more formal. Courts or special tribunals may appoint patient "representatives"; some institutions, especially ones dedicated to mental health, have patient "advocates" whose role is to inform patients about their rights (see Chapters 6 on capacity and 11 on end-of-life decisions).

There are often limitations as to what a surrogate may consent to on behalf of an incapable patient. In 2007, the UK implemented the *Mental Capacity Act* recognizing the authority of others to make decisions on behalf of an incapable patient. A patient can refuse treatment or participation in research by an advance directive which, if clearly stated, must be followed by the patient's surrogate. Advance requests for treatment, however, are "not binding if in conflict with clinical judgment." Whatever decision-making powers the surrogate has depends on what is specified in a "lasting power of attorney" document that must be registered with the Public Guardian before it can be implemented.[21]

DISCUSSION OF CASE 5.3

The question in this case is: does the mother understand what is being asked of her, that is, to accept or reject the vaccine? It is clear after a few minutes of observation that this patient cannot do so and accordingly cannot give a valid consent. Another person (this may or may not be a family member) has to make this decision for her (see Box 5.4). Of course, practically speaking, if she is very resistant and cannot be cajoled into accepting the vaccine, its very modest benefit is not worth the struggle.

BOX 5.4

Practically speaking, if a patient is incapable as regards to a particular medical procedure, then that patient can no longer make his or her own choice about that procedure. Someone else must make it for him or her.

3. Who is responsible for obtaining consent?

The patient's treating healthcare provider is ultimately responsible for obtaining consent. A physician may delegate the responsibility to others, such as nurse practitioners, physician assistants, or medical trainees. As well, these healthcare providers and others—be they physiotherapists, emergency responders, occupational therapists, x-ray technicians, phlebotomists, or psychotherapists—all have an evolving and increased responsibility for ensuring informed patient choice for what they do. Physicians cannot, should not, and do not bear responsibility for all aspects of a patient's consent, whether in hospital or out.

If other hospital staff or trainees will be obtaining consent later, the attending clinician should make sure that those designated to obtain the actual consent do so in a way with which he or she is comfortable. Most jurisdictions disapprove of medical trainees—such as nursing or medical students—obtaining patient consent for surgical procedures, as they may ill understand the intricacies of the decision that has to be made.[22] Where trainees exceed their authority and seek consent on their own, the responsibility for the adequacy of the consent may still rest on the shoulders of the most responsible clinician, if he or she leaves them undersupervised.

Similarly, those designated to obtain consent should ensure they fully understand the nature of the plan of treatment for which consent is being obtained. If not, they should seek guidance from others rather than obtaining a faulty or invalid consent. An improperly obtained consent increases the legal jeopardy and ethical problems for all concerned and makes it impossible for the patient to participate properly in the decision-making process.

4. What should be disclosed?

Providing enough pertinent information detailing the essential qualities of the proposed treatment is sometimes a worry for clinicians. What must I disclose? What does the law say? What is critical to true patient choice is to realize it requires a *process* (as opposed to a single act) of information exchange. An ongoing *conversation* between healthcare practitioner and patient is what lies at the heart of consent.[23]

Patients need information for choice
Patients' needs for and expectation of information have been well established (see Chapter 4 on truthtelling). In general, studies show that patient standards are generally much higher than what physicians attempt or achieve. (The reason some practitioners get away with poor disclosure is that it often fails to cause patients easily litigable harm and, where it does cause harm, families and patients often avoid the courts.[24]) When it comes to proposed interventions, *patients need the relevant information that will allow them to choose among the alternatives in a fashion consistent with their own values and beliefs*. This is what clinicians must tell patients in order to achieve concordance ("shared decision-making")—information that is not rote or routine but tailored to the patient and his or her needs and expectations.

Does this model of concordance mean the clinician must agree with the patient's choice? Not necessarily. But it should be a choice with which the clinician can work.

CASE 5.4 MORE SURGERY WANTED!

Ms X, a 60-year-old woman with early stage breast cancer, accompanied by her 25-year-old daughter, has come to see Dr D for a second opinion. The breast surgeon explains that, as far as surgery goes, fortunately all she needs is breast conserving surgery (BCS). Ms X does not look relieved. With her daughter translating, she replies, "That's what the other doctor said, too. But that's not what I want!" Her daughter explains her mother wants a modified radical mastectomy. Ms X has no confidence in BCS as one of her friends had a recurrence of breast cancer after this.

Dr D is a little confused. She usually finds herself in the opposite position of trying to convince some women to have any surgery at all. Although Dr D describes the morbidity associated with radical surgery, Ms X remains unconvinced. Her daughter explains this view of BCS is common in their culture.

Should Dr D go along with the request for more radical surgery than is indicated?

DISCUSSION OF CASE 5.4

In Ms X's community of origin, it is common, according to at least one study, for women to reject BCS for the very reason she cites.[25] At least in this case, her request for a modified radical mastectomy is aligned with the standard of care. It is much harder to convince some women who prefer alternative medicine to accept any surgical option. If Dr D cannot persuade Ms X to change her mind, it would not be inappropriate to go along with her request for more surgery. In this case more surgery may not be better than less surgery but is better than none at all.[26]

Reasonable-person standard

The modern standard for medical disclosure is not telling patients *"everything"*—nor is it telling patients merely what other clinicians do or don't tell. The standard instead is *what would a reasonable person in the patient's situation wish to know about the treatment before deciding whether or not to accept it?* It is up to the patient to decide whether to accept or reject the proposed intervention or plan of care (knowing the potential hazards). A duly informed patient not only makes a free choice but also, generally, assumes upon him or herself the (non-negligent) risks of the agreed-upon intervention.

It is particularly important to discuss with the patient the various treatment options (including the option of no treatment at all, see Box 5.5) and to explain the likely risks and benefits of the various options. The risk/benefit assessment should take into account the patient's particular circumstances (e.g., occupation). Values or beliefs that a patient feels to be especially crucial, such as a refusal of blood products or surgical versus non-surgical options, ought to be discussed, as they almost certainly will have an impact on which choice is best for the patient. The prudent clinician will tell the patient not only what a reasonable person would want to know, but also what this particular patient wants to know.

BOX 5.5

Whatever alternatives are available to patients, it is helpful to remind patients they always have the "zero option"—the opportunity to do nothing.[27]

Material risks

Specifically, the clinician ought to discuss with the patient, in an appropriate and respectful way, his or her prognosis with and without treatment, the treatment alternatives, the success and failure rates of the various treatments, the "material risks" of treatment (common and serious risks inherent in a procedure that a reasonable person in the patient's circumstances would want to know), any related matters the patient wishes to discuss, and the clinician's recommendation regarding treatment (see Box 5.6). The patient should not be buried under tons of detail but be enlightened and empowered with the most pertinent facts discussed in an accessible manner. One can be pithy, and not paternalistic.

BOX 5.6

Informed choice requires discussion of

- the exact nature of the proposed treatment;
- the alternative(s);
- the prognosis with and without treatment;
- the risks and benefits of the treatment and of alternatives;
- serious risks, even if unlikely; and
- any questions the patient may have.

Serious risks (such as death and permanent disability) should be disclosed even if they are very unlikely to occur. Common and, therefore, required-to-disclose risks are those with a more than 1/200 chance of occurring while not-mandatory-to-disclose risks have a less than $1/1 \times 10^6$ chance of happening. (These figures are not meant to be precise but are a rough guide to consent.) Dr Hughes's non-disclosure of a "material risk" of the procedure (serious, 1/7 chance of happening) failed to meet this requirement and was therefore suboptimal.

By contrast, the "one-in-a-million" chance seems a good cutoff for disclosure of even serious risk. "Reasonable patients" would be unlikely to make a medical decision based on such remote risks. Whether this applies by law to all procedures is hard to know, but doctors have been found free of negligence, for example, in not warning a surgical patient of the remote risk of necrotizing fasciitis.[28] The courts might find remote risk information more germane to less "medically necessary" procedures such as liposuction. Any possible serious adverse outcomes, such as death, might make reasonable people think twice about less necessary procedures. Important here is not so much the precise risk of an adverse event occurring but the provision to patients of the information that may make a difference to their decision-making.

BOX 5.7

"In the case of elective surgery, there can be no justification for withholding information."[29]

While one should not unduly alarm patients with every possibility, one should also not falsely reassure them or "sell" them on surgical interventions or pharmaceutical products. This is especially so for those cosmetic or experimental interventions not required, strictly speaking, for the patient's well-being.

Patients must be given the opportunity to express their sensitivities and exercise their idiosyncratic preferences. Ironically, the anxious patient who worries about potential but rare side effects of a treatment may well be the one patient who ends up suffering those very adverse effects if not forewarned by the clinician. Disclosure for consent purposes should be complete, "adequate," and not designed to prevent a patient's emotional responses to information. Of course, it is quite appropriate to try to understand and address a patient's unusual beliefs or emotional reactions to proposed interventions, so that lack of patient–practitioner concordance or potential threats to patient welfare can be anticipated and addressed beforehand.

Some legal decisions have suggested even minimal risks (the one-in-a-million risk) for elective procedures and all possible risks for cosmetic ones (see Box 5.7) must be disclosed. Such disclosure requirements go far beyond those for ordinary necessary procedures, as mentioned above.[30] Because clinicians may have a financial interest in patients' undergoing procedures (especially those outside of medicare), it is important to ensure that decisions are not influenced by the doctor's opinion. Some physicians performing cosmetic procedures have suffered serious consequences (e.g., loss of the licence to practise) for being less than exemplary in obtaining informed consent.[31]

The process of obtaining consent is part of the caring process. The prudent clinician shows an interest in and a genuine concern for a patient's choices. These choices will have implications not just for the patient but likely for his or her family and significant others as well. Where the clinician feels such choices should be explored further, with the patient's consent, try to involve those close to him or her as well. (See Chapter 11 on patients who refuse life-saving care).

BOX 5.8

"Treat the patient as though he [or she] were your best friend and you are telling him [or her] all about the proposed treatment."[32]

Treatment alternatives

Must clinicians inform patients about treatment alternatives? Yes—especially if the alternatives are truly different and this patient would want to know about these alternatives to make an informed choice.

Important options should be disclosed to patients—whether or not the consultant performs them. Because patients may not be sufficiently well informed to know to ask about options, clinicians should not wait for them to inquire before discussing these. Even locally unavailable options ought to be mentioned if they might better meet a patient's interests. Unusual or unproven therapies—such as homeopathic remedies—do not require disclosure if they do not conform to a reasonable standard of care. The latter clearly changes with advances in medicine, so it behooves practitioners to keep up with their discipline (and now increasingly with options discussed on the Internet).

5. How should consent be obtained?

Deciding just what and how patients should be told can be tricky. Professionals should organize their time so that effective communication with patients can take place. "Effective" means, in this context, communication habits and tactics aimed at targeting patient perspectives and successfully incorporating them into any treatment plan. Doctors, in particular, should strive not to dominate the discussion or interrupt

patients "30 seconds or less" into the consultation.[33] Healthcare professionals need to ask their patients these patient-focused questions that
should only take an extra few minutes per patient visit:

- What are your concerns?
- What else would you like to know?
- Does this make sense to you?
- Is there someone else that you would like to talk to about this?

Patients should be given all the time they need to make their decisions.
Taking time *to talk with and listen to* patients (and their families) will help
ensure that they are truly agreeing to a procedure and not simply going
along with "professional opinion."

Help with complex decisions

While medical care has become more complex, the conversations
between healthcare professionals and patients and/or their families
have not always kept up. The typical 6-to-10–minute medical consultation remains unchanged, time that is often inadequate for any serious
discussion of treatment alternatives and their risks. If conversation is
the "future of healthcare," as has been claimed,[34] clinicians may be too
rooted in the past. Fully informed of the possible harms and benefits
of a treatment, patients tend to opt for the less invasive and the less
prescription-drug-dependent course of action.[35] One author has written
that "the goal is changing to become one of informing people, enabling
them to make their own choices, regardless of whether this reduces risk."[36]
But this is too extreme a view of patient autonomy; at some point the
virtuous prudent clinician *must* be concerned about the risks to which
a patient, by his or her choices, exposes him or herself. (If so, does this
undermine the ethical commentary given in Case 5.4?)

Consent forms

It is often asked whether prescribed hospital consent forms, signed by
patients, would protect healthcare professionals from litigation regarding
consent. Although the short answer is no, they can be helpful. Consent
forms are simply evidence that a discussion of the procedure in question
took place. If no such discussion took place, a signed form is worth little.
Of course, if such prescribed forms are available, they should be used, if
only for their evidentiary role and to comply with institutional protocol.
(They should also always be used in any significant medical research.)

Research reveals many patients do not recall much about the contents
of consent forms—if they read them at all. As well, certain factors, such as

advanced age and impaired cognitive functions, can impair the quality of a patient's consent.[37] In such circumstances, physicians have an obligation to help the patient understand, as much as is reasonably feasible, the proposed interventions. Relying on consent forms is a poor substitute for having an open conversation with patients about the proposed treatment (see Box 5.9).

BOX 5.9

Help patients understand medical procedures by

- explaining matters simply;
- defining the decision and the options clearly;
- wording patient information materials carefully;
- providing written information or other media decision aids;
- having patients bring a relative to the discussion;
- encouraging patients to ask questions;
- offering the option of a second opinion;
- ensuring appropriate interpretive services are used if needed;
- ensuring ample time for decision-making; and
- asking patients to repeat in their own words what they have understood.

Patients who withdraw consent

CASE 5.5 "STOP THE TEST!"

A 58-year-old woman agrees to undergo a colonoscopy by a physician. During the procedure, despite mild sedation, she suddenly experiences severe pain and cries out, "Stop! I can't take this anymore!"

Ought the physician continue the examination?

The doctrine of consent gives the patient the definitive right to refuse medical interventions. Such refusal may conflict with other important goals, such as the expectation that medical care ought to prevent needless suffering or avoidable death, but it is nonetheless to be respected. What if, however, a patient withdraws consent during a medical procedure? Must such refusals always be heeded?

The answer is yes, but, of course, it also depends on the circumstances. In a case that came before the Supreme Court of Canada, this question was discussed in some detail.

Giovanna Ciarlariello was an Italian-speaking cleaner diagnosed at age 49 with a sub-arachnoid hemorrhage. To find the source of the bleeding, a cerebral angiogram was done after several explanations to obtain consent were made by radiologists and an intern at two adjoining hospitals. After an explanation with a family member present, the patient's daughter signed the consent form. During a second angiogram, the patient seemed to hyperventilate, lost some power and feeling in her limbs and, when calmer, said, "Enough, no more, stop the test." Temporarily stopping the test, the physicians noted an improvement in the patient's condition and recommended continuing the test since it was almost complete. The patient agreed. During the final dye injection the patient was unfortunately rendered quadriplegic and later died.

Her estate sued the physicians, arguing, among other things, that it was wrong to continue with the angiogram when the patient had withdrawn her consent.[38]

Halt unless serious harm

At issue in this case was the nature and extent of disclosure owed by a doctor to a patient who withdraws consent for a procedure during its administration. In general, *if consent is withdrawn, the procedure should be halted unless doing so might seriously harm the patient.* In this case, however, the patient appeared to consent to the test's completion. Was her consent valid? The court felt it was because (1) the patient had previously consented to the same procedure, (2) the risks had not seemingly changed, and (3) the patient seemed to understand what was being asked of her in the procedure room. As her consent was valid, the physicians had not erred in completing the test.

Onus borne by clinician

If a patient appears to withdraws consent during a test, and if the procedure is continued, the onus is borne by the clinician, who must ensure that the patient has understood what is happening. In particular the clinician may have to demonstrate later that the patient understood the explanation and instructions given to continue the procedure. If this cannot be done, especially if the material risks to the patient have changed, the test should not be started again. While the entire consent process does not have to be repeated, new material risks must be divulged, and the patient must have the capacity to understand them. If the patient lacks this capacity, he or she therefore cannot give valid consent to continue the procedure; it would be wiser to stop unless the patient would be put in undue danger by stopping or interrupting the procedure. (Of course, substitute consent could be obtained so long as it is not used as a vehicle to override that to/ from which the patient would have consented/dissented.)

DISCUSSION OF CASE 5.5

The physician would be unwise to continue the examination. He or she should, of course, try to determine why the patient felt pain and attempt to relieve it. The patient should have the risks and benefits of continuing the procedure explained. If she is adamant about stopping and understands its implications, despite sedation, her wish should be respected. (Of course even a seemingly less rational wish should be respected if the pain could only be relieved by withdrawing the colonoscope.) A physician was found guilty of battery for continuing with a sigmoidoscopy in spite of a patient's cries to stop due to pain. In that case the patient suffered a punctured bowel after the doctor had been asked to stop.[39]

V. Exceptions to Consent

There are circumstances that sometimes allow an exception to the duty to seek informed consent from a patient (see Box 5.10).

BOX 5.10

Exceptions to requirement for consent:

1. patient waiver and "delegated consent"
2. mental incapacity of patient
3. emergencies
4. therapeutic privilege

1. Patient waiver and "delegated consent"

Patients may "waive" the normal consent process by, for example, asking the doctor to "skip the gory details" about a particular intervention. Such a request should be examined further by the clinician. Why does the patient not wish to be informed? Is the patient truly capable of giving consent? Many patients may trust doctors to make decisions in their best interests, and may waive information from doctors. Others, while wanting to be *generally* informed, may not wish to know the details unless absolutely necessary.

When it comes to a particular medical plan of treatment, a patient waiver may or may not be acceptable. Patients need to be apprised of certain information to be properly prepared for a procedure. For example, patients undergoing some cardiac surgeries need to know they will likely wake up on a ventilator in the intensive care unit and so should be informed as to what this experience might be like. They may need to be reminded of the possibility of needing blood products or that their throat will hurt after intubation. For elective or cosmetic interventions, specifically because they are optional, the practitioner is within his or her rights not to accept a patient who requests to be left ignorant of the risks faced in such interventions. If the clinician is prepared to accept the patient's waiver, it would be wise to document this discussion in case of some adverse event.

"Delegated consent" occurs when a capable person appoints another person to make medical decisions for him or her. Although the patient has the capacity to consent, he or she wishes another person, for whatever reason (lack of interest, lack of will, illness, etc.) to act as he or she would. This, as with waived consent, is not usually morally contentious. Patients should be told that consenting to one treatment may implicitly involve agreeing to a sequence of other procedures and, if so, what these might be. Patients who delegate consent may still wish to be informed about the "big picture." (This may make it unlike waivered consent.)

However, dangerous or risky procedures, especially if new and bordering on the experimental, are particularly ill-suited to "waivered" or delegated consent. And, of course, waivers should not be accepted from incapable patients; by contrast, capable persons may select their delegated decision-maker in advance. (For incapable patients who have not named someone, the appropriate substitute decision-maker should be sought.)

2. Mental incapacity of patient

Incapacity of a patient is not a true exception to the consent rule except in an emergency (see Box 5.11). Consent must still be sought, but from a substitute decision-maker who has been properly informed as the patient would have been if capable. In certain situations where the patient retains some decision-making capacity, the health professional may choose to inform that patient about an impending medical intervention or treatment plan. This allows the patient to participate in the decision as far as he or she is able. (One may be surprised at how much the patient is able to understand the intervention.) It may also help the patient co-operate with or adhere to treatments and prepare for whatever consequences, such as pain or disability, that might follow from the procedure.

BOX 5.11

If a patient is incapable, consent is still required, albeit from a substitute decision-maker. Except in emergencies, healthcare professionals cannot act as decision-makers for their incapable patients.

3. Emergencies

This is the most common exception. Consent need not be obtained when the patient is at imminent risk of suffering serious injury (severe suffering, loss of limb, vital organ, or life) and obtaining consent is either not possible (e.g., the patient is comatose), or would increase the risk to the patient.[40] The assumption is that in emergencies most patients would want the care necessary to rescue them from serious harm or severe suffering (see Box 5.12). Efforts to obtain consent could jeopardize the patient's safety by wasting time, thus unreasonably delaying life-saving care. In such circumstances, consent is "implied."

BOX 5.12

The emergency rule is a kind of "social insurance" rule: it is assumed that most people would want to be saved in an emergency.

There is an exception to this exception to the consent rule: where the competent patient had previously refused the emergency treatment normally offered. Under such circumstances treatment may not be administered. (See *Malette v. Shulman* in Chapter 2 on autonomy.) Suicide notes, by the way, do not set comparable limits to treatment; for a further discussion, see Chapter 7.

4. Therapeutic privilege

CASE 5.6 AN UNSTATED RISK

A 45-year-old man is advised to have a radiological test as part of a work-up for haematuria. The radiologist does not warn him of the possibility of a serious allergic reaction to the contrast dye because this might cause the patient undue anxiety. Unfortunately, the patient has such a reaction to the dye during the test and nearly dies.

Is the withholding of information for fear of a patient's emotional state acceptable?

The failure to inform patients of some material information on the grounds that it might harm them (by increasing their anxiety) is an outmoded and paternalistic exception to consent and disclosure, even if done out of benevolent intentions. Sometimes called "therapeutic privilege," it is often neither. It is not just a "privilege" to give the patient information, it is a professional responsibility. Withholding information is also rarely "therapeutic" —quite the opposite, as the uninformed patient can be made more worried and worse off in not knowing.[41]

DISCUSSION OF CASE 5.6

The patient was wronged in not being informed of a remote but serious risk. No matter how well intentioned, the lack of disclosure is a clear abrogation of the disclosure and consent rule. As a result of risk disclosure, patients may, in the healthcare professional's opinion, "irrationally" choose not to undergo tests that are medically indicated, but that is their right (see Chapter 6 on capacity).

"But for" 18 minutes

What if the patient *had* been told the relevant information, consented to the procedure after being made aware of the risks, but then suffers a serious reaction due to the practitioner's negligence? Does the patient's consent *absolve* the practitioner of liability? The answer must be, usually, no. A patient's foreknowledge is not an excuse for a bad outcome that would not have occurred "but for" the substandard actions of the practitioner.

A case before the Supreme Court of Canada in 2013 involved a child who had suffered a severe hypoxic brain injury at birth.[42] The obstetrician had attempted but failed to deliver the infant using a high-risk mid-forceps delivery. Inability to deliver an infant is not unusual with this maneuver but, as such, the doctor must (a) inform the mother beforehand of the riskiness of the procedure and also (b) have in place what might be needed if the forceps delivery fails—the preparations for an emergency Caesarian section, such as an anesthetist on standby. The doctor did neither.

In this case the only anesthetist available was busy with another life-saving surgery. This resulted in an 18-minute hypoxic delay in the delivery of the infant. The Court found that, although the obstetrician did *not* properly obtain consent for a mid-forceps-delivery-that-might-become-a-Caesarian, this issue was not considered relevant to the issue of compensation. He was already found negligent in not being prepared for the need for the Caesarian section.

The Court awarded the estate of the child, now a severely disabled 15-year-old, over $3 million in compensation. So, even if consent to the attempted delivery by forceps *had* been obtained, it would not have been consent to an ill-prepared and dangerous delivery. "But for" the obstetrician's ill-prepared intervention resulting in a critical 18-minute delay in delivery, the hypoxia and resultant injury to the infant would not have transpired.

Patients not always suggestible

It is sometimes thought that giving more information to a suggestible patient about the potential negative outcomes of a treatment may *itself* produce negative results, thus harming the patient's well-being. Anecdotes aside, research, albeit conflicting, does not entirely bear this out. For example, giving patients detailed information about the risks of hernia surgery did not increase their anxiety.[43] Warning patients about the potential side effects of certain prescribed drugs (antihypertensives, antibiotics, and anti-inflammatory pills) did not make it more likely they would experience such side effects.[44] In this same study, however, greater information disclosure to advanced cancer patients did not increase poor patient outcomes but *did* increase their anxiety levels, especially if patients were encouraged to make decisions concerning their *own* care.[45] Participation by patients in their own care can, of course, be anxiety-provoking especially if the decisions are difficult ones and novel to the patient. Anxiety about making good/best decisions for oneself or for an incapable person is understandable. Much may be riding on the decision, including one's survival or, even more importantly, another's.[46]

Thus, one should not assume that sharing information with patients and their families is easy or straightforward. It is the healthcare provider's responsibility to give information in a sensitive manner, striving to assist patients with coping skills and anxiety management strategies.

Conclusion

High standards are expected of modern healthcare professionals when it comes to consent for medical care. Patients who do not receive important information in a comprehensible and timely way may have grounds for concern and grievance. Many "failures to communicate" are simply resolved by assiduous attention to language—avoiding jargon, spending time with patients, listening, and accessing good interpreter services. Informed choice is not merely a matter of respecting someone's choice. It is also about acting in ways that are helpful to, and experienced as helpful by, patients—in other words, to be kind and to *care* about the decisions your patients make.

Knowing how best to help and how far you must help a patient is part of your professional role as a caring professional, learned through experience and good mentoring. If, as a healthcare trainee from *any* field, you fail to learn the skills and attitudes of how to be kind and helpful in this way with patients, something so fundamental to our patients and to being able to "do right," there is something seriously amiss with your training. When you do find good role models for caring (and you will, there are many), latch on to them as long as you can.

Cases For Discussion

CASE 1: IT'S MY LIFE!

Mr R is a 46-year-old man with a 10-year history of Rheumatoid Arthritis which has become very disabling, his small hand and finger joints barely usable despite numerous corrective surgeries. Pain control has been a significant issue. Mr R is taking 300 mg of morphine a day but is still in pain. He comes to see you today as he needs more painkillers and to talk about methotrexate, the only drug he has found at all helpful in remitting his symptoms. He has been taking the drug longer than recommended; there are signs in his lab work of damage to his liver. You have advised him several times to stop the methotrexate but Mr R refuses. "It's the only thing that helps me! Damn the liver, I just want some relief!"

Questions For Discussion

1. Give reasons why the physician should or should not do as the patient requests.
2. Does Mr R's request satisfy the requirements for informed choice?

CASE 2: USE OF FORCE

You are working for a medical NGO (Non-Governmental Organization) in an impoverished region of the developing world. There is a wave of diphtheria in your region as the recent vaccine campaign did not reach many of the smaller villages. A number of the cases went untreated with several children dying of the illness, something quite preventable had there been early diagnosis and prompt treatment.

You are visiting a family at their house in an affected small town. The youngest child in this family, 5-year-old Ahna, has developed a fever and refuses to swallow. Does she have the grey membranous web on her posterior pharynx, pathognomic for diphtheria, you wonder? She defiantly refuses to open her mouth. No amount of arguing, bribing or cajoling by you or her parents will budge her.

You decide, with the parents' consent, to hold Ahna down and force her mouth open. She is fierce in her resistance. When you finally are able to look, there is a grey web to be seen at the back of her throat. Exhausted and sweaty from the struggle, you fall back into a chair. Ahna stares at you in anger. You ask yourself, "What did I just do? What kind of person am I?"[47]

Questions For Discussion

1. Who should make decisions for minors?
2. Were the actions of the clinician reasonable ones? How would you characterize them?
3. Were there other options that could have been explored?

6

The Waning and Waxing Self
Capacity and Incapacity in Medical Care

The policy of the law is that where a person, due to mental illness, lacks the capacity to make a sound and considered decision on treatment, the person should not for that reason be denied access to medical treatment that can improve functioning and alleviate suffering.

Chief Justice McLachlin, 2003[1]

T his chapter will examine the healthcare professional's complex responsibilities regarding the care of incapable patients—whether they are elderly, young, or in-between. The duty to provide effective medical care and protect vulnerable individuals from harm must be balanced against respecting the right of competent persons to make their own decisions, even if these are considered "bad" choices. Challenges exist in deciding who needs protection from themselves and how far a clinician and/or others can go in protecting patients with diminished or impaired capacity. However, mental maladies, as we shall see, are not synonymous with incapacity.[2]

I. Attending to and Assessing Capacity

CASE 6.1 "TALK TO ME, NOT MY DAUGHTER!"

A geriatric psychiatrist, consultant to a local nursing home, is asked to see Mrs Q, an 87-year-old woman with advanced Parkinson's disease, who is suffering from frightening visual hallucinations. The patient has marked rigidity and is quite unstable when walking, but there is no obvious evidence of dementia. It is unclear whether her psychiatric symptoms are secondary to her medications or the illness itself; her medications cannot however be reduced because of the severity of her physical symptoms. Mrs Q has partial insight into her psychotic symptoms. She and the psychiatrist agree these are distressing enough to warrant a trial of an atypical antipsychotic. She is warned about the potential for worsening of her Parkinson symptoms with antipsychotics and agrees to the novel antipsychotic least associated with such side effects at a low starting dose.

A note is left in her chart recommending this medication. The attending physician at the nursing home accordingly authorizes the order. As is common in many nursing homes, the protocol of routinely obtaining consent from relatives for any medication changes is followed and so Mrs Q's daughter is contacted. She refuses consent for the antipsychotic, downplaying her mother's symptoms but also expressing concern she may become overmedicated. When the psychiatrist returns the next month for his regular visit, he discovers the order for the antipsychotic has been cancelled by the attending physician.

Was the attending doctor's action appropriate?

DISCUSSION OF CASE 6.1

Told the reason she did not get the medication, Mrs Q responds angrily, "What's my daughter got to do with it? I'm the one who's going to be taking it! If I get side effects, then I'll let you know and we can stop it!" Indeed, she is right to be upset. The patient is capable of comprehending and making a decision about antipsychotic medications. Mrs Q might be old, infirm, and incapable of meeting all her physical needs, but this does not mean she cannot make an informed choice about the treatment of her hallucinations. The daughter is not the person to make the final decision about medications for her capable mother. With the patient's permission, the psychiatrist calls the daughter, as a matter of courtesy, to inform her as to the reasons for the medication and as to her mother's capacity. After some discussion, the daughter agrees a trial of medication seems reasonable. Even if she disagrees, however, the medication can be ordered, because Mrs Q has already made an informed choice.

Competencies, not competence

When we speak of competence or capacity (throughout this book, I use capacity and competence interchangeably), we are talking not about a *global* ability but rather a person's *capacity* or *ability* to perform some *specific* task or to make a *specific* decision. Different domains of competence include the ability to make a treatment decision, manage one's financial affairs, make a will, appoint a lawyer for personal care, drive a car, stand trial, or decide whether to enter a long-term care facility. Within each domain are specific decisions to be made. Whereas in the past competence was conceptualized as "all or nothing," we now talk about domain-specific competence and decision-specific competence. Only some patients, such as infants or those in a coma, may be considered globally incompetent.

More commonly, an individual may be competent in one domain and not another (although marked incapacity in one domain may often signal incompetence in others). Even here, the presumption of global capacity for all decisions within a domain may not be correct; there is often a hierarchy of decisions within each domain, ranging from the simple to the complicated. Competence is better conceptualized, then, as a *set* of capacities.[3]

In most developed societies, a person is presumed to be competent unless there are reasonable grounds to suspect otherwise. The onus is on others to prove incapacity rather than for the individual to prove competency. Capacity assessments may be done under a variety of circumstances, both informally and more formally. Whether a more formal assessment is required depends on the decision to be made. How serious is it? What are the implications of the decision for the patient and others?

Frequently, and probably most commonly, informal capacity assessments are done by clinicians every day; more formalized assessments are generally required only for decisions of greater importance. For example, risky experimental interventions or refusals for life-sustaining care need more exacting assessments of capacity.

Surveys have shown incapacity to be extremely common in acute care hospitalized adult patients but frequently unrecognized.[4, 5] While doctors may overestimate the actual functional capacity of their patients,[6] they may also underestimate the enabling measures (such as using decision aids or addressing factors that impede capacity) that could help patients to be more capable and self-directing.

Competence operationally defined

Many operational definitions of competence have been proposed but none has universal acceptance. The US President's Commission on Ethics in Medicine suggests that competence requires all of the following:

- a set of core personal values and goals;
- the ability to communicate;
- the ability to understand information;
- the ability to reason and deliberate;
- the ability to choose; and
- consistency between one's choices and one's underlying values.[7]

A lack of any one of these elements does not mean someone should be considered incompetent; it depends on the circumstances, such as how the patient is actually functioning in the decision context and what choice has to be made. Competence is a spectrum varying with the task and the decision. Moreover, a patient may be only temporarily incapacitated by drugs or illness and retain an underlying ability to perform the requisite task. Other patients can look incapable but still have an ability to make a competent decision. As we make judgments concerning someone's capacity (in order to know whether or not to abide by his or her wishes), we cannot avoid establishing thresholds or protocols for specific capabilities. Practically, however, rules around determination of capacity for particular tasks can vary in different jurisdictions. Although different capacity assessment tools are available, none, to date, are universally accepted or consistently used.[8]

> **BOX 6.1**
>
> Competence is not a diagnosis but an assessment of functional capacity.

Tests of competence

Five tests of competence to consent to medical treatment have been proposed:

1. Expressing a choice
2. Expressing a "reasonable" choice
3. Expressing a choice based on "rational reasons"
4. Showing an ability to understand the information necessary to make a decision
5. Showing an ability to appreciate one's situation and its consequences[9]

Test 1 is the least restrictive but the least helpful because it authorizes any choice made by a patient. Test 2 is inadequate in failing to recognize the patient's autonomy and privileging medically desirable outcomes, the "best interests" of patients as defined by healthcare professionals. Although a patient's refusal to consent to something others would see as necessary or beneficial often triggers a competency assessment, this does not in itself necessarily imply incapacity.

Test 3 is more acceptable as it looks less at outcomes and more at the process by which the patient arrives at a decision. It threatens to collapse into Test 2 if the set of "rational" reasons is too circumscribed. Many developed countries recognize the right to make decisions on the basis of idiosyn-cratic or unusual beliefs, especially if deeply held. This test would be more acceptable if it simply applied a consistency-processing standard: a patient is deemed less than fully competent if his or her goals do not follow consist-ently from underlying beliefs or values. Yet inconsistency is not necessarily a mark of irrationality. We all are less than consistent in our beliefs and prac-tices—but this does not mean our choices should be ignored or overruled.

Tests 4 and 5, including some variant of Test 3, are the most frequently used criteria for competence.

No one criterion will accurately predict all patients who are incom-petent. Taking into account a person's environmental supports and func-tional demands, Gutheil and Appelbaum suggest the key prerequisites for competence as

- being aware of the nature of one's situation;
- having a factual understanding of the issue(s); and
- being able to manipulate information rationally to make a decision.[10]

Each element represents a different aspect of capacity, that is, appre-ciation, understanding, and reasoning. All should be met in some fashion for persons to be considered capable in their own environment.

CASE 6.2 BEYOND HELP?

You are the primary care provider for Mr I, a 20-year-old second-year college student with a past history of depression as a teen. For several weeks, he has confined himself to his small garret-like flat, refusing visitors. Mr I's best friend was killed two months previously when a car struck his bicycle. According to others in the house, he has not been carrying out his day-to-day tasks, appearing disheveled when glimpsed. He can be heard crying and shouting day and night.

After Mr I misses several appointments, you decide to visit him at his home. Reluctantly, he lets you in. He admits stopping the antidepressant he was prescribed at the university's health service as one of his housemates told him it was a "psychiatric poison." He looks ill-kempt and admits to being very sad. Mr I acknowledges that pills and therapy are interventions that might help some people—indeed, his own episodes of depression responded to them in the past. Nonetheless, he refuses them now on the grounds that "I've seen Jesus and he can't help me. I am, as he was, as we all are," he cries, "under the control of a higher power."

What should you do?

DISCUSSION OF CASE 6.2

You would, of course, ask Mr I what's going on and carefully examine his competence to stop treatment. If, after thorough examination, he appears to have a major mental break such as "melancholia" or mania with delusional features, he may be unable to appreciate what treatment has done for him in the past and might do for him in the present and future. If so, although he might admit to being unwell, Mr I's refusal of treatment cannot be considered a capable one. If he dismisses all treatment alternatives and hospitalization, he needs careful monitoring. In cases such as this, it is the persistence of strong delusions and the overwhelming emotions that will affect and undermine the patient's ability to appreciate.

Appreciate and understand in the law

BOX 6.2

When accepting or refusing a medical treatment, a patient, to be considered capable, must demonstrate the *ability* to understand:

- his or her condition;
- the nature of the proposed treatment;
- alternatives to the treatment;
- the consequences of accepting and rejecting the treatment; and
- the risks and benefits of the various options.[11]

In most parts of North America, legislation uses very similar language in describing capacity (see Box 6.2). Under legislation in Ontario, for example, a person is considered capable of making a treatment decision if "able to understand the information that is relevant to making a decision concerning the treatment and able to appreciate the reasonably foreseeable consequences of a decision or lack of decision."[12] *This compound standard for competence to consent corresponds to the most clinically relevant tests of competence.*[13,14] For any particular task or decision, one must have certain knowledge ("understanding") and be able to apply this knowledge to oneself ("appreciation"). Applying compound standards for assessing competence will more accurately reveal a person's true decision-making capabilities. Studies have shown, for example, that hospitalized adult patients who do well on the understanding criterion of competence may ultimately be considered incompetent if they are unable to appreciate their situation or to reason properly.[15]

BOX 6.3

To demonstrate the "ability to appreciate" needed for decision-making capacity, a person must:

- acknowledge the condition that affects himself or herself;
- be able to assess how the various options would affect him or her;
- be able to reach a decision and adhere to it; and
- make a choice, not based primarily upon delusional belief.[16]

The ability to understand one's situation is one aspect of competence that can be most readily assessed, for example, by having the patient recite back the risks and benefits of treatment or no treatment. Less easy to assess are those patients able to recite the facts but whose reasoning is so clouded by strong emotions or delusions that they cannot truly appreciate the meaning of the facts in relation to themselves. Such impairment of mental faculties can be subtle and require careful consideration.

For example, certain patients can appear glibly competent but actually be incapable of deciding on their treatment because of denial or hopelessness.[17] Some patients, because of brain injury or inadequate development, may lack the cognitive capacity to make decisions. Other patients may suffer hallucinations or delusions that can interfere with their ability to apply their knowledge. Some patients with serious mental illness will be incapable at times, but often they will not be. If their symptoms materially affect the mental ability required to make a specific decision, such patients should be considered incapable—but only in relation to those specific tasks or decisions.

CASE 6.3 STILL CAPABLE

Mr G, a 24-year-old man with an active and untreated paranoid disorder, presents to the emergency room with a comminuted fractured arm.[18] His injury and the surgery proposed to correct it are explained to him. He's willing to have surgery and gives consent. Nonetheless, the surgical resident wonders if his mental disorder prevents him from giving valid consent and pages the resident on call for Psychiatry to see the patient.

You are the psychiatry resident on call. Given this patient's psychiatric history, should you see him before the surgery?

DISCUSSION OF AND FOLLOW-UP TO CASE 6.3

The surgical resident is not wrong to think about capacity even in the case of someone who goes along with treatment. In theory, all patients with possible impairments of decision-making capacity should have their capacity assessed whether or not they consent to treatment. In reality, it is often only refusals of treatment that trigger such assessments. The resident's query, however, had to do with the patient's mental status. That a mental disorder is present is not the most important issue but whether this significantly affects the specific treatment decision to be made. If the patient can understand and appreciate the decision, then his consent to surgery should be considered valid.

As such, a psychiatry consult is not mandatory before proceeding to surgery. The surgical resident's assessment in this case should suffice as the Surgery service is the one proposing the treatment. However, if he is requesting a psychiatric opinion because of uncertainty about the patient's current reasoning, then the referral should be considered reasonable. Although the surgical resident may be erring on the side of caution, better he be worried than blithely assume the patient's capacity.

As it turns out this patient was delusional but not in regards to his injury or the surgeons whom he felt were on his side. Despite his disorder, he was able to weigh the risks and benefits of surgery. He was considered competent for the purposes of the consent for surgery.

Consequences of decisions

You should be particularly vigilant about a patient's mental capacity when he or she puts him or herself in (avoidable) harm's way *and*

- there is evidence of confused and irrational thinking;
- the person cannot retain information;
- the patient's wishes and/or alertness fluctuates;
- the person is suffering so much that understanding is or would likely be impaired; or
- the person is so under the influence of drugs or alcohol that judgment is impaired.

Notice that we have not said such patients are incapable. These circumstances are red flags calling for a careful assessment of their choices. How strong must an emotion be or how poor must a person's cognitive faculties be to make his or her judgments unreliable? There is no simple answer. In part, it will depend on the importance of the decision.

CASE 6.4 "I'VE SEEN WORSE!"

You are the attending physician at a chronic care facility. One of the residents, Mr T, an 84-year-old war veteran with no living relatives, unable to look after himself owing to physical frailty and mild cognitive decline, develops gangrene in his foot due to poor circulation; it does not respond to medical treatment. Advised to have the foot amputated, Mr T refuses, saying, "My foot will get better on its own. I've seen lots worse during the war!"

Should you accept his refusal of treatment?

DISCUSSION OF AND FOLLOW-UP TO CASE 6.4

You should examine Mr T's process of reasoning in refusing life-saving therapy. To be deemed capable, he must not only be able to understand that he has gangrene but also be able to appreciate that he will most certainly die without surgery. The prudent clinician will examine whether there are any reversible factors that may have an impact on his decision to reject treatment. If so, these factors should be addressed, if possible.

The clinicians involved in his care—hopefully, a multidisciplinary team of doctor, nurse, social worker, occupational therapist, physiotherapist—should make every effort to see the situation from Mr T's perspective, ensuring that there are no countervailing factors, such as loneliness or abandonment, making his choice a less than voluntary one. His capacity should be carefully assessed by the right people. In most jurisdictions, the clinicians proposing the treatment would be responsible for the evaluation; others may be called in as necessary.

Mr T did deny he had gangrene. Despite this, he was able to acknowledge he would be, in his own words, "a fool to refuse surgery" *if* he did have gangrene. That was what the team looking after him thought, too, as his quality of life was quite reasonable. The patient didn't reject the healthcare professional's view altogether—he was prepared to admit that the clinicians just might know better than he whether or not he had gangrene (although he really didn't believe them). He was, in other words, willing to trust the professional opinion. As this was thought to be a capable delegation of consent (see Chapter 5 on "exceptions" to consent), no substitute decision-maker was needed. A team meeting was held, after which, with much encouragement, Mr T agreed to amputation and survived for several more years.

A patient's competence may wax and wane depending on illness and other circumstances. For example, cognitively impaired individuals may worsen with a change of setting or with the time of day (the "sundowning" phenomena). Many clinicians assess patients based only on a small window of time. A patient on a "good day" may then be falsely determined to be competent (similarly, a patient could be incorrectly deemed as incompetent if assessed while delirious). Serial assessments over time will be more likely to uncover a reliable and consistent pattern of behaviour and abilities that could be determined as either capable or not (see Box 6.4).

BOX 6.4

Circumstances that do not on their own warrant a finding of incapacity but may interfere with the exercise and the assessment of capacity, include the following:

- advanced or very young age;
- poor education;
- physical disability, such as impaired ability to communicate;
- different cultural or religious background;
- idiosyncratic or unusual beliefs;
- psychiatric illness, including disagreement over diagnosis; and
- refusal of treatment.

One of the better tools for assessing medical decision-making capacity is the "Aid to Capacity Evaluation"(ACE), developed by Ed Etchells, an internist in Toronto.[19] Available online, it is designed for clinicians to more reliably determine whether a patient is capable of making a particular decision.[20] ACE assesses a patient's capacity by seven simple questions. (See Box 6.5.)

BOX 6.5

A. Is the patient able to understand the following:

1. The medical problem? ("What problem are you having right now?")
2. The proposed treatment? ("What is the treatment for your problem?")
3. The alternatives? ("Are there any other options for you?")
4. The option of refusing treatment? ("Can you refuse/stop the treatment?")

B. Is the patient able to appreciate
5. The consequences of accepting treatment? ("What could happen to you if treated?")
6. The consequences of refusing treatment? ("What could happen to you if not treated?")
7. That he or she has depression/delusion/psychosis that affects the decision? ("Can you help me understand why you have accepted/refused treatment? Do you have any hope for the future? Do you think you are being punished? Do you think someone is trying to harm you?")

An independent assessment of the patient is recommended by Dr Etchells if the patient's incapacity is based on "delusional" thinking alone—presumably because it can be difficult to distinguish delusions from idiosyncratic, bizarre, eccentric, or unusual beliefs.

CASE 6.5 RE-EXAMINING "NO"

Ms L is a 20-year-old woman, mentally challenged and living in a group home, who presents to the Emergency Room with buccal cellulitis, a serious but treatable bacterial infection of the face with a small risk of intracranial spread and death. This cellulitis typically requires several days of in-patient treatment with intravenous antibiotics. She refuses admission as she is fearful of needles and hospitals. She wants to go home and is willing only to take oral medication. The resident doctor in Emergency, to whom she expresses her wishes in a vociferous way, is reluctant to treat her with the necessary intravenous antibiotics. He reasons that the patient's wishes are a clear expression of her autonomy and should be respected despite the history of mental disability. Mental disability, he says to his mentor, does not mean incapacity.

How ought Ms L be treated?

DISCUSSION OF CASE 6.5

The resident's reasoning is quite right: mental disability is not a necessary indicator of incapacity. However, while Ms L could somewhat understand she had an infection and the kind of treatment recommended, she couldn't appreciate how serious a threat it was to her well-being. As well, her vociferous resistance to the proposed in-patient treatment was based on irrational fears of being abandoned and dying in hospital. Clearly, the patient's competence should be carefully assessed. The ability to express a choice is not a sufficient criterion of capacity, especially when death may result without treatment. Ms L had a history of initially refusing various interventions in her life and her actions were often not consistent with her wishes (she would, for example, verbally protest putting on a coat in the winter but would readily co-operate once in the cold and handed her coat). Due to the limitations in her reasoning and her failure to appreciate the seriousness of her state, Ms L lacked the *ability* to make a capable choice.

In the current circumstances, one should not be distracted by her strenuous objections. "Autonomy" does not trump "beneficence," especially when the patient's autonomy is impaired. A decision about treatment with intravenous medications should be sought from a substitute decision-maker (SDM) due to Ms L's incapacity to make the treatment decision. As this patient could not have prior expressed capable wishes, the SDM will be responsible for ensuring the course of action that is in her best interests. Of course, her fears must be addressed, too, by compassionate care and by involving her as much as possible in the treatment plan. She can be reassured and treated in a respectful and medically appropriate way.

II. Substitute Decision-Makers (SDM)

Competence assessments must be done carefully because their conclusions will have a significant impact. *If a patient is found incapable, he or she loses the authority to make his or her own decisions.* An SDM must then be found. In most jurisdictions, such substitutes are required when decisions are to be made for the incapable patient. Sometimes, as in Quebec, a formal court order must be obtained to be appointed as the SDM.[21] In the US and Canada, healthcare professionals should ask whether there is an advance directive stipulating who is allowed to make decisions if the patient is incapable of doing so. If none exists, a hierarchy of substitute decision-makers is usually specified by law and ought to be followed. However, you can challenge a substitute decision-maker if you think that he/she/they are not acting on principles for acceptable substitute decision-making.

CASE 6.6 "I CAN'T LET HER DIE!"

An 88-year-old married patient, Ms W, is admitted to hospital with community-acquired pneumonia. Although she initially responds to antibiotics, she rapidly declines. Going into respiratory failure, she experiences a prolonged episode of cerebral hypoperfusion, resulting in a persistent vegetative state. She is unable to swallow and receives nutrition through a gastrostomy tube. Her spouse insists that "everything be done" to keep her alive—including cardiopulmonary resuscitation and return to the ICU should she deteriorate even more.

When asked how his spouse would respond if she could see her present state, her husband replies, "Oh, Beth would be appalled. She always told me she never wanted to go like this, all these machines and so forth. But I can't just let her die!"

Guides for the role of substitute decision-makers

Substitute decision-makers for incapable patients are usually family members but can be anyone appointed by the patient or by a court or tribunal. When patients are deemed incompetent for medical decision-making, what standards should guide those making decisions for the patient? The unimpaired prior expressed wishes of the mature and capable patient, applicable to the circumstances in question, take precedence. If unknown or not applicable (for example, wishes expressed when a child), the patient's "best interests" should be weighed. This includes a consideration of (1) the patient's values and beliefs when capable if they might pertain to the decision about treatment, and (2) the patient's well-being in relation to the proposed treatment and its alternatives. (Will the proposed treatment reduce the patient's risk of disease or death? What are the alternatives? What are the possible benefits and disadvantages of each option for the patient?)[22, 23, 24]

DISCUSSION OF CASE 6.6

Ms W's husband is not making a decision based on his wife's prior expressed wishes but wants her treated according to *his* needs. He needs to be reminded of the ethical basis for substitute decision-making—in a gentle and compassionate way of course. He needs time to grieve the loss of his wife so a decision to withdraw care ought not be made in an abrupt way. Nevertheless, his wife's prior expressed wishes were clear and should guide him and the healthcare professionals looking after her now. You could gently ask him, "Isn't time we thought about what Beth would have wanted and to let her die naturally . . . ?"

This case suggests the professional has yet another responsibility in looking after an incapable patient: ensuring the suitability of the substitute decision-maker. If the practitioner believes the SDM is acting neither on the patient's wishes nor in the patient's interests, there is a moral rationale for challenging the SDM's decision-making. (The legal option of challenging a patient's substitute decision-maker varies from one jurisdiction to another.)

CASE 6.7 RISKY BUSINESS

Ms R is a 70-year-old widow, hospitalized with cognitive impairment and advanced Parkinson's disease. No longer able to swallow without aspirating her food, a gastrostomy feeding tube has been placed with consent from her 40-year-old son, her only relative. On several occasions, however, he is found secretly feeding his mother by mouth. Moreover, after a weekend visit to her home, she returns to hospital with bruises sustained in falls when he went out and left her alone unsupervised.

What ought her clinicians do?

DISCUSSION AND FOLLOW-UP OF CASE 6.7

One assumes and hopes that Ms R's capacity has been appropriately assessed with the team having determined she is no longer capable of making decisions about her treatment, form of nutrition, place of residence, etc. Assuming she is not capable, the clinicians involved in her care must determine the appropriate substitute decision-maker. They must carefully assess her son's ability to make decisions in her best interests. In this case, protecting her airway and physical safety are paramount to her best interests. There appear to be reasons to suspect he is acting inappropriately so the team may consider challenging his role as her substitute decision-maker.

As it may not be easy to find someone else to accept responsibility for decisions about Ms R, the team should work with her son to help them understand his motivations. Why is he feeding her despite her being "NPO" (*nothing by mouth*)? Why is he taking her home and leaving her unattended? With further discussion, it becomes apparent he does not appreciate just how impaired she is. He sees continued oral feeding and home visits as "quality of life" issues for his mother. The son is motivated by feelings of guilt and of compassion. With education from health professionals and by joining a family support group for relatives with Parkinson's disease, he is better able to act in his mother's best interests but also accept the reality of her decline and not feel guilty he can no longer care for her at home.

III. Treatment of the Vulnerable

The professional duty of care for patients with reduced capacity is clear. One legal authority wrote some time ago: "As a general rule it may be accepted that a higher duty of care to avoid acts of negligence is owed to a person of unsound mind, than to a person of full capacity. The extent that the duty is increased must depend on the circumstances of the case and the nature of the incapacity."[25] I take this to mean clinicians have to exercise particular caution in the care of their patients who have impaired capacity and are unable to comprehend, and so authorize, the consequences of their decisions.

The consequence of removing an individual's right to make his or her own decisions about healthcare is sufficiently important that a fair process must be followed in arriving at that conclusion. Where it is not, healthcare providers may find their decisions challenged and overthrown in judicial proceedings, as it was in the following real-life case.

CASE 6.8 A FRACTURED HIP, A BROKEN MIND

A 76-year-old reclusive single female, Ms D, is admitted with a fractured hip to a large tertiary hospital. When told surgery is required, she refuses to consent, explaining she does not believe she is in a "real hospital," as people had been rude to her and she had noticed dust on the X-ray machine. Ms D says she doubts she has a hip fracture as she is not in that much pain. "Just send me home with a wheelchair," she exclaims. "I want to discuss this with an old ladies' organization."

The resident, finding her line of reasoning a bit unusual, deems her incapable. In contrast, the anesthetist in his pre-operative assessment writes in her chart that he found her "entirely competent" to refuse surgery, specifically highlighting the patient's score of 30/30 on the MMSE (Mini-Mental State Examination—a brief battery of tests that assesses orientation, recall, and concentration) that had been part of the resident's evaluation.

A psychiatric evaluation is therefore requested. On the basis of several visits to Ms D, the psychiatrist concludes that while the patient superficially understands the nature of hip fractures, she is unable to grasp the different approaches to hip fractures and their demonstrated benefits in the elderly,[26] apply that knowledge to herself and acknowledge that, if she had a hip fracture, surgical treatment might help her. She is deemed incapable on those grounds. Told she can challenge the finding of incapacity before a regional quasi-judicial review board, Ms D does so. Following advice from her solicitor, she does not appear before the review panel. The review board finds the patient capable as there is conflicting evidence in her chart from various professionals about her mental status.

BOX 6.6

"The focus should be not only on consent but on *capacity* to consent."[27]

DISCUSSION OF CASE 6.8

This case clearly illustrates the onus is on health professionals to prove incapacity rather than patients to prove their capacity. Ms D was not required to attend the hearing, as a patient need not give evidence "against herself." This is a disturbing aspect of this case, however. While this kind of review process provides an administrative way of resolving capacity disputes, it seems ill-designed to capture the intricacies of real-world capacity evaluations—such as evaluations regarding "the ability to appreciate." The anesthetist's focus on the MMSE seems to have swayed the board into thinking there were some grounds to doubt the finding of the incapacity. While the MMSE has its uses, it has nothing to do with testing a patient's capability to make treatment decisions (unlike the ACE tool mentioned above).

Before going to a review board, a team looking after an incapable patient should first make certain its own house is in order, that is, ensure there is a clear answer to the question as to whether the patient, fully and properly informed, has the *capacity*, the ability, *to consent*. This means clinicians need to assess, not just whether the patient appears incapable at this time, but persists in being incapable despite all the appropriate supports for linguistic, cultural, ethnic, and individual differences (such as deafness or even intellectual deficits requiring extra efforts at comprehension).

At this juncture, the health professionals could conduct another assessment of Ms D's capacity. They could ask for a new hearing before the review board or court armed with better evidence. In Ms D's case, the finding was not challenged as the clinicians were fed up and the hospital did not want to squander more resources on the issue. Somehow, Ms D trundled home, in a wheelchair, with an unfixed hip. She refused follow-up care.

IV. When Not to Rescue

Dr Russell Fleming is the chief psychiatrist at one of Canada's main forensic facilities, and so his name appears frequently in public accounts of cases of involuntary treatment of the seriously mentally ill. One story concerns that of Messrs Gallagher and Reid, involuntary patients at Penetanguishene Medical Health Centre with histories of schizophrenia and criminal behaviour. They were determined by Dr Fleming to be incapable of consenting to treatment with antipsychotics. On the grounds of their best interests, he requested authorization to treat them with such medications despite their wish, expressed to their lawyer, not to receive such drugs. Both patients had previous experience with the drugs and considered them to be non-beneficial or harmful. (It is not clear, however, whether they were assessed as capable at the time of their refusal. This was before the enactment of the Ontario *Consent to Treatment Act*.)

Right to refuse reaffirmed

These cases reached the highest court in Ontario where, along the line of reasoning given by the same court in the earlier decision of *Malette v. Shulman*, it was decided that mentally disordered patients may not be administered treatment they refused while competent. The court wrote

> With very limited exceptions, every person's body is considered inviolate, and, accordingly, every competent adult has the right to be free from unwanted medical treatment. The fact that serious risks or consequences result from a refusal of medical treatment does not vitiate the right of medical self-determination. The doctrine of informed consent ensures the freedom of individuals to make choices about their medical care. It is the patient, not the doctor, who ultimately must decide if treatment—any treatment—is to be administered.[28]

This judgment seems clear enough: by the doctrine of consent, the right of choice (consent or refusal) must extend to psychiatric patients. The paradoxical result is that the principle of autonomy—self-determination, the right to refuse—is being used to maintain a person in a non-autonomous (the untreated schizophrenic) state. In effect, such refusals of treatment are "psychiatric living wills." Serving as a "reverse Ulysses" contract (see the discussion of Case 1.4, "To Feed or Not to Feed"), based on the principle of autonomy, such advance directives allow capable persons to reject psychiatric treatment and subject themselves to the risks of untreated psychosis. Unlike

Ulysses who had his men tie him to the mast so he could not suffer self-harm under the influence of the voices of the Sirens, a reverse Ulysses contract says, in effect, "I don't want to be saved, even if incompetent and suffering." This is a hard contract for health professionals to abide by as it may lead to avoidable harms and preclude the restoration of autonomy and free choice.

Implications of right to refuse

Allowing psychotic patients to refuse psychiatric treatment based on their prior wishes means patients who may be a grave danger to others can be committed to an institution but not be treated, resulting in prolonged incarceration in a psychiatric facility. This "made no sense to Psychiatrists," as the American psychiatrist Paul Appelbaum has written. [29] Psychiatrists would effectively become jailers. As well, allowing such patients greater freedom to refuse medication may lead to problems in psychiatric hospitals such as greater use of restraints or solitary confinement and increased rates of assaults.

Respecting a psychiatric patient's prior wishes to refuse treatment may seem, in principle, no different than not transfusing a Jehovah's Witness patient hemorrhaging to death. But the logic behind the treatment of psychotic patients is not just to protect them as well as others, but also to attempt to restore their autonomy. Most psychotic patients are not a danger to others. Who will be at greater risk of death—by accident, illness, or altercations with police—from this form of the "right to refuse" are those psychotic individuals who refuse medication but are not institutionalized. Deinstitutionalization policies have meant many are released into the community without adequate supports. Gone is the old idea of "asylums" as places of "inviolable" refuge for the ill and the vulnerable, those too sick to care for themselves.

A cruel world: *Starson v. Swayze*

This is the sad story behind the complex and long drawn-out case of Scott Starson. It illustrates some of the challenging and conflicting responsibilities in assessing the capacity to make medical decisions.

Described variously as a brilliant autodidact in physics and as a troubled paranoid schizophrenic, Mr Starson has been in and out of psychiatric hospitals for over 25 years because of his propensity to utter death threats and appear menacing to others. When he refused antipsychotic medications, complaining they "dulled his mind and reduced his creativity," judicial leave was sought for him to be treated against his will. This battle went all the way to the Supreme Court of Canada (scc), which, in a surprise to some, found in favour of the patient and against the judgments of lower-level tribunals that had seen Mr Starson give testimony in person. Interestingly, while other courts have allowed psychiatrically ill patients to refuse drugs on the basis of a prior competent wish, the majority for the court viewed Mr Starson's *contemporaneous* refusal as sufficient for such purposes.[30]

There are many reasons why this judgment was made, but one is critical. Central to finding someone capable is the requirement that the person acknowledge his or her illness and how treatment will impact him or her (the "appreciation" test discussed above). In *Starson v. Swayze*, the Court found it sufficient that he admitted he was "different." It was not necessary for him to acknowledge he had a mental illness. While denial of illness on its own is not evidence of incapacity,[31] it needs to be taken into account along with other features the patient may exhibit (such as delusional thinking, hallucinations, threatening behaviours). The SCC's view that the self-admission of "difference" is sufficient acknowledgement of serious disorder is a very low bar indeed. Denial of mental illness is all too common in those with disorders of the mind. "[R]oughly half of patients with active psychotic illness lack insight into their disease."[32] It is hard to see how a refusal of treatment based on Starson's view of his situation could be an informed refusal, unaffected by distracting issues.

The Court's view would find a psychiatric patient to be capable of refusing treatment when he or she would fail every criterion proposed and supported by the courts for capable medical choice. This allowance and the downplaying of the usefulness of psychiatric treatment ("the cure proposed by his physicians [is] more damaging than his disorder") suggests a poor appreciation of the benefits of psychiatric treatment and perhaps more than a whiff of an anti-psychiatry stance—that mental illness is all "in the mind" (of the physician)—at the Supreme Court level. The pluralism of values in capacity assessments, indeed, the relativity of such assessments, that the Court's majority view espouses has not garnered much implementation at lower court levels.[33] All one can say to health professionals working in this area is be meticulous in charting, be transparently clear in your reasoning, and gird yourself for the possibility of judicial review.

Patients such as Starson may end up "warehoused" or jailed because they do not receive active treatment for their illnesses. Empirical studies done in the United States suggest that only a small percentage of patients refuse their psychiatric medications (less than 10 per cent on most wards, but up to 75 per cent on forensic units, where the patients may be trying to avoid being jailed).[34] One reason the number remains small is that difficult patients who refuse treatment may be discharged early to "roam the streets," even though they are "just as ill" as before.[35] The homeless and psychiatrically ill are sometimes romanticized but, denied the benefits of modern medicine including modern psychiatry, their reality is often a harsh and cruel one. Or, as Hobbes would have said, it is a world that is "nasty, brutish, and short." This is hardly a triumph of autonomy, more the triumph of *anomie*.

Limits on the right to refuse?

It is not yet clear what this Canadian judicial recognition of an involuntary patient's right of treatment refusal will mean in practice. In the United States, although committed patients may refuse their treatment, most get it anyway.[36] Their refusals are usually overridden by review boards or courts that accept the physician's view of appropriateness.

In Canada, there may be similar deference to professional wisdom. As well, there is federal legislation allowing the courts to order treatment of the mentally unfit accused so that the accused may come to trial.[37] Thus, there are other social interests—such as the administration of justice— that limit a patient's right of treatment refusal in specific circumstances. Also, patients may be treated without their consent in emergencies or when they are endangering themselves or others. (See Chapter 5.) Finally, "community treatment orders" are now, in various jurisdictions, a less restrictive voluntary therapeutic option for patients with a persistent and serious mental disorder.[38] This allows patients to receive care while remaining in the community.

V. Failure to Care for Self

Patients can fail to care for themselves for many reasons but a common scenario is that of cognitively impaired elderly individuals living at home on their own.

CASE 6.9 DO NOT GO GENTLY INTO A GOOD NURSING HOME

An 88-year-old widow, Ms S, is hospitalized after a neighbour finds her unconscious in her home. The house itself is in a state of extreme neglect, obvious evidence Ms S is failing to look after her basic needs for food and hygiene. She presents as confused in hospital and is discovered to be suffering from anemia and pneumonia. Once medically stable, the patient demands to be released to her rundown home. This, the medical team is reluctant to do, fearing she will be returning to an unsafe environment as she still appears quite cognitively impaired. The team strongly recommends she be discharged to a long-term care facility or a nursing home but Ms S refuses: "You can't make me go! If I have to die, I'd rather die in my own house!"

What should the team do?

DISCUSSION OF CASE 6.9

Before trying to place a resistant patient into a long-term care facility without her permission, a careful assessment should be made of her capacity to make a residential decision. Even if Ms S is at risk in returning home to independent living, her choice should be honoured if she is able to understand and appreciate the option of so doing. This can be a distressing choice for her healthcare providers who have her best interests at heart and foresee she will likely get into trouble again. Nonetheless, if Ms S can make a capable choice about where to live, they are obliged to accept this decision. This is not to say that the patient should now be abandoned to her fate. As much as possible, the treating team should attempt to put as many community supports in place to allow this woman to live as safely as possible, given her physical and cognitive limitations.

There is legislation, in various jurisdictions, that could authorize this patient's confinement to a long-term care facility without her consent so long as (1) she is not competent to decide about her living arrangement and (2) there is consent from an appropriate substitute decision-maker.[39] Such decisions are really no different than any other medical treatment decision—if the patient is not capable of making the decision, the SDM must then make a decision based on the patient's applicable prior expressed wishes or on the patient's best interests—usually, it is the latter.

Many incapable, vulnerable patients remain in the community, perhaps because it otherwise requires someone to identify and care about such persons at risk. As well, the current concern for "patient rights" (to be left alone) can lead practitioners to forget their professional skills and do only what they think the law requires. There is no "duty to attend" the suspected ailing patient at home. This can leave vulnerable patients without care.[40] Public health legislation sometimes provides powers to authorities to "search and remove" persons incapable of personal care,[41] but this is not often exercised in cases of patients with dementia.

Looked at ethically, the decision to institutionalize incapable citizens can be difficult—whether or not they will go voluntarily.[42] If cajoling doesn't work, is it better to let "nature take its course" or to bring the patient to hospital under the auspices of mental health legislation? How forcefully should one pry the reluctant person out of his or her home? The question "What good will it do?" inevitably arises, especially in the care of the very old. This attitude is no doubt in part age-biased—one would have few qualms about trying to rescue a younger person. But, it may also be a realistic appraisal as to what the elderly patient would have wanted and the limits as to what aggressive treatment can do. This is a balancing act that only a good clinical assessment of the patient's ailments as to what is treatable and of the patient's contextual factors can answer. For example, has the patient refused care before? What other illnesses does the patient have? Is there anything obviously wrong that could be addressed at home? Would extra home services be of use? The right answer is to consider the options carefully, hopefully with input from others (such as a visiting nurse, a community practitioner, a social worker from a home service provider, a geriatrician, and obviously family members).

VI. Cases Involving Minors

Children may make their own decisions about the medical care they receive, if the child has the capacity to understand and appreciate fully the consequences of consenting or not consenting to the various medical options.[43] Rather than age, what is important is the child's mental competence regarding the proposed procedure. The process of assessing capacity of minors to make treatment decisions is no different than that for adults.

There are regulations in various jurisdictions setting an age limit to capacity ("a minor is anyone under the age of 18 . . ."), especially for purposes of contracts, estate ownership, drinking, and voting. However, there is also well-developed case law permitting those under 18, who are capable, to make decisions about their own healthcare. At common law in some jurisdictions this concept is called the "mature minor rule" (although thought to be common, less than a quarter of US states recognize this doctrine).[44] Where this rule does apply, if a minor is living independently, he or she may also be considered capable (as are, for example, adolescents who have left home and/or are married, yet are still under 18 years of age). In such jurisdictions, no parental consent is necessary. This concept was first introduced in the British case of *Gillick v. West Norfolk*: "As a matter of law, the parental rights to determine whether or not the minor child below the age of 16 will have medical treatment terminates if and when the child achieves sufficient understanding and intelligence to fully understand what is being proposed."[45]

This leading UK case on consent in minors established that children, as they become more capable of understanding what is involved in making treatment decisions, acquire greater rights to make those decisions autonomously. By this guidance a doctor, for example, may accept a young teen's informed decision about birth control if she does not want her parents to know. However, a prudent physician would still seek to obtain the parents' involvement, where possible and with the competent child's consent, for procedures that are of great import for the minor's health and welfare. The involvement of other healthcare professionals could be helpful for understanding a child's unwillingness to involve his or her family. Are they not going to find out at some point anyway? If a child refuses parental involvement, the physician should fully discuss the implications of such refusals before following the minor's wishes.

Right of minors to refuse life-sustaining treatment

Despite the *Gillick* ruling, British courts have generally not permitted a minor to bring about his or her own death by refusing treatment.[46] In Canada, the courts have not been so unanimous. In New Brunswick, Canada, in 1994, 15-year-old Joshua Walker, a Jehovah's Witness with acute leukemia, was allowed to refuse life-sustaining transfusions.[47] The Court of Appeal found him to be extremely capable and therefore able to be the author of his own actions. New Brunswick and Ontario, unlike some provinces, have codified the capable-minor doctrine into law.

In a case involving another young Jehovah's Witness, an Ontario Provincial Court in 1985 allowed a 12-year-old girl with acute myeloid leukemia to refuse life-sustaining care. When she refused further blood transfusions, the Children's Aid Society sought court protection for the child. This application was denied because the court found that previous transfusions had infringed upon a "capable girl's right to security of the person" and the right not to be discriminated against on the grounds of age and religion, both guaranteed under the *Canadian Charter of Rights and Freedoms*.

The patient had "wisdom and maturity well beyond her years" and "a well-thought-out, firm and clear religious belief." The court ruled she ought to have been consulted before the transfusion. In the eyes of the court, the hospital's proposed treatment dealt with the disease only in a physical sense and failed "to address her emotional needs and religious beliefs; it fail[ed] to address the whole person." The patient died two weeks later.[48]

Different fact situations have led to different decisions by the courts. A 16-year-old Jehovah's Witness in Alberta who refused blood transfusions on account of her beliefs was ordered to have them anyway.[49] Although found by psychiatric examination to be capable, the court found her decision to be non-voluntary as she was considered to be under the "undue influence" of her Jehovah's Witness mother. This undue influence was in part due to false information provided by her mother.

Adult-like capacity not enough

The important feature of juvenile consent is that the criteria by which we judge adult capacity—the cognitive and emotional capacity of the individual to consent to treatment—may *not* be sufficient to establish a child's capacity.[50] Children are obviously developing at very different speeds and directions emotionally, physically, and neurologically.[51] No matter how smart they can be, they can be in a vulnerable position vis-à-vis adults, more readily influenced by them on account of their lack of power, their emotional bonds in the family, and their inexperience. One wonders, for example, whether a 12-year old can independently grasp the nature of a decision such as the non-provision of life-saving care. What sources of support for such a decision could a child have? Wouldn't we want and expect the child to look to and rely on his or parents? If so, this natural dependency should make us look long and hard at a child's volitional and informational autonomy before one follows a child's choice regarding treatment. Some authorities—and the *Civil Code* in Quebec—recommend that children be at least 14 before being allowed to make major treatment decisions.[52]

It may be difficult for clinicians to know when to abide by refusals of care by children—especially those on the cusp of adulthood. Teens can be volatile and hard to mollify. On the other hand, even very young children can be surprisingly capable of understanding and, by the principle of respect due persons, deserve to have their opinions, fears, and wishes taken into account. It can be argued that their assent to treatment should be sought even if the final authority for the decision is not theirs alone.

Conclusion

Despite the importance of patient autonomy, healthcare professionals are still expected to exercise their professional judgment and carefully assess and protect mentally incapable patients who are in harm's way. More difficult for clinicians to manage are situations where such patients refuse to be helped and seem to do so for inappropriate reasons.

The extent of healthcare professionals' obligations to rescue or help will be examined in the subsequent two chapters on beneficence and professionalism.

Cases For Discussion

CASE 1: A REFUSAL TO EAT

Ms C is a 58 year-old-woman with an unremarkable medical history who was apparently well until she stopped eating approximately three weeks ago. She had worked as an accountant until the birth of her children, now 21 and 25 years old. Both parents are deceased, her father having died in a farming accident when she was a child and her mother in her late 50s due to a rapidly progressive dementia. Ms C has repeatedly said she does not want to die as her mother did, in a nursing home, incontinent, lacking in dignity. "Better to die with your boots on," she has told her family.

Ms C is now quite ill. She is dehydrated and her electrolytes out of whack. She seems unconcerned but looks pale and seems withdrawn. She explains she would like to eat but cannot, due to an upset digestive system. She plays with her food and says she'll maybe eat tomorrow if her stomach feels better. "I need to cleanse out my intestines and liver," she says to the nurse looking after her. She says she's done this before and does not believe she will die. She refuses any artificial hydration and nutrition, specifically, an IV and nasogastric tube. She wants to go home. Her husband is not much help. "She's stubborn all right. She'll do whatever she needs to do," he shrugs in an offhand way. "I think we'd best go home," he adds.

Questions For Discussion

1. Why might Ms C be refusing nutrition?
2. Do you think she is an autonomous person?
3. If you feel Ms C is not competent, would you go along with her husband's decision to take her home?

CASE 2: A REFUSAL OF MEDICATION

Mr M, a 26-year-old male, living with his parents in a small agricultural town, was diagnosed with paranoid schizophrenia at the age 15. He is often aggressive, and does not trust his parents or doctor. He says the medicines prescribed to him make him "mad." Mr M has stopped taking them for the last two months, and resists all attempts by his parents to take him to see his psychiatrist. While on his medication he was able to work as an agricultural labourer, but now has spent the last six weeks wandering around the town and returning home to sleep when he feels tired. His mother is worried he will be assaulted or jailed if he becomes aggressive. She confides her fears to her son's doctor, and is advised to give him an antipsychotic mixed in his coffee. She takes this advice and her son quiets down and starts working in the fields again. Every time Mr M's parents bring up the subject of his treatment he shouts he will run away from them if he is forced to take pills again. His mother continues her deception, concealing his medicines in his coffee or other food.

Questions For Discussion

1.   Is Mr M's refusal of pills a capable one?
2.   Was his doctor's advice appropriate?
3.   Can you foresee any problems with the mother's actions?

7 Helping and Not Harming
Beneficence and Non-Maleficence

Regard your patients as human beings, while never forgetting they are your patients.

Michael Balint, 1959[1]

It is common for helping professionals to feel responsible for meeting their clients' every need . . . it can be difficult indeed to sort out the differences between a "healthy" giving, born of our deepest desires to love, and an "unhealthy" giving, springing from unfulfilled psychological needs—for approval, for achievement, to appear more saintly than we really are.

David Hilfiker, 1994[2]

Beneficence is the commitment of all healthcare professionals to the well-being of their patients. Once a practitioner takes on an individual as a patient, that person is owed a special duty of care. For that duty to be fulfilled, the clinician is expected to meet the standard of a competent practitioner's care and skill in similar circumstances. However, beneficence in medicine involves more than competence in caring for one's own patients. It also entails a commitment to professionalism (explored in Chapter 8). Beneficence requires knowing what it means to help and to harm patients, when to offer to help or "rescue" others and when not to do so.

CASE 7.1 A THEATRE PERFORMANCE

You are out on the town with your friends, celebrating your successful completion of medical school. Now, others can call you "Doctor." At the theatre that night, just as you are settling into your seat, a plea comes over the loudspeaker, "Is there a doctor in the house?"

How would you and should you respond? Is there an ethical dilemma here?

I. The Principles of Beneficence and Non-Maleficence

The Oath of Hippocrates directs physicians to use all their skills to benefit patients and keep them from harm. The principles of beneficence and non-maleficence are the oldest and most important guiding tenets of medicine. The Canadian Medical Association's Code of Ethics, like many other healthcare professional codes, directs doctors to "Consider first the well-being of the patient."[3]

Beneficence means doing good, showing active kindness to, or assisting others in need. For the medical professions, helping others is not an option ("Hmm . . . shall I help my next patient get better or not?") but a role-mandated requirement. At a minimum, by their interventions— meant to make people better or to prevent harms and setbacks to patient interests—health professionals should not make patients worse off than they were before the interventions. This principle of "non-maleficence" or "doing no harm" expects health professionals to refrain from doing evil or making anyone ill.[4]

There are standards for practice that all healthcare professionals—whether trainees, doctors, nurses, or physician assistants—are expected to meet:

> Every medical practitioner must bring to his task a reasonable degree of skill and knowledge and must exercise a reasonable degree of care. He is bound to exercise that degree of care and skill which could reasonably be expected of a normal, prudent practitioner of the same experience and standing.[5]

DISCUSSION OF CASE 7.1

If you have the skills to intervene, must you identify yourself as a doctor (or any other trained health professional)? The answer is no and yes. In the UK and most North American jurisdictions, there is *usually* no legal requirement for practitioners to intervene in emergency situations. In these jurisdictions, Good Samaritan laws protect interveners from being sued if things do not go well for the injured party. Simply put, a stranger in distress is not your patient and you owe him or her no duty of rescue from a legal point of view. However, from an ethical point of view, the answer is likely to be yes— especially if one has the skills and confidence required to respond to the emergency. The skilled clinician should offer to help, assuming there is no evident danger in doing so, because he or she may be the only person capable of helping.

Why might a duly qualified practitioner not help? The most common reasons would be not feeling he or she wants to "work," thinking someone else might respond, and/or fear of legal liability.

A duty to attend?

This is quite distinct from Quebec and European Union countries that require physicians and, indeed, all citizens (it is not, then, a duty for physicians alone), passing by an emergency or an accident, to stop and provide medical aid. This requirement derives from European Civil Law Codes, which impose certain duties of social assistance on its citizens (as opposed to Anglo-American jurisprudence that frees citizens from social encumbrances). One author has commented that "the failure to act on behalf of a person in peril is regarded to be a crime and thus a public wrong on the European continent, while it is only a matter of individuals in English law to decide not to intervene."[6]

Professional responsibilities may be more exacting, however. A Canadian physician was found in breach of professional standards when, despite having completed his regular shift, he failed to attend to a patient in the ER.[7] An Australian doctor was found negligent for refusing to attend to a person, not his patient, who collapsed outside his office.[8] In each of these cases the courts felt there was some professional requirement—in emergencies—for doctors to attend to patients if it could be done at no great personal cost and if what seems to be required is within the physician's sphere of competence. The force and scope of this retrospective court-mandated "duty to attend," however, is not clear legally. They appear to be, at this time, exceptional cases.

So, when the call goes out, "Is there a doctor in the house?", those who respond do so now largely out of moral sentiment or professional engagement.

Risks to the professional

Is there a requirement to act when this would put oneself, as the medical professional, directly in harm's way? There can be situations—during epidemics, wars, and disasters—that exceed the dangers of ordinary civil life. In such circumstances, because of their commitment and special training, it is expected that healthcare professionals may have to put themselves in harm's way *to some degree*. Nonetheless, extreme situations can tax a professional's commitment to serve patients and the public. What about an outbreak in town of a potentially lethal, and transmissible by humans-to-human, disease? Is exposing oneself to such increased hazards morally required or simply allowable? What if it entails some risk to your family? Certainly, healthcare professionals are not required to sacrifice themselves—and ought not allow this to happen to themselves (or their families, needless to say)—whether in emergencies or not. A patient waving a gun in the ER is a job for the police, not the medics.

Healthcare professionals cannot avoid taking on some extra risk, but just how much risk is hard to quantify. They are also expected to take "reasonable precautions" to look after their own safety (such as not re-capping needles to prevent exposure to contaminated fluids).[9] They should be prepared to shoulder small risks to themselves, such as getting vaccinated against influenza, to prevent harm to others.[10] Risks of great magnitude are another matter. Whether one stays if there were to be a serious infectious outbreak nearby, for example, would depend what treatments were available and what precautions one could take. This balancing of the risk to self versus the risk to others is, at times, a difficult one. In natural disasters and other calamities, members of the public and the profession often put aside utilitarian calculations of risk and seek out the injured, to help as they can.

The quality of care

In any circumstance, in exercising the duty of beneficence, medical professionals are expected to offer only *proportionate* treatment—treatment whose likely good outweighs the risk of harm. If the stakes are high, the treatment should offer a magnitude of risk of harm that is not greater than the anticipated chance of benefit. However, medical interventions, despite their therapeutic potential, almost always entail *some* degree of risk of harm to the patient: drugs can harm unpredictably, surgeons can wound unintentionally, hospitalization can expose patients to dangerous "superbugs." Weighing the hazards against the benefits is something that must in large measure turn on patient preferences. Quality of life issues for the patient are frequently unavoidable and may involve considering issues that are difficult to quantify, such as the possibility of restoring the patient's independence, maintaining ability to relate to others, capacity for happiness, satisfaction, and the ability to maintain dignity.

BOX 7.1

The principle of beneficence requires the healthcare professional to consider the following:*

- the patient's pain and suffering, both physical and mental;
- the standard of care, its attendant risks and benefits;
- the possibility of death and disability;
- the possibility of restoration of health and functional status;
- the patient's quality of life as seen from the patient's perspective; and
- the patient's expectations regarding treatment.

(*This list could go on and on, but covers some major issues to be considered.)

CASE 7.2 NO SURGERY WANTED

You are a surgeon with an 81-year-old female patient, Ms R, just diagnosed with pancreatic cancer, a malignancy usually leading to death within a year of diagnosis. Surgery is the only option that might be life-prolonging but involves a risk of morbidity and short-term mortality. Informed of the diagnosis and treatment options, the patient refuses the operation. Ms R explains she has always been terrified of surgery and adds that she feels she has lived a full life. She declines surgery.

Should you accept Ms R's refusal of surgery?

Although beneficence towards the patient is the standard that should guide medical practice, this does not mean doing everything conceivable. One should do and recommend what seems "right" for the patient, all things considered—and central to that must be the kind of life the patient has led and wants to lead.

The "best interests" standard

Beneficence is not quite the same as the "best interests" standard. The latter suggests there exists some objectively right course of action most likely to help the patient. For example, it is in the patient's "best interests" that a certain medication be taken or a specific procedure carried out in order to alleviate threats to his or her well-being. Matters are nonetheless not always so simple. At a minimum we presume something is in a person's best interests if it minimizes pain and suffering and prevents untimely or premature death. Just how these outcomes should be weighed against quality of life factors will depend intimately on a patient's personal values, something that a healthcare provider (and often family members) cannot always predict for a patient. It is this subjective side of beneficence that makes well-being dependent on the principle of autonomy (see Box 7.2). To avoid paternalism, it must take into account the patient's views of suffering.

BOX 7.2

In deciding what is beneficent, healthcare professionals must take into account not only whether the proposed medical intervention is actually likely to improve the person's condition, but also the person's values, beliefs, and expressed wishes regarding his or her condition.

Doing nothing is sometimes better

Sometimes, when the chance of harm is high and likelihood of benefit low, it is better to recommend the patient do nothing, recalling the adage "Don't just do something, stand there!" Judging when one should just stand there can be difficult, often because of uncertainty and the lack of evidence regarding outcomes. Nonetheless, because it involves risks of its own, doing nothing should not be confused with non-maleficence. For example, watchful waiting is an acceptable option in early stage prostate cancer but carries the risk that, despite proper vigilance, the patient's cancer may advance to an incurable stage. Some people are prepared to take this risk in order to avoid the more immediate risks of active treatment.

DISCUSSION OF CASE 7.2

Although the only possibly curative option for Ms R is surgery, how far should you push this? If you push too far, it might be at the expense of her views. In your role as Ms R's advocate, you must consider not only her best interests but also her preferences. This role requires leaving no stone unturned in exploring both her expressed wishes—especially where they might put her in harm's way—and the various treatment options.

First of all, is the diagnosis correct? How good was the pathology opinion? Should you recommend the patient consult with another colleague? As an octogenarian, what are Ms R's chances with surgery? Does she appreciate her limited lifespan without surgery? Is there any evidence she might not be competent to make this decision? Further questioning should be directed at why Ms R is so afraid of surgery. Has she had some bad past experience with surgery preventing her from appreciating its benefits now?

The discussion should ultimately target what would be accomplished by the proposed surgery and whether such goals are consistent with the patient's preferences. For example, Ms R's physicians might consider it a "success" to prolong her expected lifespan of eight to twelve months by four or six months. Would this gain be sufficient to offset the risks and harms of major surgery? What quality of life does she desire? Has Ms R discussed her situation with other family members and thought about the impact of her decision on them?

From the perspective of some patients—especially those who feel they've lived a full life—the option of a "natural death," free of medical procedures, is a powerful one. While one must respect an informed and competent patient's wishes, even if not "optimal" medically, one also must guard against "ageist" assumptions on anyone's part (the family doctor, the family, and even the patient) that might deny an elderly patient beneficial care.

Respecting autonomy

Healthcare is most successful when it combines the illness experience of the patient with the disease perspective of the healthcare practitioner. This requires time for negotiation or compromise, but shared decision-making is the way to go. Objectives for the healthcare professional—increasing a patient's "disease-free survival," for example—may be meaningless to the patient if accompanied by more isolation, dependence, disability, or suffering. One ought to be humble about these matters—the patient is usually the best judge of which choice is best.

Rescue can harm

Inexperience or unrestrained therapeutic zeal can sometimes cause clinicians to do "too much" good.

CASE 7.3 TOO MUCH OF A GOOD THING?

It is the last day of the last week of a resident's training program. He eagerly looks forward to becoming a full-fledged doctor in one week. On his last half-day, he is happy to see two of his favourite patients, Mr and Ms P, both in their 80s, on his list. They appreciate the resident's attention to them and his diligence. On that day, he decides to examine Ms P's circulation because she has coronary artery disease.

He is surprised to hear a bruit over her carotid arteries. Although Ms P has never had stroke-like symptoms, he decides to send her for neck Dopplers (ultrasound) to check on the patency of her arteries. These reveal a close to 90 per cent bilateral carotid artery blockage. As a major stroke is possible with this degree of blockage, he recommends an endarterectomy, to which Ms P reluctantly agrees. "Oh, do I have to, Doctor?" (In hindsight, it is not clear whether the patient appreciated the true risks or whether she just went along so as not to disappoint her doctors.) The surgery is successful and blood now flows through her carotid arteries. She is sent home four days later.

On her third day at home, Ms P suddenly collapses and is unable to be revived. A post-mortem reveals she died of a massive cerebral hemorrhage.

Was anything wrong done here?

DISCUSSION OF CASE 7.3

The resident is distraught over this outcome. Trying to be a good and thorough clinician, he had, he feels, sent this patient to her doom. Hardly a predictable outcome (but it does happen in 1/400 cases of endarterectomies—due to the high flow of blood rushing through old arteries), he nevertheless feels responsible for Ms P's death.

The resident should be reassured that just as it is hubris to believe he can save everyone, so it is arrogance to think he, as the medical professional, is always responsible for deaths of patients under his care. Some people just have "bad physiology," others have plain ill luck, and yet others die because of bad disease. There was nothing "wrong" done in this case, but such outcomes remind us that the urge to use medical interventions is a two-edged sword. One way of managing the uncertainty of benefit and the use of dangerous weapons is through shared decision-making and concordance about therapeutic goals in the context of the compassionate care.

Clinicians—and Case 7.3 would apply to any healthcare trainee or professional—need to learn to deal with and accept limits, for themselves and for their patients. This, too, is part of the uncertain art of medicine—knowing when the most beneficent thing to do is to do nothing. It is easy to be wise after the event, of course (see Case 7.3).

Perfection not expected

It is expected that clinicians will follow what is "approved practice" or what a "substantial" number of practitioners would do.[11] Unanimity of practice and good outcomes are not expected of any clinician but, where the outcome is poor (the patient suffers serious harm) or where their practices are deviant, clinicians may have their practices scrutinized by the courts or peer organizations to see if they have tried to act in the patient's best interests. One UK court opined: "A doctor is not guilty of negligence if he has acted in accordance with a practice accepted as proper by a responsible body of medical men. [A] doctor is not guilty of negligence merely because there is a body of opinion that takes a contrary view."[12] This is a broadly accepted legal standard of care for all healthcare practitioners.

Thus, the courts recognize that the appropriate exercise of medical beneficence must allow for different diagnostic and therapeutic interventions, the choice among which may be determined by professional judgment. Nonetheless, even choices of clinicians following the profession's "standard of care" can be and have been found negligent where they would be judged egregiously unsafe in the eyes of an ordinary person.[13]

II. The "Duty to Rescue" the Patient

The "duty to rescue" is one encapsulation of the healthcare professional's obligation to serve the needs of patients—better to call it the duty to *offer help* to patients in harm's way. Healthcare professionals are not obliged to roam around looking for people to help (although they might do so in emergencies such as in the aftermath of terrorist bombings, earthquakes, or floods). Usually, clinicians wait for patients to come to them by ambulance, with family assistance, or by walking into their office, clinic, or emergency unit. While the emergency or casualty room best exemplifies the obligation to help or rescue those in distress as a role-mandated duty, medical professionals every day offer treatments to try to alleviate the harms or threats to their patients. The practical dilemma for the clinician in a clinic, office or ward is to know when one should not attempt a "heroic" rescue, when an action is disproportionate to the duty (such as trying to "rescue" a patient imminently dying, already "in the article of death," *in punto di morte*) or, by contrast, when one should go out of one's way to save a person at risk (such as the person at risk of renal or respiratory failure). One can go overboard for one's patients by doing too much or, alternatively, one can abandon them to their fate by doing too little. A good practitioner learns how to devise a fine balance between these two extremes.

CASE 7.4 NOT LIKE HIMSELF

You are a visiting public health nurse called in by social services to do a house call on Mr W, a 90-year-old, previously independent and somewhat reclusive widower, who lives alone in his own bungalow. Neighbours are used to seeing him shoveling snow, raking leaves, bent over, not complaining. In recent weeks, Mr W has taken to his bed and, unlike his usual self, now seems somewhat pale, disoriented, and disheveled. After examining him, you feel he is seriously ill due to anemia of unknown cause and should be admitted to hospital for further investigation. This, the patient adamantly refuses to allow. "It's my heart," Mr W exclaims, "I'm ready to die at home." You respond, "Well, yes, it might be your heart, but I think your hemoglobin is well below normal and maybe we can do something about that . . . "

How can you best help the patient?

Patients can have mental and physical disorders—delirium, dementia, and depression—that impair their ability to be autonomous and act autonomously. As a result, they may be left vulnerable. The principle of beneficence implies a limited "duty to rescue" such individuals under an acceptable (indeed, a praiseworthy) version of "paternalism"—a "weak paternalism"[14]—taking "due care" of those suffering and vulnerable, such as a young child or an adult with developmental delay, ill and in harm's way. This duty authorizes healthcare professionals to act in a patient's best interests without that person's consent (so long as the patient is incapacitated relative to the decision regarding a treatment, pending the identification and arrival of a substitute decision-maker).

This is the role of "implied consent": if you put your arm out for a vaccine, your consent to getting it is implied by your action. Similarly, if you come to the ER, your consent to being treated is implied by your act of coming to the ER. You can leave the ER anytime, of course (unless you are incapable and/or a danger to self or others).

DISCUSSION OF AND FOLLOW-UP TO CASE 7.4

Should you simply accept Mr W's "right to refuse" treatment? Obviously not—at least, not yet. You should explore his situation further. He is able to tell you his wife had died some years before; they had no children and their families all perished in World War II. The only evidence he'd ever seen a doctor is a 15-year-old half-empty bottle of pills for blood pressure and some over-the-counter constipation remedies. Where patients are *capable*, practitioners may try to persuade patients to accept appropriate medical care. (Indeed, some argue that it is an ethical *imperative* to persuade patients to do the "right thing" when there is good and convincing evidence for one option over another.[15]) Where patients are *incapable*, healthcare professionals have added obligations: to work to prevent foreseeable harm to such patients and to try to restore their autonomy. Once, and if, their autonomy is/can be restored, such patients can again be self-determining.

The question that needs to be asked here is: is *this* patient's refusal of treatment reasonable, or merely eccentric, or does it reveal someone whose illness is so severe that it undermines his ability to make an informed choice regarding treatment? If the patient's competence is impaired and no substitute decision-maker can be found, the decision as to how to proceed cannot depend on his wishes alone.

Mr W's command of English is quite poor, so a translator is involved. After much cajoling, the patient reluctantly agrees to go to the ER. It turns out he is extremely anemic due to a large tumour in his colon. His condition stabilizes but no amount of discussion can persuade Mr W to agree to surgery.

It is questioned at the time whether his refusal of surgery is a capable one, owing to his language problems and his seeming denial that he had a tumour (he insisted he only had a kidney problem). Despite this, his refusal is respected—probably in part because of his advanced age, and perhaps also due to a feeling of futility—and he returns home one month later. He dies there of metastatic colon cancer the next year. In retrospect it can certainly be asked whether Mr W should have been more carefully examined for his decision-making capacity and whether his "rescue" was not prematurely truncated.

III. Endangering One's Self

It can be difficult to help some people. They can seem to deliberately put themselves in harm's way—as if stepping into the path of an oncoming bus—and challenge the professional as to when and whether to intervene. Here is an example.

CASE 7.5 NO FOOLS ALLOWED

Ms E is an 84-year-old patient who is as fiercely independent as she can be—she's outlasted several husbands and considers most men incompetent fools. An inveterate smoker, Ms E likes nothing better than lying in bed in silken pajamas, imbibing her single malt scotch, reading magazines, and smoking cigarette after cigarette. To make a house call on this patient is like taking a trip back in time to some smoky 1950s lounge bar. The patient also hates most aspects of aging—she cannot stand the way it has gradually stripped away her dignity, her smooth complexion, her muscle strength, her stamina, her joie de vivre, and now her memory. Most frustratingly, she is finding it difficult to cope with the requirements of living on her own. Bills are accumulating, papers and magazines are in piles everywhere, the bathrooms are filthy, food is rotting in the fridge, stale air hangs like a thick haze about her house, and cigarette burns have punctured her bedroom carpet, her sheets, and even her usually immaculate pajamas. Will she accept any help or consider moving? No way. Ms E is, in her view, "perfectly fine."

What should her primary care provider do?

What can be done about the refusal of care by a failing individual at home? There may be legislation that allows one to rescue free-ranging seriously-at-risk vulnerable adults. This can provide an administrative solution to patient "intransigence." Such laws vary in different jurisdictions and so medical professionals should confirm their possible legal options. In Ontario, for example, if one is concerned about a cognitively impaired elderly person's ability to live safely on his or her own, one could (1) use mental health legislation to force such a patient (under a "Form 1") into a hospital ER for assessment (by virtue of dementia being considered a mental illness and the patient being in imminent danger to the self); (2) arrange to have an evaluation of that person's capacity to make a long-term care decision and enable his or her placement in a long-term care facility on an urgent basis, if he or she is found incapable; or (3) as a last resort, access the Office of the Public Guardian and Trustee which can, under guardianship legislation, be appointed in some cases by the court to temporarily make decisions for the individual.[16]

Taking these steps requires much effort and also deprives people of their liberty at a time in their life when much has already ebbed away. Whom are we going to institutionalize against their will?—all people who don't bathe regularly? (Hardly—unless there is evidence of a broader failure of self-care); the inveterate hoarder? (Maybe, if at risk of dying under a mountain of garbage); a gun-toting angry reclusive? (Likely—especially if there have been acts or threats of violence in the past). A healthcare professional must make judgments about how grave and imminent the dangers are in order to justify the revocation of a patient's liberty.

DISCUSSION AND FOLLOW-UP OF CASE 7.5

Obviously an evaluation of Ms E's capacity to make a decision about her place of residence needs to be made. As well, an overall assessment of her mental status is called for. How imminent are the risks to her well-being? Can any supports be put in place that would minimize these risks and allow her to stay home? Can any family members assist with this? The goal is to seek the least restrictive alternative that will protect her while preserving her liberty.

Many avenues are explored but the patient's fierce independence slows the whole process down considerably. Everyone bends over backwards to try to accommodate her. She agrees to have help and then does not let the help in; she agrees not to smoke in bed and new burn marks are later found; her driver's licence is revoked and she is seen driving anyway. She is just capable enough to barely cope and . . . Then one day Ms E fails to answer the door. The police are called, break in, and find her lying at the bottom of the stairs with a broken arm and hip, barely conscious. She now cannot resist being carried away. She is admitted to hospital and later discharged to a nursing home. There was something inevitable about her ultimate fate. It is unlikely that any other course of action would have had a better outcome. What Ms E needed that money couldn't buy was someone to care for her. There is only so much that healthcare professionals can do.

The suicidal and the reckless

There are many things patients do that clinicians cannot control. Those who live in a democratic system are allowed to live and do as they wish, within limits, and not as others want them to. They can live recklessly and make poor choices but, so long as this affects only themselves and they are capable, they can do as they wish. There is one limit to this allowance for personal choice that seems fairly well set: patients who are actively suicidal are treated as ill and incapable, and may be hospitalized without their consent. Is suicide just another option—like deliberately stepping in front of an oncoming bus—that people can "select" if that is their choice? The answer in general is no; it is not an acceptable choice but for exceptional circumstances (e.g., in protests, war, or tragic love stories).

Suppose in Case 6.2—the depressed and possibly psychotic young man—the patient was brought by friends or the police to the ER, actively suicidal, but refused to be voluntarily admitted or to see a psychiatrist. Present-day mental health legislation in almost every jurisdiction in North America and the United Kingdom allows for the involuntary commitment of patients (1) who have a mental disorder and (2) who are at imminent risk of causing serious harm to themselves or to others.

BOX 7.3

Requirements for involuntary assessment or committal are as follows:

(1)   The patient is dangerous; i.e, the patient

• has attempted or threatened serious self-harm; or
• has behaved or threatens to behave violently towards another or causes another person to fear bodily harm from him/her; or
• has shown or is showing a lack of competence to care for him/ herself.

And

(2)   The patient suffers from a mental disorder likely to result in

• serious bodily harm to the person; or
• serious bodily harm to another person; or
• imminent and serious physical impairment of the person.

Legislation allowing involuntary admission and assessment is sometimes interpreted narrowly by physicians, who may have too restrictive an understanding of such terms as "mental disorder" or "imminent harm."[17] Imminent means "more likely than not" that it will occur—for example, a serious threat of harm to another that can be alleviated only by an urgent medical intervention, such as an emergency assessment. People with "mental disorders" include not only those who are acutely depressed or psychotic but also individuals with personality disorders or who are delirious or are irreversibly cognitively impaired. Morally, it seems preferable to protect patients or others from serious harm rather than allow an individual to refuse necessary care because of a mistaken desire to respect "patient autonomy." (See Chapter 3 on the "duty to protect.")[18]

CASE 7.6 AN ILLICIT REQUEST?

A 33-year-old woman, Ms Y, suffered a high C-spine fracture two years ago in a diving accident. She can breathe on her own but is quadriplegic other than having some limited mobility of her fingers. She became depressed after the accident and never has adapted to her injury. She hates her life and has more than once evinced to her friends a wish to die. Ms Y is not religious, has a live-in boyfriend who helps her, and two dogs who are devoted to her. One evening she is brought to the ER by her boyfriend, after being found comatose. Ms Y has somehow taken an overdose of tranquillizers. There is a suicide note, saying she is sorry but "can't take it anymore," and a document declining treatment.

What should the healthcare providers do? Should the dictates of her suicide note be followed?

A suicide note cannot be considered a form of "living will." In modern medicine, suicide is considered the product of a mind unbalanced by a serious mental malady, such as depression, and attempted in a moment of despair. "Suicide should be considered the response of someone, whether suffering from mental disease or not, who is unable to find a solution to a relational crisis."[19] A suicide attempt is often a cry for help—not a competent refusal of care or an inevitable reaction to difficult circumstances. "Only 10 to 14 per cent of persons commit suicide over the decade following a failed attempt, suggesting that in most suicidal persons, the desire to die is transient."[20]

DISCUSSION OF CASE 7.6

It would be appropriate to ignore the suicide note and do what is needed to save Ms Y's life. This may be a hard decision due to the sympathies staff may feel for Ms Y's plight. This sympathetic response should not restrain the therapeutic efforts needed to "rescue" Ms Y from harm. That she initiated the death-inducing event by ingesting pills distinguishes it from refusals of life-sustaining care. That she does not have a terminal illness also distinguishes it from morally less problematic (in some people's eyes) cases of assisted suicide. The fact she did this on her own without foreknowledge of friends and family suggests she made the decision to end her life in unsupported isolation. Perhaps she has had an under-treated depression or needs more social supports.

Rational suicide?

Can suicide ever be a rational choice? Perhaps, but it is not a choice to which one should quickly assent.

There is a long history, since Socrates and the Stoics, of viewing suicide as a noble and thoughtful gesture by an autonomous agent in the face of undignified circumstances. In the contemporary world, however, suicide could be seen as an acceptable rational choice in the very special medical circumstances of "assisted suicide." (Assisted suicide is discussed at further length in Chapter 11.) More morally troublesome are cases, like this one, where the main suffering is mental (albeit occasioned by extreme physical debility).

In the end there is only so much you can do for patients. As long as you make careful assessments of patients when they seem to be in despair and you have a good therapeutic relationship with them, you can only hope they will let you know when they need more help.

Professional's liability

In looking after and assessing their depressed patients, clinicians some-times worry about being held liable if they miss the seriousness of a patient's wish to die. In general, such fears have been unwarranted.[21] Where the courts have found a professional liable, the circumstances have usually involved a failure to follow appropriate clinical practice—such as neglect-ing to look over available medical records for evidence of past attempts at suicide or failing to re-examine a patient before discharge. Such rulings have also considered the harmful outcomes as "foreseeable," had the pro-fessional taken into consideration all the relevant factors (e.g., having a gun at home), This is clearly the crux of the matter, since predictions of patient suicide are far from certain. As long as healthcare professionals perform comprehensive and careful assessments of their patients, they are unlikely to be held liable if one of their patients succeeds in suicide.[22] Prognostic error, in this area of medicine as with other areas, is allowed so long as clinicians have exercised "due skill and care" in their assessments.

IV. In the Best Interests of Minors

The care of young children is another area where the best interests prin-ciple, shorn of some of its patient-preference-centred roots, comes to the fore as a guiding principle. Recommended treatment ought to reflect the course of action entailing the most benefit and the least harm to the juven-ile patient. Infants and very young children, of course, have no wishes that can direct care. Although slightly older children may also not be able to express *competent* wishes, they may have very strong *preferences* that should not be ignored. In the care of young children, as opposed to adult medicine, the striking difference is that healthcare professionals usually cannot have independent, if any, recourse to the young patient's wishes in deciding what to do. The child's parent (or guardian or trustee) usually makes the decision for the child.

In cases of conflict between a healthcare professional and the child's representative as to what is in a child's best interests, whose view should prevail? How should the young child's preferences regarding others' views about his or her best interests be taken into account?

What is seen to be in the juvenile patient's best interests can vary depending on the perspective of the beholder. The interests of a minor would seem to be inextricable from those of the family—it may be hard to determine what the child wants or even needs except through the filtering lens of the parents. Parents have important cultural, religious, and ethnic beliefs and customs that may influence how they and their offspring view the various medical options.

Parents, for example, may refuse what seems to be the best medical therapy for their child. Is this acceptable? The brief answer to this question is yes—but only under certain conditions.

Discretionary therapy

Medical therapy is discretionary if it is not required to save a child's life or prevent serious injury or disability. Parents can take the physician's recommendation under advisement. (An example would be whether or not to take antibiotics for an ear infection.) Even if we think parents' choices for their children are poor, we do not usually interfere. For example, we allow parents to enroll their children in hockey leagues or other contact sports, even though we know that every year some children are seriously injured in this type of sport. Refusal by parents of "ordinary care," such as childhood immunization, is allowed in many jurisdictions, if the refusal is an "informed" one. (While parents may refuse vaccination, this decision may have an impact on the child's eligibility for school.) Clinicians should make attempts to educate parents and voice their professional opinion as to what they think is in the child's interests (such as being immunized). However, only if parental refusal of best treatment seriously imperils the child is there legal authority to intervene. Child welfare authorities may also be called in for assistance in situations of lesser gravity—poor parenting skills—to help parents cope with the responsibility of raising children.

Necessary treatment

Where medical therapy will, on best medical evidence, prevent death or serious injury to the child, the parental power to refuse treatment is reduced. In Canada, the United Kingdom, and the United States, legislation obliges parents to provide their children with the necessities of life. If parents, whether by design or through neglect, mistreat their children,[23] the children can be removed by the child welfare authorities so that the needed treatment can be given.[24,25] Where the situation is a true emergency, healthcare professionals should not wait for formal judicial approval before instituting emergency care.[26]

Children cannot be martyrs

The limits to parental authority were at issue in 1923 in a leading US case, *Prince v. Massachusetts*. In that case, a Jehovah's Witness was charged with violating child-labour laws in allowing her nine-year-old niece to sell religious pamphlets on the street. The court held that the rights of parenthood are limited by the state's authority to act in the interest of children:

> The right to practice religion freely does not include liberty to expose the community or the child to communicable disease or the latter to ill health or death . . . Parents may be free to become martyrs themselves. But it does not follow that they are free . . . to make martyrs of their children before they have reached the age of full and legal discretion when they can make that choice for themselves.[27]

This much cited decision serves as the basis for limiting the right of parents to refuse treatment for their children. Thus, while adult Jehovah's Witnesses may refuse necessary blood transfusions for themselves, they may not do so for their children. In January 1995, the Supreme Court of Canada unanimously upheld the judgments of lower courts that a Jehovah's Witness couple had no right to refuse a blood transfusion for their infant (see Box 7.4).

BOX 7.4

"A parent may not deny a child—even for religious reasons—medical treatment judged necessary by a medical professional and for which there exists no legitimate alternative."[28]

Where parents refuse therapy—typically, life-saving—statutes and legal precedent exist to allow the authorities to apprehend the child and provide the treatment. (In some cases, the child is not physically removed from the parent's custody; rather consent for needed treatment is given by a temporary court-appointed guardian.) Criminal charges may also be laid if necessary. For example, in the United States, Christian

Science parents who have allowed their children to die of treatable diseases by foregoing medical care in favour of prayer have been charged with manslaughter, felony, child endangerment, and reckless endangerment.[29] A well-known Canadian case raising this entire issue in a more complex way was the Stephen Dawson case.

The Dawson case: parents not free to expose child to risk of permanent injury

Stephen Dawson was a seven-year-old boy, severely mentally and physically handicapped as a result of infantile meningitis. At the age of five months, a shunt had been inserted to drain off excess cerebrospinal fluid. The child was blind, partly deaf, and incontinent and could not feed himself, walk, stand, or talk. He suffered seizures and, to his parents, seemed to be in pain. When his shunt became blocked, his parents refused consent for remedial surgery on the grounds it would be better to allow Stephen to die than to prolong a life of suffering. The child was apprehended by the child welfare society and the British Columbia Supreme Court authorized the surgery.[30]

The court accepted medical evidence that life was not so gloomy for the child, that he was happy despite his handicaps. It did not believe that Stephen would be better off dead: "This would mean regarding the life of the handicapped child as not only less valuable than the life of a normal child, but so much less valuable that it is not worth preserving."[31] Troubled by the seemingly "imponderable" quality of life issue, the court was also worried that without surgery an even worse fate might await the child. Without the shunt he might continue to live but with more pain and disability. In allowing the surgery the court followed the UK judicial principle "not to risk the incurring of damage to children which it cannot repair."[32]

Even on the best odds, mandated therapy may not guarantee success. While parents "are not obliged to provide the best and most modern medical care for a child, they must provide a recognized treatment that is available."[33] A treatment less likely to succeed and requiring more suffering on the child's part may be seen as within the parent's discretion to refuse.

Experimental treatment not mandatory

In 1989, the parents of a seven-month-old child with biliary atresia refused authorization for liver transplantation. At that time, of the children who received this treatment, 65 per cent lived at least five years.

Representatives of Saskatchewan's Ministry of Social Services sought legal authorization for the treatment on the grounds that not doing the surgery might constitute child abuse.

However, at trial, a majority of the doctors who testified defended the rejection of surgery as a reasonable option because of its long-term uncertain outcome and the burdens it would impose upon the child. (With improvements in transplantation care, such refusal might be less acceptable today as the chances of survival are so much better.[34]) Although recognizing that it might save the child's life, the provincial court judge refused to order transplantation, agreeing that the parents' refusal was "completely within the bounds of current medical practice." He believed the parents' rejection of treatment was not a rejection "of the values society expects of thoughtful caring parents" but based on their concern for the child's best interests.[35]

There is thus some discretion allowed in deciding when parents' rejection of treatment is inappropriate.[36] Refusal by parents of life-saving care is clearly not an option, unless defensible by a "reasonable body" of medical opinion. In general, where the treatment is complicated, the "right" (or best possible) decision should be made consensually by parents and healthcare providers and should take into account not only technical factors but also the practical, psychological, and emotional aspects of the situation. In particular, close attention must be paid to the child's informational and emotional maturity and independence. The closer the child is to adult capabilities in these regards, the closer the decision taken ought to cleave to the child's preferences (see Chapter 2 on autonomy).

Child abuse and neglect

CASE 7.7 FASTING UNTO DEATH

A nine-year-old child was placed on a 40-day fast for chronic otitis media by her grandmother, who was her caregiver. A child protection agency worker found the child severely emaciated, crying, and vomiting. The agency asked a general practitioner to attend the child. He did so with some delay, diagnosed the child only as mildly dehydrated, and failed to consult a specialist despite the worries of the child protection worker. The latter did subsequently call in a pediatrician, who hospitalized the child, assessing this as a clear case of child abuse. Unfortunately, the child died of meningitis. The general practitioner was found guilty of professional misconduct for failing to attend properly to the child.[37]

By contrast with the previously discussed difficult decisions—made with the child's best interests at heart—child neglect or abuse means not looking after the basic needs of children and directly harming them or putting them in danger of readily avoidable grave harm. The health-care professional's moral and professional responsibility in *suspected* cases of neglect and abuse is to notify the child welfare authorities. (See Chapter 3 on confidentiality for further discussion of mandatory reporting.)

DISCUSSION OF CASE 7.7

The general practitioner was lucky not to be suspended, since his failure to protect this child was implicated in her death. The requirements of beneficence entail clinician responsibility to take some measures to help protect those patients under their care, such as children, who are vulnerable and dependent.[38]

This is not to suggest that parents are held to be solely responsible when bad things happen to young children. The ability to care for and look after the interests of young children is culturally and environmentally dependent. Canadian courts, for example, have been instructed to take into account, when it comes to Aboriginal defendants facing trial, the ongoing impact of "the history of colonialism, displacement, and residential schools."[39]

Judicial notice of such matters has had an impact on the legal resolution of cases of serious child neglect—even negligence leading to death.[40] There is no sacrifice of legal principle behind these cases ("it is unlawful to allow avoidable harm to come to a child under your care"), but there is also a recognition that what one does or is able to do has a great deal to do with local factors ("case-specific information") which need to be elucidated for justice to be done.[41] (See Chapter 9 on the meanings of "justice.")

V. Parental Requests for Treatment

What about the opposite situation: may parents *choose* whatever therapy they wish for their dependent children? The answer is, in general, yes, but only if the therapy is medically appropriate and consistent with the best interests principle. The leading Canadian legal case suggesting limits to parental choice was *E (Mrs) v. Eve*. As Eve's mental age was that of a very young child, it would seem the ethical principles behind this decision would be applicable to the care of young children generally.

CASE 7.8 *E (MRS) VERSUS EVE*

Eve was a 24-year-old mentally handicapped woman with a communication problem, looked after by her parents, but quite capable of interacting socially with others. The parents, who felt that she (and they) would not be able to cope with a pregnancy, requested she be sterilized for contraceptive purposes. Eve was considered by the courts too handicapped to give consent and unable to express her wishes regarding sterilization. The Supreme Court of Canada believed the parents were requesting the sterilization for the convenience of themselves and not for the benefit of the patient. The court ruled in 1986 that sterilization could never be authorized for such non-therapeutic purposes. The parents' request for sterilization was refused.[42]

Was this an appropriate decision?

DISCUSSION OF CASE 7.8

This is clearly a difficult case. Lacking at trial was any medical evidence that the effect of pregnancy on Eve would be so bad as to justify preventative sterilization. There was also insufficient evidence of no other less intrusive method than surgical sterilization for preventing conception. However, the court's ruling that surgery was not in Eve's best interests, and therefore not therapeutic, seems a narrow one. While there may have been no strictly physiological benefits to this patient from sterilization, there could have been social and psychological benefits to her. From a wider psychological perspective, it is possible that she indeed could not have coped with a pregnancy.[43] As a result of the *Eve* decision, the courts require that sterilization—indeed any medical procedure—may be done on persons incapable of consenting only for clear, medically approved reasons.[44] Hailed by some as a victory for disabled persons, it may be a hollow victory due to its restricted consideration of the needs of Eve as a whole person. The needs of a disabled person and their fulfillment may depend on the attention of others, something that might be diverted were, for example, pregnancy to intervene.[45]

Disability and a child's best interests

In cases of elective medical intervention for children, the courts require clear evidence that the procedure is necessary for preserving the dependent child's life or safeguarding his or her health. Non-therapeutic interventions, especially ones that are irreversible and pose some risk of harm, should not be carried out on children (or other dependents) merely because the parents authorize them (see Box 7.5).

BOX 7.5

The litmus test for childhood intervention: is this intervention in the child's best interests?

Thus, parental consent is insufficient justification to carry out a medical procedure on a child. Just how far to extend the *Eve* decision is unclear. Is sterilization in the severely mentally disabled ever an option? (Probably, if all other methods fail and there is proper oversight.[46]) Is circumcision of the male permissible? (Certainly it is—the risks are small, it is an important ritual for various religious traditions, and it is defended on medical grounds by a substantial section of the medical community.) What about bone marrow donation by one sibling to another? (Probably it is—if the best-interests standard takes psychological benefit to the sibling without illness into account.) Cosmetic surgery for a child with Down's syndrome? (Suspect—is it of direct benefit to the child or to the parents? How do we weigh the importance to the child of looking like others?) What about cochlear implants for a deaf child who can sign? (Dubious—if the child does not wish it and seems happy and well-adjusted to Deaf culture.[47]) Enrolling a child in a research trial? (Sometimes acceptable—see Chapter 12.)

CASE 7.9 THE PILLOW ANGEL

A six-year-old girl has a severe and untreatable neurological disorder that has left her profoundly impaired, with the mental life and physical abilities of a three-month-old child. She is looked after by her parents at home. They inquire as to the possibility of ceasing their child's physical maturation—specifically, they would like her bone growth halted and her sexual maturation prevented by surgery to avoid menstruation and pregnancy. They argue she will never benefit from or understand her sexual development and that a smaller size will make her easier to care for (a "pillow angel") and less likely to develop pressure sores and feeding problems and require institutionalization. Keeping her small would make looking after her easier and more comfortable for all.[48]

Is the parents' request for such treatment of their child a legitimate one?

DISCUSSION OF CASE 7.9

This real-life case elicited a storm of public controversy. Is it in this child's "best interests" to be kept small and immature so others can look after her more easily? On the other hand, if her parents' request were to be allowed, what are the short-term risks from the surgery and the long-term risks of medications needed to stunt her growth?

For many, the basic issue is that this child would be undergoing invasive treatment for her parents' convenience. It also suggests that the lives of the disabled are tolerated only if they conform to the needs and tolerances of the fully abled. The proposed solution seems a modern version of Procrustes' "one-size-fits-all" bed in ancient Greek mythology. Welcoming strangers into his home, Procrustes offered them food and lodging. Once on the special bed, however, the poor stranger was tortured: he was stretched if too short or, if too long, he had his legs chopped off. The message to the disabled would seem to be "you're welcome to stay but only on condition that you are easy to look after and not overly demanding."

This case is less a condemnation of the child's parents than a sad commentary as to how little support society provides for children with "special needs" and their families.

That said, these parents did an incredible job looking after an irreversibly seriously disabled child—a task emotionally, physically, and financially burdensome, which many would shun. She *would* be much better off at home, cared and loved for, than in an institution. Here is where an ethics of caring might take precedence over an ethics of "rights"; one infringes on the right to be free of intrusive interventions, the other champions the right of families to care for their dependents in realistic ways.[49]

Which do you think is better? Is it realistic to think society will accept and accommodate all persons no matter how severe their conditions are? If you were a parent with a severely disabled child, what would you be prepared to do?

Complex calculations: beyond simple best interests

Because the answers in all these situations are not entirely clear, physicians need to think carefully about parents' requests for interventions before complying with or refusing them. In complex cases, such as transplantation from one sibling to another, it is important to consider the less easily weighed factors, such as emotional benefit and family impact, in determining a child's best interests.[50]

Resist the clearly harmful

It should go without saying that one should never comply with a parental request for therapy that promises clear harm and no benefit to a child. Such is the case with all forms of female circumcision,[51] which is mutilating, always harmful, not medically justifiable, and certainly illegal under North American and European child abuse laws.[52]

In other cases of questionable—but less clearly harmful—requests for therapy, the wise healthcare professional will discuss with the parents the reasons for their requests, rather than dismissing them out of hand. It would also be important to include the child's views, if possible. It is professionally prudent and respectful of parental authority (and also respectful of the child) to try to understand their perspectives and attempt to negotiate a mutually acceptable solution. This may involve looking at other options—less hazardous and more readily correctable ones first—that will try to meet the needs and concerns of all involved. Particularly contentious disputes can be helpfully addressed by mediation and multidisciplinary teams designed to examine the ethical, legal, and medical facets of the problem.

The problem of determining what is in the child's best interests is not unique to medicine: the courts must make such determinations in child custody disputes. The wishes of the parents and child, the quality of the relationship between the child and the parents and any significant others, the child's special needs and developmental requirements are some of the factors that must be taken into account. Assessors on behalf of the court and mediators are encouraged to avoid confrontation and seek "convergent validity" by assessing the child and parents separately and together and include other perspectives as well—such as the child's teachers, other relatives, and the child's primary healthcare providers.[53]

Conclusion

Beneficence and non-maleficence are key principles informing medical care today. Relevant to all healthcare professionals, they speak to the expectations the public has of healthcare and the codes of conduct by which health professionals measure their own performance and those of their peers. In emergencies or where patients lack alternatives for care, however, there may be an evolving duty to attend even if one is not a casualty officer. Unfortunately, despite our best efforts, some patients are harmed by what we do to them. The next chapter will cover some evolving issues of healthcare professionalism: medical error and what it means to be a healthcare professional.

Cases For Discussion

CASE 1: COME BACK LATER

Mr A visits his family doctor for a persistent cough and weight loss. This is a rare foray, his last visit to the clinic being 15 years ago. He is now 71 years old and somewhat of a recluse, living alone in a small apartment, venturing out only to buy a few food items. To his family doctor he seems unwell and unkempt; blood tests and a chest X-ray are ordered.

Mr A looks like a startled deer in the headlights. "You don't think it's anything serious, do you, Doc?" he asks. His family doctor responds there could well be a problem and encourages him to get the tests done. Instead, Mr A goes straight home. He phones his doctor the next week, however, saying he feels no better. He agrees to return for the tests but never does so.

His family physician decides to make a house call. "Mr A, how are you? May I come in?" he asks through a closed door. Mr A refuses to open his apartment door. "Not now," he says, "I'll come to your office when I'm feeling better."

Questions For Discussion

1. What factors should the GP consider in deciding whether or not to agree to Mr A's request to be left alone?
2. Would it be permissible to breach his confidentiality by speaking to his neighbours or his superintendent about him?

CASE 2: A TERROR TO BE WITH

You are receiving psychological training and have an internship with the military. Unfortunately, a recent terrorist attack has set the country on edge and a number of suspects have been rounded up for "harsh interrogation." Your mentor is a psychologist in good standing, holding memberships in both the American and the Canadian Psychological Associations. She tells you that, while some members might see "harsh interrogation" as torture, she views the role of psychologist as a protector of the best interests of the detainees. "Our role," she says, "Is to make sure the military men don't go too far in their interrogation techniques." Beneficence is the principle adhered to and "without us as monitors," she continues, "the detainees would suffer more."

Questions For Discussion

1. Is this an appropriate use of the principle of beneficence?
2. Are there any circumstances where acting in this role could be defensible?

Conduct Becoming
Medical Professionalism and Managing Error

In all dealings with patients, the interest and advantage of their health should alone influence the physician's conduct towards them.

Robert Saundby, 1907[1]

There are less than optimal situations—gaps between "ought" and "is," between expectation and experience—of which a healthcare professional must be cognizant. Ethics can help provide the tools and rules to recognize and bridge these gaps. This chapter will address two connected areas, what it means to be a professional and how professionals ought to respond to error in healthcare, that should be high on the agendas of every professional and every healthcare institution and association.

I. Professionalism in Healthcare

It may seem somehow anachronistic to write about professionalism at a time of seeming "post-professionalism."[2] Expertise seems to be only a click away on the Internet. Knowledge, of course, is a necessary component of being a professional but attitude and judgment are as important, if not more crucial. A constellation of knowledge, skills, and attitudes establishes the core competencies of any healthcare professional.[3] But professionalism can be eclipsed by all sorts of distractions, from the obvious—such as the lure of money and fame—to the merely pedestrian—such as family issues and personal likes and dislikes. Buoyed by the appropriate aptitudes, trustworthy professionals, even if under siege, are like those unsinkable bath toys for kids—push them under the water as hard as you like, they always bounce back up.

CASE 8.1 AN UNEXPECTED DEATH

Ms R is a 19-year-old young woman, admitted to an urban hospital for routine gallbladder surgery. Her discharge is delayed as her bowels are sluggish and her incision hurts more than she expected. On Friday, three days after surgery, although still in some discomfort,

Ms R begs to be discharged home, a two-hour drive away, not wanting to spend the weekend in hospital. Her surgeon authorizes the discharge despite not having seen her or her parents that day. Busy all day in the OR, she reasons the nurses would have alerted her to any concerns. Ms R is advised to go to her local hospital if she develops any troubles.

On the drive home with her parents, Ms R suddenly feels short of breath. Once home, overcome by fatigue, feeling quite ill, she retires to her bed. Several hours later, she collapses. Her parents call 911 but Ms R cannot be revived.

Distraught and overwhelmed with grief, her parents call the surgeon. "If she was so sick," they angrily exclaim, "How could you have let her go home?"

How should the surgeon respond?

DISCUSSION OF CASE 8.1

There really is no ethical dilemma here. If the choice is between open communication and secretiveness, there is no ethical quandary. An unexpected death, such as this, so close to discharge, should be treated as a kind of "ethical emergency." The surgeon (and hospital representatives) should offer to see the family as soon as feasible and answer whatever questions they may have as well as they can.

Complete transparency, honesty, empathy, and avoidance of any sense of defensiveness are critical for discussions with the grieving parents. The surgeon and other staff also need to be appropriately self-aware: what can be learned from this event? What are the critical things that could have been done differently? Ought Ms R have been re-evaluated and who should have done this prior to discharge?

FOLLOW-UP OF CASE 8.1

As it turns out, autopsy results later reveal Ms R died from "DIC" (disseminated intravascular coagulation), a syndrome characterized by multiple blood clots, extensive bleeding, shock, and cardio-pulmonary failure. Usually acute and unpredictable, DIC carries a high mortality, even for hospitalized patients. The abnormalities in clotting might, or might not, have been revealed prior to her discharge if blood work had been done. Her surgeon might, or might not, have recognized her condition if she had been examined before discharge. Thus, even with the best efforts, Ms R's death might not have been foreseen or preventable. But this is not the message the family needs to hear. What they need to hear is something like this: "We (myself, the team, the hospital) are truly sorry for your loss and understand your anger and grief. We can only imagine how hard this must be for you. We will meet with you until we get answers that satisfy us all. We will review all our procedures and practices to see what we could have done better and what we can do to prevent such events in the future. Please accept our sincerest apologies and regrets for this terrible outcome."

Timely heartfelt expressions of regret and sorrow, being taken seriously—followed by appropriate corrective action—are what families often need.

Professionalism versus "doing your job"

While hard to define, almost anyone who has been a patient recognizes what is a professional attitude and what is not. Compare the surgeon who says, "The care your relative received in hospital was entirely appropriate, and what happened after her discharge is none of my concern" to one who empathizes with the family and admits the death must have been connected to the hospitalization. Compare the clinician who begins her interview with a patient by saying, "We have only 10 minutes today and so can only deal with one concern" to one who unhurriedly converses with a cancer patient by asking, "Tell me how things have been for you lately. Did anything occur that you weren't expecting?"

Something important is lacking in the attitude of some practitioners. They seem uninterested in truly understanding their patients. They will do their job, work the requisite hours, meet minimal standards for competence—the "legal" requirements for their position. But true professionals go beyond the minimum to ensure that patients receive what they are due. The professional is someone who cares about what is done and how it is done and responds to patients in ways that are reasonable, mindful, and achievable by ordinary mortals. He or she has an aptitude to focus in on the unique needs of a patient in situations where another would be distracted and stray.[4]

Professional manners

Among other things, it is the attitude to shortfalls in care that distinguishes the professional from the unprofessional provider. There is more to being a professional than knowing rules, precedents, and duties. As Peabody said, "The secret of caring is caring about the patient."[5] This requires attitudes such as civility, tolerance, patience, competence, and accountability. Professionalism is ultimately quite simple: it means recognizing and putting the interests of patients first and foremost. It is a virtue as it can be recommended to others.

Politeness and kindness are attitudes that reveal one's professionalism. Rudeness and just plain bad manners—not respecting a patient's privacy, leaving a patient in distress, failing to apologize for lateness, behavioural outbursts such as screaming at staff or patients, not saying please or thank you, not listening, not returning messages, neglecting to provide explanations to patients for clinical manoeuvers—can lead to patient disappointment and may prompt complaints to the regulatory authorities.[6] In one study a clue to malpractice actions was the failure of the surgeon to convey to patients, in the tone of his or her voice, his or her concern regarding the patient.[7] Firmly shaking hands is preferred by most patients and a sign of mutual respect in many cultures.[8] Other expected behaviours include making the patient feel prioritized by sitting at the patient's bedside, making eye contact, talking with a friendly smile or appropriate gravitas—all ways to lessen the patient–professional distance in an age of technology and anomie.

CASE 8.2 BELLY UP

You are on call one weekend with a resident, covering several wards of adult Internal Medicine patients. It is busy and both you and she have been up for much of the night admitting patients from the backed-up ER. It is now Saturday morning and time to round on all the admitted patients. The resident turns up a half-hour late, dressed in an outfit that includes a short top revealing her lower torso and her bejewelled navel. As you round on the patients, most of them fix their eyes on the resident's exposed belly.

Should you say anything to the resident?

DISCUSSION OF CASE 8.2

Other than address the issue of lateness (which may indicate a lack of full concern for others), many people would not say anything to the resident about her attire. After all, we live in a diverse and modern society and people should be allowed to dress in any way they see fit. Others would argue that, as professionals, we should be concerned about the impact of what we say or how we behave upon our patients. In this case an argument could be made that the resident's attire is distracting and interfering with the work that has to be done. As the attending staff, you should say something—tactfully explore with the resident whether she is aware of the impact her clothing has upon others and whether something a little more modest might be better suited to the clinical setting. Empirical studies suggest that the style of dress of clinicians is important in establishing confidence and trust. Studies from the UK,[9] the USA,[10] Hawai'i,[11] and Korea[12] have all shown a preference of patients for doctors to wear white coats. More professional dress such as semi-formal clothes under the white coat were also preferred in all but the Hawai'i study.

It's a simple matter, but also a matter of professionalism, to dress in a way that shows respect for patients and that encourages respect from the patient for the professional.

Respect for self and colleagues

Respect for patients must also include respect for oneself and one's colleagues. Perfection is something we often expect and look for in others. It's hard to come by as mistakes can be made by anyone, even in the best of circumstances.

CASE 8.3 TIME AND WOUNDS

Mr V is an active 62-year-old married man who has developed exertional dyspnea. His daughter, Dr W, herself a cardiology resident, arranges an urgent consultation for him at her teaching hospital. Her father's exercise stress test is abnormal, suggesting ischemic heart disease. Coronary angiogram demonstrates an occluded right coronary artery as well as significant blockages in his left main coronary artery. The date of surgical intervention is delayed so the patient can donate two units of his own blood. Alarmed by her father's high-risk finding, Dr W's intuition tells her, "This is ominous, he needs urgent surgical assessment." "He should have urgent surgery, shouldn't he?" the daughter anxiously inquires of her mentor, a well-respected cardiologist. "No hurry," is the response, "It can be arranged electively." Despite her mentor's reassuring words, she is still worried but doesn't feel she should try, or even has the power or experience, to push her father to the head of the line for surgery.

Three weeks into the waiting and six days before surgery, Mr V has a cardiac arrest and dies. The daughter is stricken with grief and guilt.[13]

Ethically, is there a problem here?

Medicine is not a predictable enterprise. Patients with trivial symptoms can turn out to have horrible diseases. Some, seemingly hale and hearty, die suddenly for inexplicable reasons. Others despite multiple morbidities surprise us with their resilience. Trainees need mentors to teach them how to parse the difference. Wrong prognostications, being unable to trust one's intuitions, a temporary loss of focus can overwhelm the unprepared, who can respond by harsh self-criticism or disappearing into silence and despair. They can develop wounds that time never heals—especially if the patient is your parent, spouse, or child.

DISCUSSION OF CASE 8.3

In this case Mr V's care was "hurried up" by his daughter who, worried, had him seen in the best hospital by the best specialist. She would, no doubt, feel some responsibility for her father's untimely demise—"If *only* I had intervened more, if only I had trusted my intuition." But she did do all she could—she opened doors until she came up against the wall of reassuring experience. But experience can be wrong and intuition right.

Some might think that Mr V's doctor daughter was unfairly "gaming the system" but who could argue against seeking, if you can *and any way you can*, urgent care for your loved ones? Anyone in the position of the daughter, loving her father as she did, would and should have acted as she did *without* hesitation. As the late English philosopher, Bernard Williams, would famously claim, to think otherwise is to have "one thought too many."[14] Favouritism, in defense of one's family (at least to some reasonable degree), is no vice.[15]

A new charter

In response to the concern that modern medicine was in danger of losing its moral mooring, a "new professionalism" initiative was launched in 2002 by various internal medicine societies for physicians. The American Board of Internal Medicine (ABIM), American College of Physicians–American Society of Internal Medicine (ACP-ASIM), and the European Federation of Internal Medicine (EFIM) adopted the "Medical Professionalism in the New Millennium: A Physician Charter." This charter is based on the three principles underpinning the practice of medicine, namely, the primacy of patient welfare, patient autonomy, and "social justice." The charter is intended to "promote an action agenda for the profession of medicine that is universal in scope and purpose."[16]

The charter's principles could, quite frankly, apply to any of the healthcare professions. According to the charter, physician obligations include a series of commitments (see Box 8.1).

BOX 8.1

Medical professionals shall exhibit or strive for the following:

- professional competence;
- honesty with patients;
- patient confidentiality;
- maintaining appropriate relations with patients;
- improving quality of care;
- improving access to care;
- a just distribution of finite resources;
- scientific knowledge;
- maintaining trust by managing conflicts of interest; and
- professional responsibilities, such as regulating members and setting standards.

There has been remarkable uptake of the Charter in the 10 years since it was introduced.[17] Its themes and principles are ones this book has tried to iterate. Not all the Charter's themes—avoidance of conflicts of interest, honesty, or aiding in the just distribution of care—are easy to achieve. Conflicts of interest are common, complete honesty is rarely achieved, and some argue clinicians have no special social duties. Professionalism in healthcare is a work in progress.

The crux

Medicine's ability to help and to heal requires an atmosphere of trust, something the courts remind us time and again. In a case that came to court, the judge wrote that "the essence of a fiduciary relationship . . . is that one party exercises power on behalf of another and pledges . . . to act in the best interests of the other." This is the crux of professionalism and of ethics in medicine. The judge continued that the clinician owes his or her patient: "loyalty, good faith, and avoidance of conflict of duty and self-interest."[18]

It is said that Hippocrates refused to attend to the sick of the Persian Empire—at that time at war with Greece—despite being offered a considerable recompense by the Persian emperor. One can take this as a tale with a favourable moral: a clinician ought not be swayed to treat patients by the lure of money alone. This is not to say healthcare professionals should not receive adequate or even generous payment for what they do, but only that it should not be—cannot be—their sole motivation. (This raises interesting questions about the relation between virtue and doing right: can one be considered to have done the right thing if one acts out of self-interest? Is self-interest always an unethical motive?) On a less generous interpretation, Hippocrates refused to treat patients in need because of a morally irrelevant reason—they were not Greek citizens. While a country's citizens are not duty-bound to help those of another country, even on the battlefield the modern army medic tends to the wounds of enemy soldiers as well as those of his or her own country's combatants.[19] This is true professionalism—it is not money or nationality that should motivate clinicians but the needs of the wounded before them.[20] In the professional's unbiased eyes all those who are suffering are humans, equally deserving of care. (See Chapter 9 on justice.)

Nowadays, it is not emperors and regal potentates who seek to influence healthcare professionals but private industry and large pharmaceutical companies. It is "Pharmageddon" time, as one author has chillingly described it.[21]

II. Professionals and the Drug Industry

CASE 8.4 SUPPING WITH THE DEVIL

You are a clinician with an older clientele. You have a particular interest in hypertension and are willing to try new drugs in your patients with resistant hypertension. One such drug, Syperia, is released following a large international drug trial showing it to be at least as safe and as effective as the leading drugs in this area. The pharmaceutical representative from the new drug's manufacturer offers you an opportunity to take part in a Phase 4 research trial. (This is a drug trial undertaken after a drug has been approved for use.) For every patient you enrol, you will receive $100 per year and an extra $100 at the study's completion. All you have to do is make a switch to Syperia and assess the patient's response to treatment every three months.

Is there anything of concern with your participation in this research?

DISCUSSION OF CASE 8.4

Your eyebrows should at least be raised. Is this true research or just veiled marketing? This type of "study" is purported to assess the effectiveness of such a drug in "real-life" patients. But it is often a not so subtle attempt to influence practitioner prescribing patterns,[22] a practice that has attracted widespread condemnation.[23] This is sometimes called a "seeding" trial whose main purpose is not knowledge but marketing on the part of pharmaceutical companies. If in taking part in a trial you recommend a patient switch to this new drug, are you doing so for the patients' interests or for your own? Even if you convince yourself you are prescribing the drug for the patient's benefit, many people would not see it that way. Notice it is not the amount of money that is at issue but the perceived lack of independent judgment—"a conflict of interest"—that triggers concern.

Clinicians can avoid (or at least ameliorate) conflicts of interests by: [24]

- disclosing their recompense to their patients;
- ensuring patients understand the research component to what they are doing;
- ensuring that patients and their families appreciate what the research entails;
- accepting only reasonable compensation for work actually done and avoiding gifts from private industry; and
- carrying out only bona fide research that
  - has been vetted by a trustworthy research ethics review board; and
  - passes the credibility test: will it contribute more to the fund of usable knowledge or more to your wallet?

The above "study" of a drug that is equivalent to current alternatives (i.e., no-better-than-but-probably-more-expensive-than) may not pass these criteria; however, if the new drug might be more effective or cheaper than the alternatives, better tolerated by some patients, or have fewer side effects, then one could try it. But why accept payment for what you would be doing anyway?

You can "sup with the devil," to paraphrase an old saying, "but use a long spoon."[25] Concerns about health professionals' relationships with private industry have led to formal strategies to make the spoon longer and the meal a more open table. In the US, the Pews Prescription Project aims to improve physician prescribing patterns and reduce undue pharmaceutical influence by supporting legislation curbing inappropriate relationships with private industry.[26] For example, included in the to-be-enacted in 2014 US *Patient Protection and Affordable Care Act* (PPACA) is a provision (the Physician Payments Sunshine Act) that requires drug and medical device companies to report payments worth more than $10 to any physician or other prescribers and make this public on the Web. This includes stock options, research grants, knickknacks, consulting fees, and travel to and from medical conferences.[27]

This kind of legislation is encouraged by the public's perception that prescribers are "on the take" from the drug industry. Indeed, literally tens of billions of dollars are spent yearly by the drug companies on physician-directed gifts, ads, and various other promotional efforts to influence their prescribing patterns.[28] The upside is that such influence may encourage the early adoption of beneficial drugs. The downside is that prescribers may prematurely turn to unproven or expensive drugs. A further downside is that it can be seen to eclipse the independent judgment of health-care professionals, a bad outcome for all.

Similarly, in Canada, the Canadian Medical Association has supported guidelines for physicians' relations with private industry.[29] The drug industry has been obliged to adapt to these guidelines, which strictly limit the kinds of events that can be supported by the private sector. Nowadays every speaker or writer must disclose their relations with pharmaceutical companies. Conferences must be organized for independent educational reasons. Gone are the fancy dinners and private holidays. Whether these regulations will reduce "Big Pharma's" influence is anyone's guess. They do help reduce the advantages of money and largesse of the pharmaceutical industry and may help increase the weight of evidence and appropriate prescribing by clinicians.

CASE 8.5 DRUG REDUX

You decide to join the Phase 4 Syperia® trial, confident you are immune to any untoward influence of the study on your practice. There are many alternatives for refractory hypertension but the new drug's apparent lack of side effects and once-daily dosing may make it a valuable alternative in your "resistant" patients. You see the rep from the pharmaceutical company before your clinic, accept drug samples for use with your patients, decline the $100 offer but agree to attend an educational dinner at a pleasant restaurant with a speaker on resistant hypertension, sponsored by the same company.

Are you doing anything unprofessional here?

DISCUSSION OF CASE 8.5

Many doctors routinely see drug representatives—many think they get useful, if biased, educational information from them, many like having samples to use with their patients, and many would attend a drug dinner sponsored by a reputable company. Such educational sessions are rarely simply advertisements for new drugs—speakers have their independence and attendees are not stupid. On the other hand, maybe we are kidding ourselves. Studies have shown time and again that clinicians and trainees who accept certain relations with industry are more likely to use their drugs.[30] The drug companies aren't stupid either.

You should periodically monitor your drug prescribing patterns to ensure their true independence from the industry. Comparing your prescribing habits with the recommendations in evidence-based guidelines will help ensure your integrity and also lessen your reliance on industry for your education. Forming a reading group with other prescribers is another check on perceived drug company influence.

Conflicts of interest

Conflicts of interest occur when the clinician's primary commitment (doing what is best for the patient) takes a back seat to the interests of the clinician or of some third party (such as the state, a pharmaceutical company, or the hospital). This can threaten to overwhelm (or be seen to overwhelm) the health professional–patient relationship.[31] For example, what if a physician sends a patient for blood work to a laboratory located in the same facility in which she works? (This should be fine, assuming the physician receives no financial kickbacks, such as nice gifts or reduced overhead, from the facility). What if a clinician sends patients to the pharmacy in his building in exchange for reduced rent? (This is unethical as there is a clear financial conflict). What if a physician sells exorbitantly expensive unproven drugs to desperately ill patients? (A no-brainer. Go straight to jail or the discipline committee of the regulatory authorities if caught.[32])

The determination of appropriate boundaries with third parties such as the drug industry is an important aspect of the New Charter for professionalism mentioned above. Just as important is the setting of appropriate boundaries with patients.

III. Boundaries and Crossings

How far can one go and must one go in helping a patient? Can a practitioner do too much? The answer is yes: clinicians can indeed go too far in trying to aid and "rescue" patients. (Consider Case 7.3 for a benign example of this.) The next case from Newfoundland received much publicity.

CASE 8.6 A BOUNDARY TOO FAR

A 33-year-old physician, Dr T, was in a Newfoundland jail awaiting extradition for the murder of her ex-boyfriend in the US. Apparently estranged from her family, she had no one to put up the $60,000 for her bail set by the Newfoundland and Labrador court. In desperation, she called her psychiatrist, pleading with him to help her. Concerned about her mood, he cancelled a half-day of patients to attend her bail hearing and provided the surety for the bail.[33] Dr T was released from jail and later would drown her infant son and commit suicide.

Was the doctor's action a breach of professionalism?

Serving patients

The professional relationship suffers and patients can be harmed where safe therapeutic boundaries are not recognized and respected. Among other things, professionals run the risk of treating some patients differently from other patients—either favouring them as "special" patients or shunning them if things turn out badly. Patients, in turn, may either develop inappropriate expectations of help from the clinician or, if things go badly, become mistrustful of all healthcare professionals.[34]

Crossings and violations

Transgressions of such boundaries fall into two categories: violations and crossings.[35] "Crossings" are minor infractions of a boundary. These are deviations from expected professional behaviours, such as accepting tokens of appreciation from patients or attending a social function held by a patient. (Is attempting to get urgent care for a loved one—as in Case 8.3—just such a crossing? If so, it is an understandable one.) "Violations" are more serious boundary transgressions, whether by intent or by the deed itself, that compromise the professional encounter, such as having sexual relations with a patient. A violation undermines the patient-centred, "best interests" therapeutic nature of the clinician–patient encounter and replaces it with a situation where the healthcare professional's needs displace those of the patient. Some of these occurrences may be attempts to be helpful to patients. These situations may speak more to the clinician's personal need to be the "rescuer" than the patient's need to be rescued.

Gifts from patients to professionals

Boundary violations go beyond the sexual to include other forms of personal and inappropriate infringements on the therapeutic relationship. Excessive gift receiving by healthcare practitioners can encroach upon the appropriate distance between clinician and patient. Gifts of a small nature are usually acceptable so long as they remain simply totemic representations of the therapeutic encounter; small gifts can be, for example, respectful and courteous "thank you's" from patients and not necessarily intrinsically wrong.[36] However, even seemingly trivial gifts, if driven by the wrong motives, may degrade the professional relationship and undermine the quality of care provided.[37]

Gifts from professionals to patients

> ### BOX 8.2
>
> "Physicians might feel compelled to give money to a patient because, fundamentally, physicians are compassionate and empathic professionals who care for and about their patients."[38]

What about "gift giving" *by* healthcare professionals *to* patients? The existing literature deals with transactions such as giving patients bus fare to go home or providing them with the money to buy needed drugs they cannot afford. While frowned upon, giving money to or doing favours for patients is nowhere considered unethical *per se* by regulatory authorities. (Providing patients with free samples of needed drugs is usually considered a good thing.) What about more significant gifts donated by a clinician to his or her patient?

DISCUSSION OF CASE 8.6

Unfortunately, fate is unkind to many patients, dealing them blows of ill fortune and harm. It is not usually the job of healthcare providers to assist patients in avoiding all the harms and stressors that non-medical ill fortune—from stock-market crashes to job losses—hands them. Healthcare practitioners may help patients cope with the outcomes or impact of such events on their lives but they do not, in general, seek to intervene in the private lives of their patients to prevent such bad events from occurring.

The psychiatrist's action in providing surety for Dr T's bail went far beyond what is reasonable or expected professional behaviour. He was either naïve or extremely misguided about this patient. In any case the psychiatrist's action was a serious and unprofessional boundary violation.

Other observers might see the psychiatrist's actions as entirely understandable. His motivation seemed therapeutic and not obviously self-serving. At worst he may have been motivated by an overwhelming desire to rescue Dr T—a mistake in judgment, for sure, but not a crime deserving of punishment.[39] That he sought no supporting peer opinion as to what he was doing suggests he acted impulsively and thought little about the implications of his actions. (Of course, one can say the judge seriously erred in even allowing Dr T bail.) Psychiatrists, in particular, must be careful not to allow their boundaries to become blurred: to go too far in trying to rescue a patient undermines the requisite therapeutic space needed for patient independence and healing to take place.[40]

When faced with an unusual or inappropriate request from a patient, the astute clinician should ask for the opinion of others, such as his or her peers, professional insurers or professional and regulatory authorities. This advice can help ensure that one's actions do not go beyond the normal clinical interventions used by professionals. Unusual or personal favours for patients can have pernicious results for the therapeutic encounter and can damage the reputation of medicine generally.

Bottom line: clinicians must exercise prudent judgments of proportionality in doing the right thing. The further removed an action is from the profession's approved practice (the standard of practice of your peers), the more careful one's reasoning regarding it must be.

Sexual impropriety

While many clinicians may be uncomfortable overseeing their peers, there are some cases in which we must be our brethren's keeper. This is especially so for serious infractions such as sexual impropriety with patients.

CASE 8.7 AN UNCOMFORTABLE REVELATION

You are a primary care clinician seeing a new patient, Ms G, for a medical reason. In taking her history, you ask about her most recent medical care. She tells you she has been without a primary care practitioner for some time. She states she did not feel comfortable seeing her former doctor as he had made, on more than one occasion, sexually explicit remarks to her, even asking her out on a "date." Ms G has not told anyone else of this. As she tells you her story, you realize that you, too, have feelings for her—not just compassion for her tribulations, but feelings of attraction towards her.

What should you do?

A variety of interpersonal encounters and transactions between healthcare practitioners and patients have been traditionally disallowed or frowned upon, with the regulatory colleges of the various groups of healthcare practitioners setting out guidelines most clearly around sexual contact with patients.

As far back as Hippocrates, sexual relationships between healers and patients have been forbidden. Since then, any sexual involvement with a patient has been considered a misuse of the healthcare professional's power and prestige: "it is the doctor's breach of fiduciary trust, not the patient's consent, which is the central issue regarding sexual misconduct."[41]

This is why sexualization of a current professional relationship between patient and healthcare practitioner is everywhere considered inappropriate. Although there is some leeway with respect to former patients for general practitioners and the like (usually a year or two after the last clinical encounter), psychotherapists in particular must adhere to more rigid prohibitions. Sexual relations with former as well as current patients are forbidden indefinitely in most, if not all, codes of ethics for health professionals engaged in psychotherapy[42] (see Box 8.3).

BOX 8.3

Sexual abuse includes sexual intercourse with a patient, sexually touching a patient, and "behaviour or remarks of a sexual nature."[43]

DISCUSSION OF CASE 8.7

Sexual abuse of patients is an egregious misuse of a health professional's authority and a breach of the rule that health professionals must act only in the patient's interests (see Chapter 6 on Beneficence). The Canadian Medical Association advises physicians to take "every reasonable step to ensure that such behaviour is reported to the appropriate authorities."[44] In Ontario any member of a regulated healthcare profession must report if he or she has "reasonable grounds, obtained in the course of practising the profession, to believe that another member of the same or a different college has sexually abused a patient" and the professional knows the name of that member.[45] Failure to report could itself be considered professional misconduct.

In this case, knowing what to do about Ms G's previous practitioner is easy. If her allegations are true, his interactions with her clearly constitute sexual misconduct. You should do as the CMA suggests to its members. It is preferable that allegations be submitted with Ms G's consent. However, if she prefers not to register a complaint, you may lodge the complaint with the regulatory College of the purported offender without naming her.

The harder part is what to do about your *own* nascent feelings of attraction to the patient.[46] True, it is only the first visit and perhaps the feelings will wane with time. However, if you are not extremely careful and do not deal with your feelings, you may get yourself into trouble. You may consider transferring this patient's care to another physician. That said, all clinicians at some time develop feelings of affection (or disaffection) for their patients.[47] Rather than dismissing them all from your practice,[48] it would be preferable to acknowledge your feelings of like and dislike for your patients and try to "work through" them. Working through means exploring your feelings (How do you present yourself? Why do you think you are attracted to the patient?) and discussing them with your colleagues, with a counsellor, or in a suitable context such as a Balint group.

The new professionalism suggests we must be vigilant when it comes to clinical failings of our colleagues and, indeed, of ourselves. We have a collective responsibility to ensure the well-being of our patients and, to some degree, the public at large. Medicine in being more powerful is now also more dangerous, itself frequently the cause of patient harm. As a healthcare professional you will make your share of mistakes—it is the way in which you manage them that will test your true commitment to professionalism.

IV. The Error of Our Ways

CASE 8.8 "I'M JUST SO TIRED!" A MISSED RESULT

You are a busy family practitioner in independent practice. You are seeing Ms L, a 45-year-old corporate lawyer with two children, who complains of fatigue of several months' duration. She reports working very long hours preparing for a case and has been additionally stressed as her assistant is on maternity leave. She admits she is not eating properly nor getting enough sleep. You both agree she should strive for more balance in her life. Just to rule out other causes of fatigue, you send her that day for some basic blood tests, telling her your office will call her only if the results are abnormal. Otherwise, Ms L should come back to see you in three months.

When she returns for her follow-up visit as scheduled, you look over her chart just before entering the examining room. To your horror, you see that her blood work indicated a significant reduction in her platelet, red and white blood cell counts compatible with aplastic anemia. You have absolutely no recollection of ever having looked at the report. "Doctor, I'm still feeling really exhausted even though I'm getting enough sleep and the court case has been settled," Ms L says as you sit down.

What should you say or do?

Error, adverse events, and negligence

An error in healthcare may be broadly defined as any outcome or process that you would have preferred not to have occurred—as when one says afterwards, "Oh, that was a mistake." Errors are not always harmful—they may be interrupted before affecting anyone. For example, writing the wrong dose on a prescription may be an error but not cause the patient harm if the pharmacist catches the mistake before the patient receives the medication. Errors also usually entail some moral responsibility because one could have done otherwise—acted "better" or "differently"—in the circumstances. (If you couldn't or wouldn't, reasonably, have done differently, then there is no "mistake," only an unfortunate event.) By contrast, adverse events are incidents caused by a medical intervention that are harmful to patients or that threaten to harm (set back the interests of) patients. About one-third to half of adverse events are considered preventable and so can be designated as errors. (An adverse event would be a rash following the first-time administration of penicillin to a patient; it would be an error if the same outcome took place due to an inadvertent second-time use of penicillin in the same patient.[49])

BOX 8.4

Negligence requires:

- a duty of care;
- a breach of the standard of care;
- an injury to the patient; and
- that the injury must have been caused by the breach.

"Negligent events" refer to that smaller class of events that cause harm, are preventable, and would not have been made by a careful clinician in the circumstances in question. Perfection is not the standard of care; "reasonableness" is if the "standard of care" has been followed.[50] For example, a practitioner may make a mistake in diagnosis despite having done everything correctly up to that moment. If a mistake could be made by a reasonably careful and knowledgeable practitioner acting in a similar situation, then the mistake may not be deemed negligent in a court of law (see Box 8.5).[51]

BOX 8.5

"the standard of care which the law requires is not insurance against accidental slips. It is such a degree of care as a normally skilful member of the profession may reasonably be expected to exercise in the actual circumstances of the case in question. It is not every slip or mistake which imports negligence . . ."[52]

The scope of the problem of medical error and adverse outcomes is huge. Studies done in Canada, Australia, the UK, and the US reveal very similar adverse event and error rates.[53] Overall, preventable adverse incidents are connected with the deaths of about 1 in 200 patients admitted to hospitals. This astonishing number has been disputed, but the studies are very consistent. Whatever the exact number, adverse events in medicine are acknowledged by all to be a serious quality of care issue for healthcare. They were the subject of a major and influential US report released in 1999.[54] Research since then has shown remarkable improvements in care in some areas—surgical error,[55] acute myocardial infarction care,[56] reduction in healthcare-related infections[57]—but there remains a long ways to go.[58]

Honesty about error

Medicine is perilous and difficult. "Life is short, the art is long, judgment uncertain and experiment perilous," so wrote Hippocrates or one of his followers 2000 years ago. All clinicians can have bad days and even the best make mistakes. But what is the proper professional attitude when an error or adverse event transpires? When such bad things happen to our patients, the automatic human response is often to be defensive and embarrassed about them.[59] Professionals involved in medical mishaps must learn to tame such automatic responses and try to be open and honest about such events. Many arguments for open disclosure of unwanted outcomes have been recognized: public expectations, legal requirements, philosophical reasons, respect for patients, public trust, psychological reasons, and system improvement reasons.

Public expectations

There are few "laws" *per se* that require healthcare professionals to be honest with patients.[60] This is changing. The cases of medical harm particularly prompting patient and public ire are often those events where no one has assumed responsibility—especially if patients have been similarly harmed in the past. A perception of a "cover-up" by the professionals and institutions involved is a frequent addendum to the concerns about an unwanted outcome.[61]

The failure of professionals to be thoroughly honest about such harms or hazardous situations is a violation of professionalism, considered to be deserving of sanction. For example, damages of $20,000 were awarded in a 1999 British Columbia case in which a surgeon left an abdominal roll in the patient's abdomen. During the more than two months' delay in telling the patient, he took active steps to cover up the mistake (for example, telling the nurses not to make any written record of it). The court described the surgeon's delay in informing his patient and his deliberate attempts to cover up his mistake as demonstrating "bad faith and unprofessional behaviour deserving of punishment."[62]

Patients and families who pursue legal action are often motivated by a need for explanation and accountability and a concern for the standards of care.[63] Thus, it can be helpful to provide patients and/or their families with a full explanation of "unexpected events," even if "minor."[64] Informing patients and families promptly and honestly about harmful incidents fosters a healthier and more realistic understanding of medical care and may prevent anger.

Unfortunately, not all clinicians agree: one third of US doctors surveyed in a 2012 study did not completely agree with disclosing serious medical errors to patients.[65] More comforting is another 2012 study, this time of *medical trainees,* which showed that interns now, as compared with 10 years ago, are more open about their errors and appreciated, among other things, that honesty in regards to error is the best path.[66] Thus, habits of professionalism may be a generational issue: the new cohort of health-care practitioners may, as a result of the ongoing revolution in healthcare pedagogy, be more inclined to act in professional ways.

DISCUSSION OF CASE 8.8

You must be honest with Ms L about the missed lab report and what the abnormal results likely mean. You should tell her what you know about pancytopenia, its causes and management. Even if she fails to ask, you should tell her of last year's missed report. A lawsuit might result but, quite frankly, this should be the furthest thing from your mind. Your mind should be turned to "how can I ensure this patient gets the best care possible without further delays?" Ms L needs to understand that part of the urgency stems from the missed lab reports. It is doubly bad to compound the original mistake by attempting to conceal it. If the patient is not told and finds out later, this might result in anger over a perceived cover-up.

Reducing risk of lawsuits

Certain "facilitative" communication styles by health professionals can be protective against suits and complaints, no matter what the patient outcomes ("Do my recommendations make sense to you?" "Do you have any other concerns we haven't addressed today?" "Has anything about your illness or the treatment to date been a surprise for you?").[67] Studies suggest full disclosure of error and adverse events may reduce a clinician's malpractice relative risk by about one third (absolute risk reduction, 8 per cent).[68] Overall, legal advice sought by patients or their families in the US was more likely if an incident was not disclosed and/or had a serious impact on the patient.

While disclosure may be no guarantee against suits and complaints, honesty can reduce the punitive "sting" that sometimes accompanies judgments against clinicians. Kraman and colleagues reported on the experience in an American Veterans Administration hospital that routinely informs patients and their families of any harmful incident and then offers them help in filing legal claims for compensation.[69] This "pro-active" policy of disclosure did lead to a net increase in the number of claims made against the hospital but many more were local, out-of-court settlements. As a result, this hospital had the eighth lowest total monetary payouts out of comparable VA hospitals. Similarly, the University of Michigan Health System combined disclosure with an offer of compensation without increasing its total claims and liability costs.[70]

Disclosure therapeutic

Although honesty may be the best policy, some clinicians are still reluctant to adopt it, sometimes out of fear of legal consequences, but also because of shame and the typically high standards of perfection they set for themselves. Secrecy is counterproductive as it impedes learning from critical events and can leave clinicians who participated in the poor outcomes with a never-ending negative emotional burden of guilt and shame.[71] Case reports by clinicians remind us of the tremendous psychological strain "healers" undergo when they appear to harm the patients they serve.[72] Clinicians and trainees need to be supported as they, too, suffer when patients are harmed and when others find out.[73] Disclosure of the event can sometimes be therapeutic for clinicians and prevent the corrosive effects of duplicity on one's self-esteem as a healthcare professional.[74] On the other hand, it can be frightening for clinicians as they can feel exposed and defenceless.

When to disclose

When should a clinician disclose error or medical harm? Disclosure is a proportionate duty taking into account the preferences of patients and families, the clinical circumstances of the patient, and the nature and gravity of the incident:

- The greater the impact or harm an adverse event has or may have upon a patient, the greater is the obligation to disclose the event to the patient and/or the family.
- By corollary, "non-significant events" do not require disclosure. However, just what "significant" means may depend on individual or subjective factors that need to be taken into account by clinicians when deciding whether they ought to disclose an unanticipated outcome to the patient.
- When in doubt, it is better for clinicians and institutions to err on the side of disclosure than non-disclosure.

As a general rule, acknowledgment and discussion of an unexpected serious event should be undertaken by a trusted clinician known to the patient/family. This should take place as soon as possible after the incident has been identified and when the patient is able to understand it.

BACK TO CASE 8.8

You take a deep breath and begin to explain what happened with the lab report from three months ago.[75]

How should you make this disclosure to the patient?

How to disclose error

Establishing rapport with the patient is the first step. Express sympathy: "I am sorry to see that you are still feeling so tired." Don't beat around the bush and don't wait for her to ask. Instead say, "I have something difficult to tell you: the abnormalities were also there the last time we did blood work on you."

- Once rapport has been established, provide information and offer, "Would it be helpful for me to explain what I think happened . . . ?"
- Avoid being defensive.
- Provide a narrative account.
- Avoid placing blame on yourself or others (see Box 8.6).
- Don't speculate: if you don't know, find out. "Here's what I know now . . ."
- Empathize with/normalize the patient's feelings. Use reflective listening: "I know this must be hard for you . . ."
- Apologize for the event and be accountable for your part in its occurrence, its satisfactory management and prevention.

BOX 8.6

Using the following language has been, in the past, cautioned against and should still be avoided when discussing "error" as it simplifies what is usually a complex event.

- "I dropped the ball . . ."
- "I sure made a mess out of things today."
- "Yes, I know it is not your fault . . . it is all my own."
- "I made a mistake and now you will have to have surgery."
- "The events are entirely my own fault . . ."[76]

Although honest apologies may be protective against lawsuits, it is helpful to know many jurisdictions have passed "Apology acts" that do not make the offering of an apology an admission of liability. *The Uniform Apology*

Act in Canada also excludes, as an admission of liability, a healthcare practitioner's admission of *fault or responsibility* for an untoward outcome.

BOX 8.7

Favoured Canadian Apology Act:
"An apology made by or on behalf of a person in connection with any matter,

(a) does not, in law, constitute an express or implied admission of fault or liability by the person in connection with that matter [. . .]
(c) shall not be taken into account in any determination of fault or liability in connection with that matter."[77]

Cause and accountability

The aetiologies of error and adverse events in healthcare are manifold and well-explored elsewhere in many books and journals.[78] Suffice it to say that there are typically systemic and individual factors involved. An example of a "persons" issue is a nurse who, through fatigue or inattention, inadvertently causes the death of a patient in giving IV KCl, instead of IV NaCl. The systems issue would be the hospital stocking lookalike medications, one lethal and the other not, in the same location. The systems issue facilitated or allowed the nurse to make the error; the error was occasioned by the nurse's fallibility. As we are human, no matter how good we are as clinicians, we will make mistakes, sometimes with grievous consequences. We need safer systems that plan for human fallibility and that can encourage learning.[79]

For example, as in Case 8.8, a common error is the "missed result." Sometimes clinicians say such mistakes—resulting in omissions of appropriate timely treatment—occur because they are "too busy" to follow up on all the tests they order. The courts have not been kind to such arguments.

A lapse in care

Dr V, a hospital-based obstetrician-gynecologist, did a Pap smear on Ms B in May 1992. The patient was not informed that pre-cancerous cells were found. Not until 11 months later, when diagnosed with an advanced form of cervical cancer, did she receive treatment. Ms B died of the disease one and a half years later. Her estate sued Dr V for negligence.[80] Evidence was presented at trial that Dr V had left the country for an extended period shortly after doing the Pap smear. The hospital closed the clinic in which he worked without making any arrangements to handle his reports. As a result, Ms B's Pap smear report remained unseen by a clinician until almost a year later.

The original trial judge was tough. The "standard of care" for following up on an abnormal test result as in this case, he opined, did not involve "medical skill or expertise." Thus, this could not be a case of "error of judgment . . . Having an appropriate system in place fell within the ambit of his (Dr V's) personal professional responsibility." The judge found no direct hospital liability, ruling the failure was all Dr V's.

The higher Appeals Court thought this standard was "too high" in requiring the doctor to "ensure" such a system was in place. Instead, the standard should be "a duty upon the physician to see to it that there is a reasonably effective "follow-up system in place" as well as "a responsibility on hospitals to see to it that adequate procedures are in place to 'ensure' (but not guarantee) patient safety." "Where a patient in a hospital is treated by more than one specialty, the hospital owes a duty to ensure that proper coordination occurs and that the treatment program it offers operates as a unified and cohesive whole." The court found liability to be shared by Dr V and the hospital.

I think the Appeals Court got it right. No one would defend missing an abnormal Pap smear for a year as an acceptable error, one that a reasonable physician could make. It could not be disputed that the delay in diagnosis contributed to the patient's demise. The only open question was, who should bear liability? The physician could and should have arranged coverage for his patients.[81] The hospital also had a responsibility to its patients, so a shared liability seems appropriate.

Anonymity and co-operation

What Balint called the "collusion of anonymity" is all too often the core problem. When different healthcare professionals are involved in the care of a patient, it is easy for the patient's care to fall between the cracks and for no one clinician to feel responsible.[82] In modern healthcare, where multiple specialties and professions are almost always involved in patient care, the failure to provide coordinated leadership can have serious repercussions for the patient. The responsibility for patient welfare also does not end if one claims to be only indirectly involved in the care of a patient.[83] If ancillary professionals have some information bearing on the patient's well-being, there is an evolving duty to see that this information is received and acted upon. For example, when significantly new and unexpected findings are seen on an X-ray, issuing a timely and accurate report may be insufficient: liability may accrue for radiologists who do not ensure that the findings are acted upon.

> Where there is an unexpected finding which may affect patient management or where the severity of the condition is greater than expected, it is the responsibility of the radiologist to communicate this information to the clinical team either by direct discussion or other means.[84]

If this is so, why not other professions or specialties as well: pathologists (who detect cancerous cells in a specimen) or physiotherapists (who detect a weak leg in a person still driving)? The interdisciplinary requirements regarding healthcare, insofar as different professions are essential to the comprehensive care of patients, are growing. To meet these needs, the following recommendations for radiologists could apply to any healthcare professional.[85]

He or she

- must coordinate his or her efforts with those of other healthcare professionals involved in the care of the patient;
- must have a system in place whereby unusual, hazardous findings can be communicated to the patient and/or the treating team; and
- may have a duty to communicate directly with the patient if he or she is unable to contact the most responsible clinician in a timely way.

Large-scale adverse events

Medical errors have been recognized to affect whole classes of patients and can be particularly trying for healthcare professionals and their institutions. Large-scale adverse events are a series of related incidents or processes that increase the risk that multiple patients have been injured due to healthcare management. This has occurred, for example, due to faulty cleaning of investigative technologies, such as endoscopes or EEG leads, or due to contaminated drugs.[86] The increased risk was unanticipated by healthcare professionals, not recognized at the occurrence of the incident or process, and, even with best management at the time, may or may not have been preventable.[87] The level of risk to the population potentially affected is typically not known prior to the retrospective review, but usually more people are physically *not* affected than affected by the faulty materials.

One example: The Newfoundland Breast Hormone Assay Inquiry

In 2005 in Newfoundland, a patient with advanced metastatic breast cancer, not responsive to conventional treatment, whose hormone receptor test was initially negative, was retested and found to be positive. This was a critical harm to her as hormone receptor assays dictate the type of adjuvant treatment a breast cancer patient receives (estrogen-receptor positive women receive anti-estrogen therapy while estrogen-receptor negative patients usually do not). Retesting of 25 other hormone-receptor negative patients revealed that over half of the original tests had also "converted." Due to this unusually high conversion rate, anyone initially tested between May 1997 and August 2005 was contacted in order to be retested.

It was discovered that one third of those initially tested received incorrect results, with implications for their treatment disposition. The province's look-back confirmed that 108 of the patients who died were not receiving adequate treatment and that 383 of 1,013 patients did not receive the recommended treatment due to the incorrect test results. Fifty women, some of whom received mastectomies, were told they had advanced stages of breast cancer when they did not. External audits of the lab noted poor quality control, deficient procedures, and frequent turnover of pathologists.[88]

There should be no ethical dilemma in this case. Given the magnitude of the error and the tremendous implications for patients, there could be no defense of non-disclosure. But spokespersons for the Regional Health Authority initially appeared to be attempting to keep the findings out of the public eye. Why?—perhaps shock, perhaps uncertainty over its scope, perhaps concern over causing public panic. Unfortunately, this delay in disclosure meant many of those affected first found out about the incident through the public media.[89]

The bottom line: patients may worry if warned of possible harm by a faulty medical undertaking. However, people who have sued for the alleged psychological harms caused by such warnings have not found much support in the courts. Transparency is recognized as best practice and ought not to be punished.

Conclusion

Professionalism encompasses a broad scope of duties, attitudes, and behaviours by healthcare practitioners. Honesty, altruism, openness about medicine's limits and harms, and the importance of learning will all advance medicine. Professionalism is being reconsidered and remodelled in profound ways by the educational, regulatory, and credentialing institutions for healthcare. This renewal may help the professions maintain their patient-focused ethos in hard times.

Cases For Discussion

CASE 1: A MODERN-DAY ROBIN HOOD?

You are a healthcare practitioner working in a poor and medically underserviced area. You work long hours and have large bills to pay—alimony, children in private school, overhead on the office, mortgage on the house . . . it all adds up. But you worry more about the population you serve. Among your patients is a large group of destitute and frequently homeless men and women. With poor nutrition, minimal protection from the elements, and poor hygiene, they are sitting ducks for TB and protein and vitamin deficiency syndromes.

You feel a great deal of empathy for *les misérables*, the detritus of society. "Talk about the social determinates of disease . . ." you think to yourself as you gaze out into your crowded waiting room. "Surely, one important way I can help them is to improve their nutrition." You decide to use a regional food aid program and prescribe socially funded "special diets" for your destitute and weary patients. After all, you think, you will be helping the poor; you are really just being their social advocate.[90] Your receptionist greets you as you come in— you will see at least 50-60 patients today. She reminds you about the importance of fully billing for each and every patient you see.

Questions For Discussion

1. Is your programme ethically (as opposed to legally) defensible?
2. Why might your proposed advocacy program catch the eye of those responsible for the regional food program?
3. What changes to the program might make it acceptable?

CASE 2: THE "JULY EFFECT"

It is July and you have finally begun your internship. You are on a surgical rotation in Orthopedics and discovering it really is as demanding as you were warned. Up all night—doing a lot of scut work, but also loving the action in the OR and on the Trauma team. In a couple of days you've seen more pathology than you'd seen in all your undergraduate years. While expecting to be supervised closely, you are surprised by how much latitude you have—after just a few days on a ward where all the patients are new to you, you find yourself ordering drugs and doing procedures you'd only witnessed before.

Mr O is your next patient, a 65-year-old man admitted with a pneumothorax following a motor vehicle collision. The nurses tell you at 2 A.M. that his chest tube has fallen out and he needs it replaced—he's already getting breathless, they say. The chief resident is busy in the OR, and the attending is at home; your only compatriot is an inexperienced clinical clerk. You have done one previous chest tube insertion before under supervision and it didn't seem such a big deal. You confidently tell the nurses you can do it and ask them to get the room set up.

As you enter the room, Mr O eyes you warily, "You look pretty young," he exclaims, "I sure hope you know what you're doin'! It's July, isn't it?[91] I heard tell that's when the new fellas start and when real bad things can happen to patients. Are you one of them fellas?"

Questions For Discussion

1. How would you respond to Mr O? Are trainees obliged to disclose their inexperience to patients?
2. What about more experienced clinicians who are using a new drug or technique in their practice?

9

Beyond the Patient
Doing Justice to Justice

It was the best of times, it was the worst of times, it was the age of wisdom, it was the age of foolishness, it was the epoch of belief, it was the epoch of incredulity, it was the season of Light, it was the season of Darkness, it was the spring of hope, it was the winter of despair, we had everything before us, we had nothing before us . . .

Charles Dickens, 1859[1]

Justice is always rough around the edges.

Norman Daniels, 2008[2]

I. Justice in Everyday Medicine

It is certainly not the worst of times for medicine, but it is not the best either. It seems to be troubled times for medicine today—patients are generally doing better than ever but many are not happier for it—they are, in the words of one observer of medicine, "Doing better, feeling worse."[3] Healthcare professionals seem to share this malaise. The recent past seems to have been a time of optimism and unlimited potential, when any disease could be cured and price was no object. Now, things seem more complicated—diseases are more challenging and care is more complex, more expensive, less readily available, and can *itself* be the cause of significant medical injury. With the escalation of costs has come erosion in professional independence and questions about how, and if, decisions about limiting healthcare can be made without sacrificing the principle of patient autonomy as well as that of beneficence. Issues around cost and scarcity give rise to questions concerning fairness and allocation. Can patients expect to have every wish for care met no matter how "futile" treatment might be? In this chapter we will explore in greater detail the principle of justice and how it affects healthcare and healthcare practitioners.

Though often not consciously considered, questions of justice come into play every day in patient care.

CASE 9.1 TIME WELL SPENT?

You are the primary care provider for Ms J, a 92-year-old widow who visits you in the clinic monthly. Ms J's main complaints are fatigue and sadness connected with her experience of aging. Although she is not physically ill in any particular way, your main reason for seeing her is simply to listen to her concerns and be supportive. Although you cannot cure her sadness, the patient feels somewhat happier knowing someone is listening to her. After a number of appointments, you wonder whether the time spent with this patient is justified, given your many other patients who also need your time. Just yesterday you delayed seeing a patient with a seemingly more urgent medical problem rather than disappoint Ms J by postponing her appointment.

Should you keep seeing Ms J regularly?

Doing justice

The idea of justice is, like a diamond, multi-faceted and has many meanings, such as

- "retributive" or "punitive" justice—this determines the punishment to befit an action or an alleged crime;
- "restorative" or "reparative" justice—this repairs "the harms suffered by individual victims and by the community as a whole, promoting a sense of responsibility and an acknowledgment of the harm caused on the part of the offender, and attempting to rehabilitate or heal the offender . . . [by] restitution and reintegration into the community";[4]
- "compensatory" justice—this makes up for losses, such as in negligence cases where monetary damages are awarded as a way to compensate for or make good loss and suffering;
- "distributive" justice—this allocates goods or resources fairly;
- "procedural" justice—this follows "rules of fair play" or "principles of natural justice," such as the right to be heard or the right to be considered without prejudice.

I will focus on the features of justice that are captured in the definition from the *Oxford English Dictionary*:

to do justice to (a person or thing): to render (one) what is his due, or vindicate his just claims, to treat (one) fairly by acknowledging

his merits or the like, hence, To treat (a subject or thing) in a manner showing due appreciation, to deal with (it) as is right or fitting.[5]

This definition suggests that justice involves an individual having the
opportunity to access, and to receive, certain goods according to ways that
are "right" and "proportionate."

Practitioners' waiting rooms can be seen as testing grounds for various theories of justice. Should it be first come, first served? Or should
access to the clinician be prioritized by medical need? What exactly is
medical need and who determines it? Can more time be spent with one
patient, even if this means less time available for all other patients waiting
to be seen? Or should everyone get just 10 minutes and only one complaint per visit?

The principle of justice in medicine is intimately connected with
questions of what a patient fairly deserves to receive in a healthcare system
and what obligations clinicians have to ensure patients are treated fairly.
What the OED definition does not capture is the more morally contentious
notion that clinicians and patients must also be concerned about "the
system"—the wider set of medical and social resources that clinicians
need to access in order to help patients. But in the debate over fairness, which language will prevail: that of healing and succour or that of
efficiency and commerce?[6]

As Ms J's clinician, you do have a duty of care to her, but how far does
it extend? The patient can expect you, as her primary care clinician, to
spend the time with her that is proportionate to her medical needs. These
do not have to be physical—they can be her psychosocial needs as an aging
person. To attend to these is to show her respect as a person and is a necessary part of the effective medical care of a human being.

If Ms J benefits from these visits and your time is not so stretched that
questions of priorities arise, then you should continue seeing her. While
Ms J may consider your visits to be "chatting," you would also be careful
to assess depth of her sadness, the reasons for it, and what could be done
about it. The visits may also be necessary to help you decide what social
services or referrals are appropriate for her.

Determining what need is "more urgent" than hers is a clinical issue; if
Ms J is seriously depressed or suicidal, her need may be no less important
than another patient's. And her claim on the healthcare system is hardly
excessive. One could argue from a utilitarian perspective that a little
deontological caring (caring for her as a person) shown by her doctor may
help prevent more serious (and ultimately costly) illnesses.

More than money is at stake in debates over scarcity and justice in
medicine. Prioritizing some patients for treatment means, of course, "posteriorizing" others.[7]

Lessons from the field of battle

During war, resources are often scarce and rationing common: some people are denied resources that might help them. This is even more so on the field of battle. When not everyone can be saved, triage decisions must be made. The sickest are often treated "expectantly" (that is, left to die), while those most readily salvageable and able to be returned to combat are treated first.[8] While some might compare healthcare to modern warfare (the enemy being the country's debt or the "fiscal cliff"), it is *not* in one significant sense. Healthcare is not well organized. Even when extreme situations occur, those for whom treatment is simple, likely to work and have the biggest impact are *not* always prioritized for treatment. Sicker patients requiring more complex expensive care may still be prioritized despite their costs of care and best evidence suggesting treatment will not be effective. "Managed care" is designed to address this. But making providers into gatekeepers to the system (and reimbursed if they follow pre-designed care paths to provide economically "efficient" care) threatens to put clinicians on a collision course with patients.[9]

Awareness of the need to balance economic costs of care against the benefits of interventions is appropriate and should influence clinicians' obligations to their patients. The problem is that the clinician's single-minded focus on one patient's/family's wishes can lead to ignoring the larger context.[10] Compromises in care must be made; not everyone can get or needs the most expensive artificial hip, cheaper drugs are just as good for hypertension as the latest most expensive designer pills, generic drugs can be as effective as brand name ones. Avoiding futile, ineffective, or marginally effective, care—"wasteful care"—is one way, a less morally troublesome way, of coping with hard trade-offs in care.[11]

CASE 9.2 TO B12 OR NOT TO B12?

You have taken over the care of an independent and somewhat reclusive 83-year-old widow, Ms Q, whose family physician of many years has recently retired. She tells you she has received regular B12 injections since her husband died 10 years ago.

The chart indicates Ms Q does not have pernicious anemia, the only clear physiological rationale for B12 injections. Nonetheless, she asks these be continued because they have "kept me going all these years." She also requests a visiting nurse to give them to her at home because she is too old to get out much. You advise her that oral B12 might just be as good, but . . . this falls on deaf ears. "Oh, I couldn't do without the injections, Doctor. My old family doctor said I'd be on them for life."

> You decide to comply with her request and fill out a Home Care referral form. The next day the Home Care coordinator calls to ask how you can justify this service.
>
> *Is this a service to which Ms Q is entitled in a just system?*

II. Distributive Justice

Distributive justice renders onto others what they are "due" in the way of the distribution of social goods such as healthcare. There are ends (goods or rewards) that others should receive in ways that are "right" and "proportionate." Justice involves elements of autonomy (the right to be considered and heard without prejudice) and beneficence (the right to have one's needs met, not just "considered," depending on the available resources and what goods others are getting.) Distributive justice may be defined "minimally" as the absence of injustice and no discrimination. Alternatively, it may be defined "optimally." This requires giving a bigger boost to those who have less and are more needy, and so may entail a "reverse discrimination" in *favour* of the more deprived and historically disadvantaged.[12, 13] For example, while everyone with a foot problem should have the right to access a specialist, a young child from an impoverished area who lost a foot in a farming accident might be prioritized for treatment while Uncle Joe with a hammer toe might just have to wait a while.

A just system requires, as the most important twentieth-century political philosopher, John Rawls, has written, "a mutually recognized point of view from which citizens can adjudicate their claims . . . on their . . . institutions or against one another."[14] Rawls and his commentators argue that [15, 16]

(a) there are some "primary goods" (such as wealth, health, basic liberties, self-respect) to which all deserve the opportunity to access, so

(b) a just healthcare system must equitably distribute these goods and the opportunity to access them, and

(c) any inequalities of access or opportunities to access care are only acceptable if the most needy and the most disadvantaged also benefit. In the real world this means ongoing efforts to raise the care provided to those at the bottom of the healthcare ladder to equitable levels.

The Rawlsian view of justice is definitely "advantage reducing," as we have seen ethical theories tend to be (see the Introduction and Chapter 1). Too often, poverty, illness and disability are caused by, and in turn exacerbate, lack of opportunity to participate as fully as possible in the wider human community and deprivation more generally.

Rawls invites us to consider inventing a new society whereby "blinded observers" (who do not know where they themselves would end up) choose the kind of system they would prefer: would they prefer a system or a society where a small number of people are the recipients of the greatest amount of goods and rewards or one where resources are more evenly distributed? If rationally motivated, chances are they would choose the society with a more equitable distribution of goods. A society with a big gap between top and bottom and the majority of citizens at the bottom would increase the chance of their ending up on the wrong end of the distribution curve. Rawls' thought experiment is a test for how we are doing with "moralizing" ("advantage levelling") our societies. The less egalitarian a society, the further we are from a just system.

DISCUSSION OF CASE 9.2

The Home Care coordinator may not realize it, but she is asking a question of justice: are the resources the patient requests her due? Ms Q wishes her B12 by injection; with it she has remained remarkably well.

The B12 may have helped Ms Q because of an unrecognized vitamin deficiency or because of a placebo effect. Her use of B12, however, probably belongs to the good old days when clinicians provided a "tonic" to pick up a patient's energy. No doubt, evidence-based medicine would consider this a waste of resources. In addition, unless backed up by tests to show she cannot absorb B12 orally, its continued provision as a publicly funded healthcare service could be considered deceitful and fraudulent.

Nonetheless, it would seem reasonable or at least respectful to continue the B12—for now anyway, until you get to know her better. Then, perhaps, you can substitute your relationship with her for the B12. Balint pointed out that the strongest drug one can dispense is the drug, "doctor,"[17] but the idea can apply to any healthcare professional who tries to be with his or her patients.

III. Medically Necessary Treatment

The difficulty with achieving "optimal" justice for all—accessing the proper healthcare for all—is that resources are never infinite: individuals cannot always get what they want and trade-offs must always be made. Where and how might we fairly draw this line? More ethical healthcare systems, especially universal ones such as Canada's medicare system and the UK's National Health Service, should aim to provide all citizens equal access to (their fair share of) essential healthcare resources. Whether or not citizens have a right to *all* "necessary medical care" is another question—nowhere in Canadian law, for example, does it say to which medical care all citizens have a right. The right to access may simply mean the right to join a queue.

The *Canada Health Act* requires provision of those "services medically necessary for the purposes of maintaining health, preventing disease or treating an injury, illness or disability"; such care is "any medically required services rendered by medical practitioners." This is a very loose definition as it would cover whatever practitioners are willing to provide!

The concern that Canada's publically funded system would prevent some patients from getting what they need or want in a timely way led to a constitutional challenge to the prohibition of private insurance to cover public services. The issue, which came before the Supreme Court of Canada, centred around whether this prohibition was necessary to preserve the quality of healthcare and the equality of access to it.[18] The challenge to the prohibition was successful with the majority holding that allowing people to "buy" medical services would not threaten the system's quality while the minority argued that in so doing the *principle* of free and equal access to care would be undermined.[19] This judgment did not address the question as to which services are necessary and which are not and has yet to result in any seismic shifts in Canada's medicare system.

Necessity defined

Necessity is defined in the *Oxford Dictionary* as that which is indispensable or requisite for or to, that which must be done, a constraint or compulsion, that which is inevitable (a "necessary evil"), a thing without which life cannot be maintained ("the necessities of life") or would be unduly harsh.[20] These definitions are quite strong. It is not clear that many of the things we do in medicine are necessary in these senses.

CASE 9.3 "MISFORTUNE BEGETTING INJUSTICE"[21]

You are a practitioner who has recently joined a community health centre. One of the patients assigned to your multidisciplinary professional team is Ms D, a proud woman in her late 50s. She has had an unfortunate life, single-handedly raising her own three children and now caring for her daughter's two young children since her daughter's murder a year ago. As she hasn't been to the clinic for a while, you decide to visit her at home to get to know her.

Ms D lives in a poor neighborhood on a small disability pension, unable to work due to her multiple morbidities—disabling osteoarthritis, emphysema, adult-onset insulin-dependent diabetes, obesity, and congestive heart failure. She can't recall the name or exact profession of the last provider she saw in the community health centre but says "he seemed nice." "Life," she sighs, "hasn't turned out the way I thought it would."

In discussing her functional status, Ms D reveals she sometimes goes without insulin for a few days as she cannot get to her pharmacy easily. Even with a walker, she can negotiate only short distances. She cannot manage steps and so is confined to the front of her small house. She stopped taking the local subsidized accessible bus service when she thought she saw the driver smoking marijuana. Ms D is dependent on her two surviving children for transportation but is reluctant to bother them. She applied for an electric scooter but was turned down because the information submitted did not support its "medical necessity."[22]

Is there an ethical issue here and, if so, what are the responsibilities of her primary care provider?

DISCUSSION OF CASE 9.3

There are a number of ethical issues here but a primary one is that Ms D seems to be receiving less than her fair share of medical resources. Her poverty and social situation conspire against her receiving the aids—customized support services, an electric scooter—that would allow her greater freedom of action and improve her quality of life.

"[P]eople with disabilities are particularly susceptible to receiving substandard care,"[23] as are patients from lower socioeconomic strata—perhaps in the former case because of blinkered vision and a lack of skills on the part of healthcare providers and in the latter case, in part, due to the lack of continuity of care from one primary care provider.[24] (The clinic has had a great deal of turnover in staff and Ms D "fell between the cracks.") The burden of disability and disease carried by members of socially disadvantaged groups is closely linked to the deprivations they experience in society, creating a healthcare gradient "in striking conformity to a social gradient."[25]

This cycle of poverty, deprivation, ill-health, and injustice has so far been difficult to break but Ms D has something going for her: *you*. As the new practitioner at the clinic you can help her get what she fairly needs and deserves:

- an advocate (you and your team as a start), especially when it comes to ensuring she gets needed care (as do her grandchildren who are also at risk);
- continuity in healthcare providers, especially one primary care provider or one team, (you can be this professional, and avoid what Balint called the "collusion of anonymity"[26]);
- regular comprehensive care (suited to your multidisciplinary unit, regular home visits); and
- someone to address her inability to receive adequate supports: an expansion of "medically necessary" services to include "functional needs" (an ideal goal for your team).

One moral issue for the healthcare professional is, how obliged is he or she to pursue an amelioration of situations such as Ms D's? This will, no doubt, depend on who the healthcare practitioner is (Does he or she have the right skill set? Does the clinic have a holistic, patient-centred, chronic-disease management philosophy? Does it support and motivate the clinicians to go the "extra mile" or two for patients like Ms D?), and how tractable the social circumstances are. If there are no avenues of social support open in a very resource-limited society, there may not be much that anyone can do. On the other hand, a more resource-laden society may provide hidden assets that could be accessed by an imaginative healthcare team. This would seem to be a proportionate duty . . . the harder the effort required and the less "necessary" the resource is to the patient's sense of well-being, the less obligatory is the duty to help. Just where the line is to be drawn between obligatory professional duties of aid and rescue and "optional" or "exceptional," "saintly" tasks will depend on many local factors.[27] Recognizing what a patient needs and wants may be quite different than having access to it, but it is a first step in achieving it.

When resources are limited, clinicians may need to make extra efforts to ensure that access to such resources by their patients is fair or just. Of course, in hard times, clinicians, as with everyone else, must be concerned about the wise, prudent, and parsimonious access to and use of healthcare resources.[28] Addressing the needs of one's patients is important but must be done in a way mindful of the importance of conserving scarce resources.

Do not trade off due care

At a minimum, all patients are due access to beneficial treatment regardless of disability, ill health, age, race, gender, faith, culture, class, or sexual orientation.

Discrimination is an unjust distinction, whether intentional or not, that

- is based on grounds relating to personal characteristics of an individual or group; and
- imposes burdens, obligations, or disadvantages on such individuals or groups not imposed on others, or that withholds access to opportunities, benefits, and advantages available to other members of society.[29]

All patients deserve non-discriminatory care. Beyond that, in the way of positive benefits, patients deserve non-negligent care, care without which they will come to avoidable harm. The standard by which treatment is judged as warranted or appropriate is the "best interests of the patient," that is, the care that a reasonable professional would, under the circumstances, provide to the patient. Patients should expect to receive access to care that is proportionate to their needs (see Box 9.1).

BOX 9.1

Acceptable criteria for optimal resource allocation among patients include the following:[30]

- likelihood of benefit to the patient;
- expected improvement in the patient's quality of life;
- expected duration of benefit;
- urgency of the patient's condition;
- amount of resources needed for successful treatment; and
- availability of alternative treatments.

Unjust care

By contrast, inappropriate discrimination among and between patients was common and is still seen in medicine. There are many examples of apparent discrimination in medicine, but here are a few:

1. Age and racial bias were evident when dialysis machines were introduced in Seattle, Washington, in the late 1950s. Because these were expensive and in short supply, one of the first ever ethics committees—a "God squad"—was set up in 1962 to decide who should receive treatment.[31] Not surprisingly, those who were single, elderly, female, black, or poor were unlikely to be offered dialysis. This "odious practice," as one observer noted, did not end until 1972 when the US Congress passed a bill, Public Law 92-603, authorizing Medicare to pay for dialysis for all patients with end-stage renal disease.[32]
2. Age bias persisted in end-stage renal care. Until the mid-1990s, age limits were common for access to dialysis for end-stage

kidney disease.[33] In the United Kingdom, there was a dramatic drop-off in dialysis for patients over 55 years of age.[34] This started to change in the late 1990s with the realization by nephrologists that dialysis was a viable option in older individuals.[35] After that, to exclude the aged from dialysis would no longer be unfortunate, but unfair.

3. Gender bias seems present still in cardiac care. It has been claimed that "women with ischemic heart disease [receive] less than a fair deal."[36] For example, women presenting to the ER with acute coronary syndromes are less likely than men to be hospitalized or undergo coronary revascularization.[37]

4. Gender bias seems to occur in other areas as well. In a Canadian study of men and women presenting to physicians with equally arthritic knees, men were twice as likely as women to have surgery recommended.[38] The authors speculated unconscious biases against women might have been to blame.

These may all be examples of "Aristotelian" injustice: likes being treated as un-likes and the latter receiving less than what they are due.[39] Patients who are similar in "relevant" ways should be treated in a similar fashion. Thus, if two patients have the same burden of illness—be it depression, back pain, or arthritic knees—they should be treated in the same fashion, irrespective of gender, race, ethnicity, and so on—assuming of course that these other factors are irrelevant to the proper care and treatment of the patient. For example, the same principles of treatment should be used for any child with meningococcal meningitis, whether he or she lives in Toronto, Paris, or New Delhi. An injustice is done when a child so ill in New Delhi fails to receive the same treatment as a child similarly ill would get elsewhere.

Acceptable use of patient factors

The use of patient-specific factors is ethical and *not* discriminatory, however, when it reflects a *real* difference in patient populations. For example, it has been suggested that women with heart disease may be treated differently than men because their blood vessel physiology is "different." (I'd like to see the evidence for that, however.) It is also appropriate and, indeed, required when it accords with the patient's own wishes and values. For example, it would be acceptable to put limits on life-saving care such as dialysis for the elderly if the patients themselves choose to forego life-sustaining treatment. Indeed, when asked, the very old often do decline medical interventions, especially when accurately informed of the predictably less than positive outcomes.[40] As advanced age, on its own, nonetheless is *not* a predictive factor for a poor outcome in surgery,[41] there is a need to ensure older patients' refusals are informed ones if they choose to decline potentially helpful care (see Case 7.2).

Scarcity

Given the scarcity of resources, each individual patient may not receive what he or she "needs." In such cases, justice would require persons in need to at least have an equal *opportunity* to access that care. In creating a just health-care system, it can be a challenge to objectively evaluate need and harm—or at least in ways upon which we can mutually agree. In the optimistic view, difficult rationing decisions will be avoided by getting rid of inefficiencies and useless treatments. In the pessimistic view, even if this is achieved, there will still be insufficient resources to satisfy everyone. Pessimists compare the healthcare system to a balloon.[42] Squeeze it in one place and it simply expands in another. They believe hard rationing decisions are unavoidable and we will always have to deny some patients the treatment they may need.

Futility and justice

When hard choices of allocation must be made, the discussion about the ethics of funding care that does not "work" always arises. This should be uncontroversial, even trite. Why would anyone *offer*, let alone fund, care that cannot achieve its intended objectives? One explanation is there may be different interpretations of the goals of medicine. Futility may be to some degree in the mind of the beholder. There are also other resources in addition to healthcare, such as education, culture, national defense, which deserve funding. There must be a limit to what society can expend on healthcare and so, too, there must be limits *within* healthcare. We cannot do everything to rescue all persons from all harms, such as those who are permanently comatose or too ill to benefit. (The issue of a limit to rescuing patients is discussed again in Chapter 11.)

Just care

A just society has an ill-defined obligation to see that the healthcare needs of its citizens are met. Some, on account of illness or disability, will require more than others. This compensates those with disability and disadvantage and results in some levelling of the social playing field. Whether we become disadvantaged by birth, accident, or illness, medical care offers one oppor-tunity to surpass the "handicaps" we are handed. If equality of opportunity of access to effective care is not present, deprivation and absence of choice which often accompany illness and disability are "viewed as natural mis-fortunes," as if illness and its consequences were "just bad luck."[43] A fully moralized healthcare system would be a "*dis*advantage-reducing" system. It would ensure the opportunity to access healthcare resources is as balanced and equitable as possible. Some inequalities—of disease, of disability, of finances *within* countries—are more easily addressed. Others—such as national borders, geographic distance from a healthcare facility, genomic predisposition to diseases, situations of extreme deprivation—will require much more work to overcome.

A new system for medicine is immediately faced with difficult questions: how are we to make better, more just, decisions when the decision-making processes followed by national and regional administrators and government officials often remain hidden?[44] Using Rawls' words, what is missing is an open "system of cooperation between free and equal citizens" for making hard choices about medicine's present and future. This should not stop clinicians from trying to do better in their areas of work. There have been notable attempts at constructing just or fair systems of allocation in some areas of medicine. Below are two examples: vaccination and transplantation.

Vaccination

Vaccination against infectious diseases has been one of humanity's most successful medical advances.[45] Achieving universal vaccination has been an important principle of vaccine programs throughout the world. The permanent eradication of smallpox is the most impressive success of these programs. Dramatic reductions in the incidence of measles and diphtheria, for example, have been possible only on account of the widespread distribution of vaccines. By the same means, the eradication of polio throughout the world is now within reach.[46]

But pandemic infectious illnesses still occur with an unpredictable frequency. Often viral in origin, their spread may be prevented or ameliorated by timely vaccination. Decisions have to be made early on in the course of an outbreak, whether epidemic or pandemic, regarding who is to be vaccinated. In outbreaks of known disease, such as polio or a known respiratory viral illness, a substantial proportion of the population may already be vaccinated, the supply of vaccine adequate for the needs of the population, and no hard questions of justice are required. In novel and rapidly spreading infectious outbreaks, however, even if an effective vaccine is found, there may be an insufficient supply. In such situations, various authorities have proposed principles for access to vaccination.[47] It has been recommended that priority be given to:

- healthcare professionals who are essential to the pandemic response and/or who provide care for persons who are ill;
- those who maintain essential community services;

- all children; and
- those workers who are at greater risk of infection due to their job.

Notice the combination of utilitarian and deontological principles for allocating vaccines—first, to those essential to the vaccine's effective delivery (fundamental to vaccination programs); second, to children (respect for persons would seem to justify placing children on the priority list, having had less opportunity to experience their "fair innings" of life); and, third, to those at greater risk on account of their occupations (if we want professionals to work in dangerous jobs, we have to protect them). Further principles of distribution are not provided in this guidance document but presumably would aim for universal coverage starting with those populations at particular risk. For equally situated persons in each group, random allocation by lottery would best serve justice (as opposed to first come, first served, which would preference the swiftest).

Transplantation

Organ transplantation in North America is one medical service in which significant progress has been made around resolving the problem of distributing scarce medical resources fairly and efficiently. Impartial criteria have been established which include likely medical benefit, time on the waiting list, and urgency of need.[48] Patients are ranked according to a complicated computerized point system taking into account factors such as how close to death the patient is, how quickly the donor organ can get to the recipient, and how likely it is that the patient will survive the operation. This system purportedly does not allow for prejudice or favouritism.

CASE 9.4 TRANSPLANTATION TOURISM

A 45-year-old well-connected businessman, Mr C, has been on the waiting list for a kidney transplant for three years. He has survived on home peritoneal dialysis, but he is finding it increasingly burdensome and uncomfortable. He has no idea when, if ever, a kidney will become available for him. Mr C decides to look into buying a kidney from another country such as India. He asks for your opinion.

How would you respond?

Organ transplantation is special in being a closely monitored and relatively finite system within which there is a great deal of agreement about the purpose of treatment.[49] Even here there are moral problems: should an 70-year-old be lower on the waiting list than a 30-year-old?

Should the alcoholic patient with end-stage liver failure not be considered a candidate? Should we always give preference to those who might benefit the most, or is some consideration owed to those who are less likely to benefit?[50] Even seemingly impartial standards of benefit, such as HLA-matching criteria for organ transplantation (absolutely essential for transplantation success by making sure the donor and the recipient have tissue compatibility), can unexpectedly result in racial inequalities in access to transplantation.[51] Racial differences in transplantation rates may not be due, as was thought, to racial discrimination. Rather, it is the result of certain ethnic groups being less likely to give consent for donation, hence making HLA-matching less likely.

Asking the public what should be done is one way of addressing the issue of who should get the available organs. Interestingly, public opinion polls do not support the position that organs for transplant should always go to the most needy or the most ill—the public thinks even those less likely to benefit should be given a chance to benefit.[52] This might indicate the average citizen cannot imagine saying no to anyone or that they may overestimate the availability of organs. It might also mean that, at some level, there is a deontological barrier to allocating organs by utilitarian criteria, a belief that anyone in need deserves a "kick at the healthcare can," even if he or she is unlikely to be successful. This attempt to balance benefit against the "right to be considered" is interesting and may be the most ethically defensible path to take since it considers need, efficacy, and opportunity. It thus takes into account the three principles of ethics (beneficence, justice, and autonomy, respectively). It may also compensate for the tendency of some patients to exhibit entitlement and others to consider themselves less worthy when it comes to receiving an organ.

All this leaves aside the fundamental injustice of transplant medicine: while organ donation and transplantation can be "fairly" carried out within advanced countries, there is never enough supply, thereby encouraging patients to look outside their borders for organs. The massive inequality in wealth worldwide results in asymmetrical purchase of organs: the well-off buy from the destitute. Some argue that impoverished people in the underdeveloped world should have the opportunity to sell a kidney if this is the only way of saving their family from grinding poverty.[53] This is a strong argument, I think, but is the practice of buying and selling organs tolerated only because it takes place a long ways away in another country? Would we tolerate an internal market in organs? What is the experience of those who sell a kidney? Do they have a shorter life span? Does the money really get them out of impoverishment? (Iran is currently the only country in the world that does not have a supply problem of too few kidneys—it allows its citizens to sell and buy kidneys, resulting in many more people willing to sell one of their kidneys than there are buyers.[54])

DISCUSSION OF CASE 9.4

You might have personal feelings about "transplant tourism" but restrain yourself. At this juncture, it would not be helpful to engage Mr C in a discussion of its morality. Only those who have been so ill and kept waiting for years on a transplant list can appreciate how emotionally and physically draining it can be.

Your first response should be one of empathy—acknowledging how hard the wait has been for the patient and his family. You should not presume to understand how he feels; your discussion should try to elicit his concerns, what life has been like for him. Next, you could reflect back to him the dangers he might face in going overseas for an operation and how much safer it might be to bide his time at home. Finally, you should discuss why the wait is so long at home and what might be done to hurry it up—perhaps a call to a director of the program, to see how far down the list the patient is, would be helpful.

Gaming the system by using the man's connections of wealth to get him moved up the transplant ladder would not be appropriate. You would, of course, want to ensure all possible supports—psychosocial, peer-based—have been mobilized for him.

Impartiality as ideal

Faced with scarce resources, will we always distribute medical services according to need? How will we ensure that those slightly less needy get their due? What about patients with difficulty advocating for themselves— the impoverished, the homeless, the very young, those without families, those rendered incapable by illness or lack of comprehension? How will their needs be recognized?

Such problems are not, I think, insurmountable. The current schemes to distribute scarce resources such as organs are better than earlier versions that made no attempt at impartiality. While perfect impartiality may be ultimately unachievable (and perhaps, as suggested in Case 8.3, not always desirable), it can still serve as a regulatory ideal that can foster the development of ethical and fair guidelines for medical practice.

IV. The Role of Practice Guidelines

Research shows that a significant proportion—close to 50 per cent—of medical care is not appropriate, may not improve a population's health and may even detract from it.[55] This is an astonishing number. It should force us—as patients and providers alike—to take a sobering second look at the value of healthcare interventions. In 2010 the US Institute of Medicine estimated that 30 per cent of healthcare costs, more than $760 billion, is wasted per year[56] and, if eliminated, would not affect the quality of care.[57] It is often not the big ticket items—CTs, MRIs—but the little ticket items—the unnecessary blood tests and X-rays—that ratchet up the cost of care.[58] Determination of the net benefit of an intervention will depend upon its cost and its significance for patients and their families. To aid such decisions, it is helpful to know the increment in cost-effectiveness and health outcomes that one intervention or test makes over another (see Box 9.2).

BOX 9.2

Five questions to ask before ordering tests:[59]

1. Did the patient have this test before?
2. Will the test result change my care?
3. What are the chances and risks of a false-positive test?
4. Is the patient in any danger if the test is not done?
5. Am I ordering the test simply to reassure the patient?

CASE 9.5 TERMS OF ENTITLEMENT

A wealthy couple, Mr and Mrs K, considered "demanding" (that is, "having a sense of entitlement"), comes to see you, their general practitioner. They have just been to the husband's new internist (his old one retired) and are disappointed. Unlike his previous internist, the new one has not ordered an EKG, a urinalysis, or a blood test for the prostate. On questioning, you discover that the 75-year-old husband has no new cardiac or prostate complaints. All the same, the couple has come to expect these tests to be done yearly and ask you to order them.

Should you comply with the couple's request?

Guidelines defined

To help healthcare professionals evaluate clinical practice and make more appropriate care decisions, there has been great interest in outcomes research and the development of clinical practice guidelines.[60] These are systematically developed statements that assist practitioners' decisions about what is appropriate healthcare for specific clinical circumstances. Guidelines or "practice policies" are meant to distinguish between what works and what does not work on the basis of the best evidence.[61] Some guidelines are consensus-based; if solely based on consensus, however, these may reflect professional biases. Better guidelines are based, as much as possible, on evidence of the benefits and harms to patients from well-conducted trials. Trustworthy guidelines are ones that are constantly updated, open to external review and public input, rigorous in their review of the evidence, and free from conflicts of interest.[62]

Patients deserve medicine that works

The principle that patients deserve medicine that works suggests part of the solution to the problem of justly allocating healthcare. Autonomy and patient preferences are critical to good medical care but cannot alone determine what is appropriate or best care. A subjective patient-preference standard for care (based on individual patient wishes) must be supplemented by a more impartial, evidence-based criterion of benefit. An intervention is appropriate and should only be employed if, according to well-conducted research, it makes a "significant difference" for patients' lives *and* has been shown to work as a cost-effective contribution to patient care. In this view of medicine, patients deserve and ought to have the opportunity to receive what has been shown to work best for patients similar to themselves.[63] This is not a plea for uniformity of treatment; the application of guidelines must take into account "the incredible variation in patient preferences and characteristics."[64] This is especially so where the evidence is unreliable and anecdotal and experience may rule the day.

DISCUSSION OF CASE 9.5

Battles over the usefulness of medical interventions are common in healthcare. Whether it's a request for antibiotics from a patient with a viral infection (see Case 1.1) or a request to perform CPR on a patient unable to experience any benefit (see Case 1.3), differences of opinion between patients or families and healthcare professionals abound. As with any other intervention, screening tests—such as an annual EKG and prostate blood test—should be done only if there is evidence they are incrementally beneficial.

Rather than simply comply with this couple's request (which is not in keeping with the standard of practice for primary care), it would be better to find out why they seem so demanding. The request should be examined. Was there a legitimate *patient-based* reason for the request? Can it be met in any other way? Is the wife overly anxious about her husband's health? Was there a failure of communication with the new internist? Try to sympathize with their fears while not denying their requests head-on. If you have time and are a skilled negotiator, you might get away with not doing the tests. Then again, the day is short and this couple may be uninterested in dialogue. If so, you may choose to battle another day and reluctantly, give in to their wishes. Just don't forget there is a war to be won even if you lose today's skirmish!

Guidelines and autonomy

With the development of practice guidelines, some worry that the autonomy and needs of the patient may take second place to society's interest in limiting healthcare spending. This need not be. Accurate assessments of benefit allow patients and their surrogates to make more realistic healthcare choices.[65] "Downstream" costs of interventions—such as routine PSA testing or routine back X-rays—may include further expensive tests and treatment of no net benefit to patients. Guidelines, as reflections of what is likely to be helpful in the way of prevention and/or treatment, can take patients' preferences into account (see Box 9.3).[66]

BOX 9.3

Guidelines are most influential if they
- incorporate the latest advances in medical research, yet not be over-awed by the new;
- allow for clinical discretion and flexible interpretation;
- are easily implemented;
- are seen as aids to decision-making and not as regulations;
- incorporate specialists' and generalists' perspectives; and
- incorporate the patient's point of view.[67]

An example of the need to include the patient's perspective can be found in the development of a protocol for the treatment of deep-vein thrombosis (DVT). In the 1980s a panel of experts recommended the ideal treatment for DVT should be a combination of streptokinase and heparin because of evidence the two together were better at preventing the common post-phlebitic syndrome than heparin alone. However, a 1994 study showed this treatment was unacceptable to patients because it involved a small risk of a devastating stroke.[68] A better and more acceptable practice guideline for DVT treatment takes the wishes of patients, who tend to be more risk-averse than doctors, into account.

A help to patients

Some scholars, such as Wennberg, believe that once we tell our patients the true, often poor, outcomes of most interventions, many will decline them.[69] Indeed, some truly informed patients will decline interventions—such as drug treatment for hypercholesterolemia or early screening for prostate cancer—that can be overvalued by physicians but are of lesser relevance to the patient. This will save the system the expense of marginally useful, possibly harmful, and unwanted interventions. If so, it would be a nice by-product of outcomes research, since refusals of treatment by patients ("patient-choice" rationing) are the most morally defensible ones. Outcomes research would thus expand, not contract, the patient's autonomy and could also save the system money.[70]

By contrast, some patients, no matter how small the likelihood of benefit, will want such tests done regularly, such as in the last case above. What should be done about patients who cannot "regulate" themselves? Clinicians in their role as professionals (see Chapters 2 on autonomy and 8 on professionalism) have to learn to just say no.

Nonetheless, adhering to guidelines will not always reduce costs as some patients may end up receiving treatment they are unjustly not receiving now.[71] But, if some current practices with less evidential basis (such as colonoscopy screening in all asymptomatic adults or mammography in women under 50) are withdrawn, this will save the system money without compromising patient outcomes.

Unfortunately, due to lack of good evidence, trustworthy guidelines can capture, as yet, only a small portion of medical practice.

V. The Health Professional's Master

Throughout the world, rationing or priority setting seems unavoidable in the foreseeable future. In tough times, medicine may subtly shift from its focus on individual patients to an emphasis on measurable results and performance standards in guideline-oriented medicine.

Guidelines a legal risk?

Guidelines might be legally risky if, in following them, the clinician loses sight of the needs of the individual patient. Indeed, a suit in the UK attempted to suggest that, in following a procedural guideline, a doctor had exhibited negligence and that the guideline he was following was "faulty and flawed." Loath to second-guess what was, on consideration of the evidence, reasonable practice, the judge found in favour of the physician: "Unless a medical procedure is patently unsafe or goes against a common practice or usage a court should not attempt to substitute its views for those of the profession."[72] In Australia, it has been likewise held: "Given their purpose and evidence-based foundation, it is unlikely that clinical practice guidelines will promote litigation. Arguably, they may well reduce it by reducing any uncertainty about what constitutes reasonable medical practice."[73]

Guidelines themselves are unlikely to increase the risk of litigation because they may be used to define the applicable "standard of care." The real test for malpractice actions will be whether, in a particular circumstance, the defendant doctor's actions deviate from a widely accepted standard of practice—something guidelines may help define, but will not capture entirely.[74] There is ample room for "expert opinion" and "professional judgment."

Principled patient care

It is less contentious if guidelines are used to limit access to non-beneficial or non-standard-of-care care. If the guidelines limit patient access to available and *better* care on the basis of cost, patients should be explicitly told this.[75] The best place for the economic evaluation of healthcare, such as cost-benefit analysis and cost-effectiveness comparisons, is at the level of social planning—at the level of society in general—where all the costs and benefits of an intervention can be seen.[76] This avoids putting the practitioner in a direct conflict of interest with his or her patients. It is at a higher level—away from the clinical encounter—that difficult healthcare choices, such as funding for new and expensive technologies, need to take place. At the bedside, shared decision-making is the way to go—especially as the scientific evidence for any course of care is often unclear.[77] Cost-effective care must also be sensitive to and reflective of patient preferences. "Nothing about me without me," as the saying goes.

CASE 9.6 AN EXPENSIVE PROPOSITION

You are a hospitalist looking after Mr U, an elderly bachelor who has come into hospital with community-acquired pneumonia. Because he has been critically ill in the past with interstitial pneumonia, you worry the drug provided by the pharmacy on advice of the Drug Therapeutics Committee is less than optimal for the patient. You would prefer an expensive third-line drug but your unit's drug budget is already through the roof. Indications for the use of this drug also require evidence of the patient's failure to respond to the recommended medication. You worry this requirement will create a further delay, by which time Mr U will be too ill to respond.

What should you do?

Clinicians' decisions regarding individual patients must be guided by reasonable professional practice standards and by reasonable patients' preferences. Where physicians' actions are constrained by choices made by others, they may be less likely to be blamed for patient outcomes that are less than ideal.

It can be difficult for healthcare professionals to recognize when such limit-setting is acceptable and when it is not.[78] Where decisions made by others seem to be at the expense of the patient's interests, clinicians should explore the rationale for such decisions. The healthcare professional acting as the patient's advocate is particularly important in managed care systems where there can be conflicts of interest between the managed care system and the patient. Fairness, not bottom-dollar-driven interests, should be the central focus of any professional working in a managed healthcare system.[79]

DISCUSSION OF CASE 9.6

You need not take the Drug Therapeutics Committee's decision lying down. You have good evidence this patient needs the more expensive drug. If the Committee is fairly constituted, it could do well by starting with Daniel's "criteria for reasonableness": its deliberations and rationale for rationing or limiting access should be transparent, with reasons recognized as relevant by "fair-minded" people, and there should be a mechanism for appealing its decisions and a mechanism for enforcing it.[80] These criteria make allocation or distributive justice decisions under conditions of scarcity more amenable to public debate and discussion, rather than being made in secret and presented as a *fait accompli*. You should advocate for your patient and hope that the "fair-minded" members are swayed by your arguments.

System constraints

A physician who provides substandard care out of concern for limited resources may be found negligent. In the 1995 case of *Law Estate v. Simice*, the Court's concern centered on an adult male patient in British Columbia who died of a burst cerebral aneurysm after a long delay in getting a brain CT scan.[81] At trial the physicians testified they felt constrained by the medical system to restrict their requests for CT scans as diagnostic tools. Although agreeing such tests were expensive and acknowledging budgetary constraints on them, the court claimed these constraints "worked against the patient's interest by inhibiting doctors in their judgment of what should be done for him." The judge was of the opinion that, "if it comes to a choice between a physician's responsibility to his or her individual patient and his or her responsibility to the Medicare system overall, the former must take precedence in a case such as this."

For the physician of a patient with a medical need, costs should recede into the background: "The severity of the harm that may occur to the patient who is permitted to go undiagnosed is far greater than the financial harm that will occur to the medical system if one more CT scan procedure only shows the patient is not suffering from a serious medical condition."[82]

In other words, where the patient may benefit from an intervention, physicians would be unwise to think of the costs to the system. Rather than act as willing door closers, physicians ought to try to obtain reasonably beneficial services for their patients. In the *Simice* case the physicians may have too readily accepted a tacit limit to care—they were not following an evidence-based guideline developed by the profession. Their failure to obtain appropriate care for the patient resulted in injury to the patient and a finding of professional negligence. Where physicians are in reality clearly constrained by decisions already made by society, they can partially discharge their fiduciary obligations to their patients by informing them of these limits and suggesting alternative treatment. Although implicit or hidden rationing has its defenders (worried about social unrest from the excluded!),[83] it seems far more morally robust to be open with patients about the limits to care that may damage their interests.

This extra duty of care can be important for patients with special needs and unique circumstances, such as those with "disabilities," Aboriginal persons, transgendered persons and others with different sexual preferences, and those who suffer from rare "orphan" diseases like progeria. Abstractly, an "equitable" theory of justice might suggest all patients be treated in the same way. But all people are "diversely different" and a more fine-tuned application of justice (both consequentialist and deontological), as we saw in the case of access to organ transplantation, should consider the special interests of *everyone*.

Interestingly, but only with glancing relevance, there has recently been a move in the criminal judiciary towards "restorative" justice. The Supreme Court of Canada requires judges to take into account the "background and systemic factors" of offenders.[84] Searching for new solutions to old problems is necessary to address the overwhelming presence of indigenous people in the penitentiary system. When it comes to punishment and sentencing, the recommendation has been made that judges consider the wrongdoer's background and the impact that colonialism, the deliberate destruction of homes and families, and severe deprivation may have had. This is all to make the punishment better fit the crime.[85]

In healthcare, patients are not punished but are meant to receive the proper treatment for their problems. Applied to distributive justice concerning healthcare, the restorative approach suggests a just society owes extra duties of care, not just to Aboriginal peoples, but to all patients who have been traditionally underserviced by society and by healthcare. Ethical rules are "advantage reducing" the benefits of those already standing on higher ground and "advantage increasing" the benefits of those who have been used to standing on lower ground. We need to take the "unique circumstances" of these patients into account to see what they are fairly due. This is a big job, not for healthcare professionals alone. Patients, clinicians, and, indeed, administers of institutions of healthcare need to develop a "shared purpose" orientation whereby the goals of improved patient outcomes and reduced costs are consonant with the primary principles of healthcare: patient autonomy, beneficence, and justice. "The challenge is to cultivate consensus on an organization's shared purpose" which all parties can see as their own.[86] The issue of the costs of care is a problem not for someone else, but for all of us—patients and providers alike.

Conclusion

"The future," the novelist Don DeLillo has written, "belongs to crowds."[87] He may be right—this could be in the cards, especially if healthcare in the future becomes faceless and demoralized. To swim against that current requires a continued reliance on medicine's traditional ethical moorings. Clinicians will often accommodate patients who badly want scarce medical resources that many healthcare professionals consider unnecessary.[88] This may not be the best move as, in a world of increasingly expensive care and limited resources, this will exacerbate problems of allocation. Better to reduce healthcare spending by taking steps to prevent illness, helping patients curb risky behaviour and increase healthy behaviour, and agreeing on the limits of care.

If a healthcare professional believes an access to care standard has been imposed solely to hold down costs, the professional should consider not adhering to that standard and may wish, if appropriate, to inform his or her patients of this.[89] On the other hand, a treatment shown by well-conducted studies to lack distinct benefit or to be only marginally beneficial should be recognized as discretionary care. A shared purpose orientation may make "us/them" conflicts over the benefits and the appropriateness of care less likely.

In the next chapter we will look at new areas of reproductive and regenerative medicine, areas that are not making decisions over the cost of care any easier.

Cases For Discussion

CASE 1: A SUITABLE HARVEST

You are helping in the design of a new program aimed at increasing the number of organs available for transplantation. Despite repeated public education efforts to increase awareness of the need for donations, there is still a tremendous shortfall in available organs. In your jurisdiction, organs are made available only upon the death of a person who has voluntarily offered in advance to donate and then only if the family consents.

Several proposals are made to address this problem. Someone suggests paying the families the cost of the funeral for their deceased relative should they consent to the harvesting of his organs. Another recommends that only those people who offer in advance their organs for harvesting (when they die, of course) would be allowed to join the transplant-needed pool should their organ(s) fail. Yet another suggestion is to allow "directed donations"—individuals who voluntarily offer their organs in advance could direct their organs to a particular person or group or away from certain others. Finally, someone else proposes a default "opt-in" program for organ harvesting in the event of death—that is, your organs will be up for harvesting upon your death unless you say no in advance.

Questions For Discussion

1. What are the merits and drawbacks of each proposal?
2. What if the same schemas were applied to living donors?—for example, scenarios in which individuals are prepared to donate a kidney or a portion of their liver and direct them to particular individuals.

CASE 2: LAW 101

This case is well-known to first-year law students.[90]

Three men were afloat in a life-raft after their ship sank in the high seas. There was no opportunity to make any emergency signaling and there were limited provisions. After 21 days at sea, close to death, the two most able-bodied sailors decided they could survive only by "hastening the death of" (i.e., strangling) their youngest, and sickest, companion, the 17-year-old cabin boy. The two survived a further week at sea by cannibalizing the boy.

The two survivors argued later that what they did was not wrong as the cabin boy was about to die anyway and it was better that two survive than none. Others argued this was simply murder.

Questions For Discussion

1. Some people compare the spending crisis to being in a lifeboat too small to accommodate all. Discuss the helpfulness and implications of that metaphor to decisions about healthcare allocation.

2. What if the cabin boy consented to their actions (as he knew he was going to die anyway)? Would this still be considered murder?

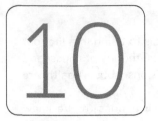

10

Labour Pains
Ethics and New Life

The best course . . . is to allow the duty of the mother to her foetus to remain a moral obligation which, for the vast majority of women, is already freely respected.

Chief Justice Lamer, 1999[1]

Among the most important moral issues faced by this generation are questions arising from technologically assisted reproduction—the artificial creation of human life.

Chief Justice McLachlin, 2010[2]

There is great diversity of opinion and unavoidable disagreements in any ethical discussion around issues of birthing and reproduction. Because it is impossible to examine all the complex facets of these issues, this chapter focuses on topics such as abortion, women's rights, fetal rights, and assisted reproduction, where some guidelines for healthcare professionals do exist.

I. Birthing and Reproductive Choice

Medical professionals are taught there are two patients in pregnancy, but are the two patients morally equivalent? How should a health professional respond to a patient's request to terminate her pregnancy? The answers to these questions vary throughout the world, but the evolving consensus in modern medicine is that practitioners must avoid putting their own views ahead of those of their patients.

CASE 10.1 A TRIVIAL MATTER?

A 23-year-old woman, Ms F, who seems happily pregnant, presents at 16 weeks to be screened for fetal anomalies. When the ultrasound reveals her fetus has a cleft palate, she requests a pregnancy termination. Her clinician considers this a rather trivial reason for a therapeutic abortion and shares this opinion with her.

> *Is it acceptable for the clinician to voice such an opinion? Or should the clinician simply shut up and fill out the referral form for the abortion?*

Modern medicine has helped make pregnancy and its termination safe and secure, giving women, at least in some parts of the world, more reproductive choice. Reproductive choice in the modern era has particularly meant that women no longer need to be enslaved by biology or be mere vessels for the fetus. Some people question whether this freedom is "natural," but progress in medicine has been about attempts to replace the "natural" course of an illness or condition with an "unnatural" and more felicitous, human-made course. Nature is sometimes cruel and unjust; one task of medicine is to allow humans more say over their destiny. As the great eighteenth-century philosopher Hegel argued, human beings, in constructing society, create a "nature above nature."[3] We must find and develop our own "laws" or rules to govern this "second nature."

The progression of medical advances in reproductive and sexual rights is not without ethical and legal quandaries. These dilemmas and disagreements should not obscure certain areas of moral consensus. For most, if not all, healthcare choices, medical practitioners should not interfere with their competent patients' right to decide for themselves, even if we personally disagree with their choices. The dominant view of morality in a pluralistic society gives citizens a right to be left alone to their own choices, especially when it comes to family planning. But what happens when a person's choice requires another person to enable it? One controversial choice is the decision to end a pregnancy.

DISCUSSION OF CASE 10.1

The clinician is not wrong to express an opinion—at least insofar as it is a professional, as opposed to a purely personal, opinion. Patients' views may be questioned or probed by their clinicians, especially if they act inconsistently. Affirming the right of a patient to access a service, such as pregnancy termination, does not necessarily require agreement with the patient or acceptance of the patient's reasoning. However, the doctor is on ethically slippery ground. Counselling should only be offered "if the woman requests it or there is a perceived need for it."[4]

It does seem curious, however, that she should now want an abortion if she was so "happily pregnant." It may be worth exploring, if the patient assents. Why should the presence of an easily correctable lesion such as a cleft palate make this patient decide to end a hitherto wanted pregnancy? What does she know about cleft palates? Is this an excuse to end a pregnancy now unwanted for other reasons? To what extent is the father of the fetus involved?

Notwithstanding these good questions, the clinician should be careful to separate out his or her opinion from "the facts": the fact is, the decision around continuing a pregnancy is ultimately the woman's to make. It is not the clinician's role to prevaricate or to oppose a woman's choice in this area.

It is argued the right to choice in pregnancy arises from the asymmetry in rights of the woman versus those of the fetus. By this view, even if one considers a fetus a person, no person has the "right" to piggy-back onto another person.[5] Just as my "right" to your blood or your second kidney depends on your consent, so the "right" of the fetus to its life depends on the pregnant woman's ongoing "consent." This is not a knockdown argument against the view that pregnancy entails responsibility. For many people, in the context of a wanted and consented to pregnancy, the woman has a moral and social responsibility to "take care" to protect her fetus during the pregnancy. A similar situation would be one in which someone who, having agreed to donate some tissue (or provide a gift) to another person, behaves in ways that imperil the donation (or takes the gift back). We would find this morally objectionable (or at least difficult to fathom—"Why would they do that?") much like breaking a promise. Such moral qualms should not, however, lead to sanctions such as refusing to respect or co-operate with the would-be donor, since the donation, like a mother's support for her fetus, is a voluntary matter. Rather, the donor's (like the promise breaker's) change of heart needs to be understood.

The rights of women to control their own bodies—the paramount ones being the right to birth control and the right to terminate pregnancy by abortion—are relatively recent ones, even in the West. For example, before 1969 in Canada, abortion was outlawed completely and an abortion provider could be charged with murder or manslaughter. In 1969, Canadian criminal law was amended to allow abortions only if a "therapeutic abortion committee" was of the opinion that the abortion was "medically necessary."[6]

Fairness in pregnancy

In 1988, this law was deemed unconstitutional by the Supreme Court of Canada in the landmark *Morgentaler* decision. As one of the judges explained, in giving the majority reasons, the law contravened the protection of "security of the person" guaranteed by section 7 of the *Canadian Charter of Rights and Freedoms*. Forcing a woman to endure an unwanted pregnancy, unless she met "criteria unrelated to her own priorities and aspirations," violated her "most basic physical and emotional condition." Moreover, the whole process was "manifestly unfair," violating "principles of fundamental fairness" because many hospitals did not have therapeutic abortion committees and some refused abortions to married women unless they were in physical danger. Since that decision, Canada has remained without any law regulating pregnancy and its termination or continuance, leaving it up to a woman and her doctor—a medical decision like any other.[7]

Similarly, in the United States, restrictions on the right to abortion were struck down as unconstitutional in 1973 in the well-known *Roe v. Wade* Supreme Court decision.[8] The court reasoned that the right to privacy protected women from interference with their decision to terminate their own pregnancy up until the point of fetal viability. The court did not, however, prohibit restrictions later in pregnancy and the door was left open to permit state regulation and prohibitions of late-term abortions.[9]

In any case, abortions beyond 24 weeks are unusual in North America—unless the mother's life is at risk or the fetus has died, has major congenital malformations, or is found to have anomalies incompatible with life, such as anencephaly. Although 24 weeks is the legal definition of fetal viability, this should not be taken as a hard and fast rule nullifying parental or professional responsibilities to a neonate. Once born alive outside the woman's body, no matter at what gestational age (GA), the fetus is a person at law and, morally, deserves the same rights as any other infant. The dangers of not recognizing this are seen in this case from British Columbia.

An abortion procedure was performed in 1985 on a woman who claimed to be in her first trimester. In fact she was in her third trimester. The fetus was born alive at about 26 weeks' gestation.[10] The baby was treated as if dead and abandoned in a recovery room. Finally discovered to be still breathing 40 minutes post-partum, the child was resuscitated but suffered severe and permanent brain damage as a result. On her behalf, her adoptive family was awarded over $8 million, one of the highest negligence settlements in Canadian judicial history.[11]

The standard of care in this area—whether one has a duty to resuscitate an extremely pre-term infant—may change as advances in medicine allow for the survival of pre-terms ("preemies") at earlier and earlier stages of pregnancy. Until recently, the definition of extrauterine fetal viability was considered to be 24 weeks, as survival prior to that point was unprecedented. Now, depending on the country, the survival of preemies born at 23 weeks GA ranges from 10 per cent in Sweden to 35 per cent in Canada and 54 per cent in Japan (part of the differences may have to with which babies are counted—all those delivered or only those who make it alive to intensive care). Of those who live, one third to one half will survive free of "severe neurodevelopmental outcomes." Because of these variable and difficult outcomes, there should be a graded approach to resuscitation of preterm infants.

The extreme preemie

The Canadian Paediatric Society has recommended that premature infants delivered alive at or less than 22 weeks' gestation should not receive active resuscitation but comfort care.[12] They should not be simply abandoned as they may continue to breathe for several days. The poor prognosis for infants between 23- and 25-weeks GA especially calls for shared decision-making with parents. The management of these infants will vary: some at 23 weeks may receive active care and others comfort care. For infants 25 weeks and over, barring other serious congenital anomalies, active treatment is initiated once they are born alive. Respect for persons means (a) involving parents in the decision-making as much as possible with the provision of proper information and (b) providing the premature infant, as with any newborn, with the best care possible. Transparency in the decision-making process regarding the critically ill infant may prevent communication failures and inappropriate processes and outcomes of care,[13] and can allow the decisions that are made to be seen as fair and reasonable by all involved.

Requests for abortion

Absolute prohibitions on abortion do not eliminate the procedure but simply drive it underground and make it much more risky. In North America where induced abortions have been made available, early and safe abortions are the general norm. It is in the developing countries, where 97 per cent of the world's unsafe abortions take place, that maternal mortality is high and is a major public health problem.[14]

If, however, a healthcare provider has a moral objection to abortion, what role, if any, must he or she play if a patient requests one?

Although abortion may be controversial ethically, in Canada it is a recognized and legitimate option that healthcare providers or others delay or impede at their own and their patient's peril. Claims of conscientious objection by healthcare professionals are sometimes acceptable.[15] Healthcare providers opposed to abortion on the grounds of conscience certainly do not have a duty to participate in it. Where abortion services are easy for patients to find, they may not even have a duty to refer them to another resource. But these stances are controversial—especially if the thinking is that as a healthcare professional one has no obligation to refer when it conflicts with one's personal morality. The practice of medicine always involves some degree of "moral risk."[16] The risk of moral harm to the practitioner's conscience is outweighed by the magnitude of physical and psychological harm to a patient should she be unable to obtain a timely pregnancy termination. Because failing to refer could put a woman at an increased risk of a delayed abortion and a bad outcome (as real physical and psychological risks for women increase, the later the termination[17]), this could be construed as negligence or patient abandonment. It all depends on the options available and known to the patient and the difficulty of accessing them without the clinician's help.

Some studies suggest that reproductive services providers allow their values to influence their clinical decisions.[18] Although this may at times be appropriate where those values are protective of the patient's interests, clinicians must be careful to refrain from making decisions that properly belong to the patient.

The bottom line: where health professionals are unable for any reason to provide an expected service, they must know to whom to refer the patient and provide that referral in a timely way.[19]

A mother's right, a father's obligation

A woman from Quebec, who became pregnant while in a two-year common-law relationship, sought pregnancy termination. The father of the fetus obtained a court injunction preventing her from having an abortion. Clarification of the rights of the father and of the fetus were sought through the appeal to the Supreme Court of Canada.

This case, *Tremblay v. Daigle*, both solidified the right of a woman to decide independently regarding her pregnancy and clarified the rights of the father. No point of English law offered rights to the fetus: "The fetus cannot, in English law . . . have a right of its own at least until it is born and has a separate existence from its mother."[20]

Specifically, when it comes to the decision about pregnancy termination, the father does not have "veto" rights: "No court in Quebec or elsewhere has ever accepted the argument that a father's interest in a fetus which he helped create could support a right to veto a woman's decisions in respect of the fetus she is carrying."[21]

That fathers have no legal say in the decision over pregnancy does not mean they are free from obligations regarding the pregnancy; would-be "hit-and-run" fathers must provide support if a pregnancy they helped engender is successfully taken to term. There is an asymmetry, in this view, between the rights of potential fathers and mothers: women have the final say over a pregnancy's continuation because it is their body; men must take (at least financial) responsibility for fathering children as a consequence, as it were, of having access to the woman's body.

These judicial rulings create a space for women to make reproductive decisions on their own. However, access to abortion services remains problematic in many parts of North America. Finding someone to perform the abortion is not difficult in most, but not all, provinces in Canada—at least in the larger cities—but can be a challenge in many American jurisdictions. Surprisingly, hospitals are not required to provide such needed services. Many in fact choose not to provide them, making access a problem.[22] Abortion committees and archaic criminal restrictions still exist in many other countries, especially in Africa and South America. Even in the UK, for example, a woman must still seek approval from two physicians to obtain an abortion, a requirement opposed by the majority of United Kingdom citizens and many clinicians as well.[23]

While abortion may be readily available in some countries, this does not mean that all such requests carry the same moral weight. A key question is who is making the request. In some countries abortion has been forced on women,[24] an obviously objectionable practice from any perspective. Sometimes, more subtle forms of coercion exist that make the choice to terminate less than free. The practitioner needs to be sensitive to these.

CASE 10.2 A RIGHT TO BE TESTED?

You are a primary care practitioner looking after a professional couple in their early thirties who have two young girls at home. The woman is in the first trimester of her third pregnancy. At low risk for congenital anomalies and accurate for time of conception, she nevertheless requests an obstetrical ultrasound or amniocentesis. Her husband admits they are primarily seeking to know the sex of the fetus. If it is a girl, he says, they will seek pregnancy termination and try to get pregnant again.

Must you help them?

DISCUSSION OF CASE 10.2

On the face of things, this would seem quite simple: the couple seeks a medical service—an ultrasound—that is readily available and easily accessed. You may disagree with their rationale for pregnancy termination but is that a sufficient reason to try to change their minds? If you were truly concerned, counselling them, being sensitive to the different ethnic and cultural opinions in this area and to not imposing your views on them, would be acceptable. If possible, it would be not unreasonable to have a discussion with the woman without the husband in the room. Does she share the same views as her husband? Has there been any pressure from her family regarding the decision? As long as the woman is making an authentic choice and not seemingly coerced by her spouse or her culture, her choice ought to be respected. However, "respect" does not mean she has an unfettered right to the test.

It may seem odd but, although abortions are allowed for any reason in Canada, certain restrictions are imposed on access to antenatal *testing* for those who simply wish to know the sex of their fetus. This is to prevent sex-selection clinics from springing up and professionals from profiting from such services. So, now that the couple has admitted the true reason for seeking the ultrasound, the cat is out of the bag, so to speak, and you have a professionally acceptable reason for refusing to make the referral. It is unlikely you would be sanctioned for this because (1) this may be an inappropriate *professional* indication for an ultrasound (sex determination unconnected with disease)[25] and (2) ultrasound services are accessible to couples by going outside medicare or crossing the border to the United States where such testing is readily available.

II. In the Interest of the Child: Being Born and Living Life

The advance of medical science creates new obligations for helping patients and families with reproductive choice. Healthcare providers are obliged to properly inform prospective parents about the appropriate tests that can be readily done to evaluate fetal health. Failing to provide accurate genetic screening or counselling (such as amniocentesis to detect birth defects) is one such professional deficiency.[26] Parents may claim that they would not have continued the pregnancy or even conceived the child had they been properly apprised of the genetic risks. Where negligence is found, damages have been awarded for at least some of the costs and losses to the parents in raising the child.[27] (Legal liability on the part of a physician can be claimed if it can be shown, for example, that the parents would have opted for pregnancy termination had they been properly informed of the potential risks to the fetus. See Case 4.2, "Not to worry.")

Wrongful birth suits have also been filed by parents when an unexpected pregnancy occurs as a result of a negligently performed sterilization. In such cases, where a healthy child is born, claims for damages—the cost of pregnancy, delivery, and the rearing of a child, healthy or disabled—have received variable recognition in Western societies. Courts have traditionally viewed awarding damages for the birth and life of a healthy child as repugnant. Laterally, however, some Canadian and UK courts have compensated simply for the negligent sterilization.[28]

The moral rationale for wrongful birth suits rests on the right of women (or couples) to decide whether pregnancies ought to be undertaken or continued in the light of all the relevant information. Especially where there may be information relevant to the parents over the continuance of a pregnancy, healthcare professionals have an obligation to see that the parents-to-be are properly informed or to refer them on to others who can provide the needed information.

By contrast, wrongful life suits are filed on the infant's behalf, seeking damages for the pain and suffering caused to the child by his or her very existence because of an impairment. The claim is made that the clinician negligently allowed a severely handicapped child to be born. Most courts in Canada and the UK have turned down such suits. The value of death over any kind of life is not something the courts are comfortable with calculating as a matter of justice and compensation in law. They see it as a matter for "philosophers and theologians."[29] (Needless to say, philosophers and theologians have not come up with an acceptable price for existence either.) Such suits seem morally suspect anyway as they devalue the lives of those with disabilities—implying that non-existence for them is preferable to life. This is not a view held by many who have survived despite hardships and handicaps.[30]

Issues relating to the health of the fetus—such as maternal activities that may harm the fetus—must be discussed with the pregnant woman, as managing these issues most effectively and respectfully depends on her informed choice and voluntary participation in risk-abatement activities.

CASE 10.3 FETUS AT RISK

You are a nurse practitioner in a small town in northern Ontario. One of your patients, Ms S, is a 29-year-old woman in her second pregnancy. Her first child suffers from fetal alcohol syndrome (FAS) and is in foster care. Ms S continues to drink heavily during this second pregnancy. Alerted to this by her common-law spouse, you are concerned for the well-being of the fetus as well as of the mother. Someone suggests you get tough with Ms S by making an urgent

> application for court-ordered protection for the fetus and seeking involuntary hospitalization away from the Reserve for the woman to ensure compliance (with a plan to treat her alcohol problem and control her alcohol intake).
>
> *Would you go along with this suggestion?*

Coercing an addicted mother into treatment risks turning healers into jailers and pits the pregnant mother against her fetus in multiple ways. Would we act in similar ways with a woman who smokes during pregnancy? What if she eats excessively or decides to take a plane trip in her third trimester? There is no practical or ethically acceptable way to intervene in any of these scenarios, lacking the mother's co-operation. Of course, it is still ethical to "intervene" with counselling, advice, even exhortations, and offers of support or assistance, referrals, and the like, all short of coercion or forcing compliance. The same is true of intervening to ensure that *fathers* make wise lifestyle choices to promote the well-being of their children. The "blaming-the-mother" attitude ignores studies showing that problems in mothering (antenatal and postpartum) can arise due to maternal deprivation and lack of support (e.g., financial, emotional) from the father.[31]

DISCUSSION OF CASE 10.3

This is a tough case in which to be involved—tough because one knows the predictable consequence of the mother's behaviour is another child with FAS, a huge problem for society but also for the child-to-be. Tough, also, because what can one do? One cannot incarcerate the mother—no crime has been committed or even considered. Concentrating on the fetus alone, such as by giving it "rights," as some have argued,[32] would be unlikely to help. The pregnant woman and her fetus are one interrelated biological unit. Although it is difficult for health professionals to watch pregnant women continue to engage in risky behaviours, imposing a duty of care on them would lead to intolerable and unjust intrusions into the everyday lives of women and would be a violation of section 7 of the Canadian Constitution guaranteeing women liberty and security of the person.

A vindictive approach will not work. You should see what other supports—financial, cultural, emotional—can be found to help the woman. You could find out what role does drinking play in her life? What has the history of indifference toward and abuse of indigenous people had upon her and her family? What resources can be mounted for her from her community? The context is one factor influencing her self-destructive behaviour and may also hold the key to helping Ms S. What seems on the surface to be an "ethical dilemma," a clash of fundamental principles or interests, may be resolved at a practical level by the skills and training of healthcare professionals working together with the patient and the resources of her local culture.

Given the serious and intimate nature of pregnancy and abortion, there seems no more legitimate and reliable person to make the decision to continue or terminate a pregnancy, and to take the responsibility for living with the decision, than the woman who is pregnant (see Box 10.1) Whether or not the fetus is considered a person (and many opinions regarding this exist), in Canada the fetus, while *en ventre de sa mère*, ("in the belly of its mother"), has no legal protection; its continued existence should depend on the woman's ongoing consent. Citizens are not obliged to have their bodies, or any part thereof, used by anyone else—be it fetus, child, or some other person—even if for "good" therapeutic ends. Forced intrusions on pregnant women are constraints on the liberty and privacy citizens expect in a free society. As such, they rarely receive judicial sanction, even in the US, and are not supported by moral or legal reasoning.[34]

BOX 10.1

"Parliament has failed to establish either a standard or a procedure whereby any [state] interests might prevail over those of the woman in a fair and non-arbitrary fashion."[33]

III. The New Age of Reproduction

No longer must women fear becoming pregnant; they can choose if, when, and even *how* they give birth. Some women opt to terminate a viable pregnancy, whereas other women go to extraordinary lengths to become pregnant. Reproduction used to be a fairly simple matter: woman, man, sex, birth, child. Infertility was less of a problem than the puerperal-related death of mother and child. As with so much else in the past century, the situation may now be much safer but not nearly as straightforward. One does not, directly at any rate, need a man to be there; one does not, except initially, need a woman to be there—well, okay, a woman's uterus is still needed but almost any uterus will do. Age, sexual orientation, infertility, a lack of sperm or eggs, even death, are all no longer limitations to successful reproduction. Sperm can be provided and joined with an ovum in a petri dish (an *in vitro* embryo); sperm can be injected directly into an ovum (Intra-Cytoplasmic Sperm Injection, ISCI); fertilized eggs, embryos, and blastocysts (early embryonic development of a fertilized egg) can be implanted in the mother's womb (*In Vitro* Fertilization, IVF); the womb may be that of a surrogate mother; gametes may be collected and stored prior to chemotherapy, bone marrow irradiation or surgery or harvested after death. Reproduction has now been "globalized" as reproduction is outsourced and unregulated from the West to Third World women with wombs for rent.

If the continuation of one's chromosomes is the rationale for evolution, then modern assisted reproduction technology (ART) has given our genes a way of replicating almost without us. Male and female gametes (sperm and ova or eggs, respectively) and a safe place to be joined and develop are all that are needed prior to implantation in a womb. ART includes the services, techniques, and technology used to assist individuals who cannot conceive on their own—from simple artificial insemination and IVF to egg donation and pre-implantation genetic diagnosis (PGD).[35] This includes all the varied techniques of harvesting, preserving, manipulating, transferring, and conjoining gametes and the technology for analyzing, storing, sharing, and using the genetic material of gametes and embryos.

CASE 10.4 WHOSE BABY IS IT ANYWAY?

A childless heterosexual couple arrange for the creation of an *in vitro* embryo from an egg and sperm donated anonymously. The embryo is successfully implanted into a surrogate mother contracted by the couple to give birth to the child, whom they intend to then adopt and raise. Although the pregnancy successfully carries to term, the contracting couple splits up just prior to childbirth. The husband now says he wants nothing to do with the birth or the child.

Who should be considered the parents for this child?

DISCUSSION OF CASE 10.4

It used to be the existence of arranged marriages that worried (and still worries) some people. Now there are arranged births facilitated by clinics where eggs are harvested, combined with male gametes and transferred into a uterus of choice. It sounds a little mechanical but assisted reproduction (AR) has allowed thousands of infertile/childless couples a chance to have children of their own. Questions with uncertain answers arise in this process, however.

Troubles may occur, for example, if the father no longer wishes to be involved or if the surrogate mother decides she wishes to keep the infant. Does it matter whether the child was conceived with

- the surrogate mother's ovum?
- donated ovum/ova?
- the husband's sperm?
- donated sperm?
- the wife's ovum/ova?

The permutations and combinations are obviously complex. Surrogacy means implanting a fertilized egg (which may or may not belong to the surrogate mother) into a surrogate's womb. In traditional surrogacy, one uses the husband's sperm and inseminates the surrogate mother. In more recent surrogacy arrangements, another woman's eggs are used to sever any genetic link between the birth mother and the child and try to forestall any claim by the surrogate that she is the "real" mother.

But what if the father, as in this case, wishes to escape from the commitment to raising the child once born? The language of the surrogate contract may make the legal answer seem easy: the contracting couple, as the "ordering" couple, is designated, by mutual agreement with the surrogate, to be the child's parents. Even without a formal agreement or legal contract, morally they have obligations to the child, once born, from which they cannot escape. Assuming the wife wishes to keep the child, the ex-husband should incur the expenses that a natural father would undertake.

Does it really matter where the gametes come from? This is unsettled in law. When a dispute arises over "Whose baby is it anyway?" some courts have deemed the baby to be the surrogate's. After all, she is the one who has endured the burdens of pregnancy and developed the bond with the child. In many places the child is the surrogate's until formal adoption proceedings are completed. Other courts have found, irrespective of gamete origin, against the surrogate mother if it seems the newborn child would be better off with the contractual parents.[36] A father may have rights of child custody if he is the source of the male gametes, but not if he donated his sperm anonymously. It is unclear whether he has any obligations if he knowingly donates sperm to, for example, a lesbian couple who later seek child support. Presumably not, especially if there was a "pre-concep" agreement limiting his involvement in child rearing.

ART create dilemmas not only as to who the parents are but also as to the status of the offspring. Are the products of ART conceptions—unborn but not implanted embryos—somehow persons with rights and interests of their own or are they mere chattel, objects belonging to the highest bidder? If the ordering parents die and leave an estate, does the estate now belong to the unborn embryo or is the embryo inherited along with the estate? No doubt these conundrums will keep the courts and lawyers busy for years.

What is a good healthcare practitioner to do in this new age of fertility and reproduction? Are there no boundaries to what is acceptable? Here, as elsewhere, there are some indicators as to what is, and what is not, ethically acceptable conduct. One thing is clear: assisted reproductive services are not for everyone. But one has to be careful about whom one excludes.

Denying choice?

In 1993, a physician directing an ART clinic, specializing in fertilizing the ova of women with sperm donated by unrelated men, decided to no longer allow lesbian couples access to the clinic's services. Several years earlier, he had testified in a child custody case involving another lesbian couple who had undergone successful insemination in his clinic. The resultant publicity had led to harassing phone calls criticizing him for inseminating lesbians; this eventually led to his decision to limit his practice.[37]

A complaint of discrimination on account of sexual orientation was laid and upheld by the Supreme Court of British Columbia.[38] The physician was found in violation of the *British Columbia Human Rights Act*. This decision might have been controversial then, but not now. It is accepted as mainstream that ART services should be available to gays, lesbians, and unmarried persons.[39] What is odd about this finding of rights violation is that the doctor involved offered the couple a referral to *another* clinic prepared to help them. Usually, clinicians who object to a medical procedure fulfill their duty to would-be patients by appropriate referral. It's not clear why this did not suffice in this case.

The upshot: physicians providing any medical services must ensure there is no discrimination in their provision.[40]

Physicians can deny any medical service if there are legitimate safety concerns, such as serious threats to the welfare of patients or society. For example, they can reject the "gift" of donation of sperm if there are safety concerns (such as, for example, infectious disease contamination) concerning the gametes. There is no "right" of donation; health practitioners and medical facilities are not obliged to accept all and any donations of blood, gametes, or organs.[41] Thus, sperm donation, governed for public health purposes since 1996, in Canada curiously only under the federal *Food and Drug Act*, can be denied on the grounds of sexual orientation, because there is a higher risk of serious disease with certain sexual practices. Can healthcare professionals deny some patients access to medical services, such as ART, if it might cause harm or less than optimal outcomes to future offspring?

What if would-be parents want to use ART services to choose for their offspring an existence that most people would not choose for themselves, for example, parents with achondroplastic dwarfism who desire to have an offspring with the same condition? Thus, while considered a less than optimal existence from a non-dwarf perspective, is the birth of such a child so bad that it should always be prevented? There is a vibrant "short persons" culture with dwarfism being quite compatible with a happy life.[42] In any case, infertility clinics are ill equipped to evaluate parental choices, such as planning for offspring. Whether people are suited to be parents or not is usually not decided by a community. Persons, "disabled" or not, can, with or without modern medicine's help, reproduce as they see fit. If the child-to-be is likely to be seriously harmed by the would-be parents, then the ART healthcare professional may be obliged not to help them.[43] Just what parental conditions would justify not offering ART (Drug abuse? Possibly, especially if the gestational-mother-to-be is drug-addicted. Abject poverty? Not on its own, but they couldn't afford it anyway. A history of child abuse and neglect? Almost certainly.) is an issue about which there is not yet consensus.

Bottom line: providers of professional services are not obliged to provide their services to patients so long as this is consonant with the professional standards of care—one such standard is preventing avoidable serious harms to others.

In the real world, the "right" of opportunity to access artificial reproductive services—or at least to join the queue to access ART—is a limited one, usually accessible only to those with financial means. There is no financial reimbursement for ART use by infertile couples or individuals in many countries, including Canada.[44] Most of these services are not covered under provincial healthcare plans. The failure of governments to reimburse such services might be viewed as treating infertility differently from other medical conditions and, arguably, infringing on the infertile person's "equality rights." Should the "right" to become pregnant be on par with another patient's "right" to be free of limitations on lying flat because of Grade IV heart failure or another's "right" to be treated for an inability to mix socially on account of a pervasive social anxiety disorder? Infertility is not one thing: it may be due to disease and injury or simply due to older age, so the preference for ART may run from the reasonable to the outlandish.

Not only is resource allocation (see Chapter 9 on justice) a political and social issue, but so are notions of disease and ill health. Briefly, illnesses are, in one broadly accepted view, deviations from the normal human range of functioning which cause harm to patients, or threaten to do so.[45] Such conditions, for which there can be some helpful interventions, are seen as unfair and tend to be reimbursed. We do not reimburse patients for the merely unfortunate experiences of life, such as being born poor or short—whether or not we can change these. Many view infertility as an unfortunate occurrence, not as an illness that renders persons so afflicted they are any less able to participate in life.

The Supreme Court of Nova Scotia has held that not reimbursing ART is a legitimate policy decision, interpreting it as a "reasonable limit" on the provision of services that is "demonstrably justified" in a democratic society as permitted by the *Canadian Charter of Rights and Freedoms*. "It would be unrealistic for this Court to assume that there are unlimited funds to address the needs of all," opined one judge.[46] This judgment misses the nuances in the causes of infertility and the rationale for seeking ART.

The proliferation of ART exists in an international patchwork quilt of regulations and regulatory vacuums. Not surprisingly, there is little harmony in this area. For example, the US does not as yet regulate pre-implantation genetic testing on embryos, whereas the UK and Canada do. The regulations are partial, in flux, poorly enforceable, and subject to bypass through "reproductive tourism."[47]

The Assisted Human Reproductive Act

Canada, similar to many other countries, has scrambled to keep up with the advances in reproductive medicine. Legislation to provide direction in this troubled area—the *Assisted Human Reproductive Act* (the *"Reproductive Act"*)—was devised and passed by Parliament in 2004 (see Box 10.2).[48]

BOX 10.2

The *Canadian Reproductive Act* is guided by five principles:

- respect for human individuality, dignity, and integrity;
- "precautionary" approach to protect and promote health;
- non-commodification and non-commercialization;
- informed choice; and
- accountability and transparency.

The primary purpose of this federal legislation was to define certain acts in the area of new reproduction techniques as criminal and others as permissible if regulated. Prohibited acts include the following:

- human cloning;
- the commercialization of human reproductive material and the reproductive functions of women and men; and
- the use of *in vitro* embryos without consent.

The permitted activities, so long as they are carried out in accordance with regulations made under the *Act*, under licence and in licensed premises, are "controlled activities":

- the manipulation of human reproductive material or *in vitro* embryos,
- transgenic engineering; and
- reimbursement of the expenditures of donors and surrogate mothers.

The *Reproductive Act* also set out the terms of a new national agency that would oversee the field and ensure compliance with regulations.[49] It is important to note that the *Reproductive Act* governs only the use of "embryos." *Once transferred into a woman, the treatment or use of the fetus is not governed by the* Reproductive Act's *provisions.*

The *Reproductive Act* addresses concerns that unregulated ART could undermine the fundamental principle of dignity and respect for persons embodied in the practice of medicine. This principle of respect attempts to exclude monetary gain as the primary motivation for the actions of healthcare professionals working in this field. For example, in an attempt to prevent commercialization of the process and exploitation of persons involved, the following would not be permitted:

- sex selection via embryo testing, except for medical reasons, such as, to prevent sex-specific disease such as Duchenne's muscular dystrophy. (This could prevent couples from testing for sex or other non-medical reasons);[50]
- payments to would-be gamete (egg or sperm) donors, except for reasonable expenses;[51]
- payments to surrogate mothers. They can be reimbursed only for reasonable costs and losses of pregnancy—this is to remove any financial windfalls to them and prevent a market-driven traffic in babies and wombs for hire. (This does not prevent generous "gifts" to the surrogate mother.)

This legislation has, however, not yet made it to the implementation stage. From the outset, its constitutionality was challenged by Quebec which argued the *Act* was attempting to regulate the practice of medicine and research, an area of provincial jurisdiction. The opposing view was that the primary intent of the legislation was to criminalize (and thus prevent) certain evil activities and only secondarily to allow (and so promote?) certain good practices. According to this view, the "pith and substance" of the *Act* was that it

> is a valid exercise of the federal power over criminal law. The dominant purpose and effect of the legislative scheme is to prohibit practices that would undercut moral values, produce public health evils, and threaten the security of donors, donees, and persons conceived by assisted reproduction.[52]

This view was not upheld. When the case was finally decided by the Supreme Court in 2010, the judges were split 4–4 with the deciding vote equivocally supporting the fundamental unconstitutionality of the *Act*.[53]

As a result, surrogacy is virtually as unregulated on a federal level as it was previously. It is now up to the provinces to devise the appropriate legislation to govern this area of medical practice. At least one province—Quebec—has done so. (Surrogacy contracts, for example, are not recognized in Quebec, as is the case in many jurisdictions in Europe.)

The right to know one's past

There is one important area remaining unresolved due to the *Act* remaining in limbo. Adopted children ("adoptees") have a right to seek access to information on file about their biological parents. Do offspring resulting from ART also have access to their parental genetic information and other health risks? It appears not—at least not yet in Canada. The *Food and Drug Act*'s regulations recommend, but do not mandate, that non-identifying information on the donor of sperm be kept on file "indefinitely."[54] The *Reproductive Act* proposed a new federal agency that would hold a confidential registry for information on gamete donors. With the donor's consent, access to this information would be granted to a donor's offspring. Lacking implementation of this legislation, however, no federal registry has been established and so there are no effective routes for donor offspring to ascertain their genetic history.

This is unlike the UK where, under the auspices of the Human Fertilisation and Embryology Authority,[55] a central registry of all gamete donors and all births as a result of assisted conceptions in licensed UK facilities has been kept since 1991. Although no unique identifying information will be provided, donor-conceived individuals 16 years of age and older can discover the donor's age, ethnicity, other children (if any), physical characteristics, health status and any other information the donor may have wished to have passed on.

British Columbia, which failed under its adoption act to provide donor offspring the same rights and protections of adoptees (among them the right to have access to donor information), was found in breach of article 15 of the Canadian Charter, the right to equal protection under the law.[56] While this goes some way in recognizing the right of donor offspring not to be deprived of access, it did not take the further step of affirming a positive state duty to provide the requisite information.[57] Without being pushed by the courts, a lack of attention to this issue by the federal government continues to exist.

It is still a time of turmoil in this area of medicine. Given the expense of these ART procedures, buyers may end up going to the cheapest and, so, probably least regulated, markets. All one can say is good luck and *caveat emptor*. Concerns about the safety of the new reproductive techniques will continue until effective national and international constraints are put in place.[58]

IV. Desperately Seeking Stem Cells

The use of human "stem cells" to enhance human reproduction and health is also controversial. Stem cells are primal cells capable of renewing themselves through cell division and also possessing the potential to differentiate into more specialized cells. Human stem cells exist in two main forms. Embryonic cells, which have been found to have the greatest differentiating capacity to date, are derived from blastocysts or early stage embryos—about four to five days old in humans. Induced pluripotent (the ability-to-differentiate-into-all-other-cell-lines) cells, in contrast, are derived from "adult" non-embryonic (somatic) tissues. There is a limited number of pluripotent stem cells present in adults (there are many in skin or bone marrow and virtually none in the heart or brain).

Stem cells have been legitimately used for over 50 years to regenerate bone marrow and blood cells in patients with diseases such as leukemia. Today, more than 50,000 people worldwide receive this form of stem cell treatment.[59] Stem cells offer the hope of definitive (i.e., disease modifying) treatment for other conditions such as heart failure, macular degeneration, Parkinson's disease, spinal cord injuries, and juvenile-onset diabetes—diseases affecting tissues or organs where stem cells are not apparent in adults. Infused stem cells could, in theory, replenish the loss of differentiated cells, such as in Parkinson's, the loss of dopamine-producing neurons. Stem cells have shown promise in regenerating certain tissues, such as cardiac tissue damaged by myocardial infarction.[60] Phase 1 trials have shown safety of intracoronary infusions of cardiac derived stem cells—the researchers noted "unprecedented increases in . . . viable myocardium" of damaged hearts.[61] This is turn may prevent heart failure, but many complex practical challenges remain.[62]

As with other scientific developments in medicine, the new reproductive techniques and stem cell therapies raise new hopes and pose formidable ethical challenges for professional societies. Unproven and unregulated use of stem cells by less scrupulous practitioners for desperate patients with other diseases is already, controversially, taking place.[63]

CASE 10.5 THE SAVIOUR CHILD

A three-year-old child is gravely ill with leukemia. Curative treatment is possible but requires bone marrow stem cell donation from a suitable donor. Without it, the child will almost certainly die when the disease recurs in several years. No suitable match is found. The parents decide to conceive a new child in the hopes that it will be a suitable donor, but they need ART because the woman experienced premature ovarian failure at age 43. The mother has a twin sister who is prepared to donate her eggs.

Is this an acceptable use of ART? What if the parents wanted the fetus's embryonic stem cells and requested the creation of multiple fertilized eggs to maximize the chances of a suitable donor fetus?

Research using embryonic stem cells has generally been more controversial than that involving adult stem cells. Some oppose using embryonic-derived cells because they seem to come with a moral tithe: the embryo may have to be created and then sacrificed to derive such cells. Because a human embryo is a potential human being, so the reasoning goes, destroying it contributes to the devaluation of human life.[64] By the same token, it seems wrong to treat gametes or embryos as mere property to be bought or sold to the highest bidder. These actions and attitudes seem morally repugnant because they treat human life as a means to an end, rather than as an end in itself. (This, as you can tell, is a deontological argument.)

Supporters of embryonic stem cell research, by contrast, point to the tremendous potential for improving the quality of human life. (This, by contrast, is a consequentialist argument.) An unimplanted embryo *in vitro* is not the same, morally, as a third trimester fetus, let alone identical to a child or an adult, they say. Most countries do not prohibit, outright, work with embryonic human stem cells. Such work, it is argued, need not be done at the expense of a respectful view of human life, if adhering to certain restrictions.

Where to draw the line as to when life begins is obviously a point of controversy. For centuries, a common view was that life began at "quickening," the point at which the woman could feel the child move in the uterus (16–20 weeks typically). Many countries try to get around religious concerns and limit the use of embryos to the pre-implantation stage.[65] However, firm proponents of the sanctity of life now date life back to the point of conception. This makes compromise and consensus in this area challenging.

Embryos are readily available as by-products of IVF procedures. Many end up not being used and are, in effect, abandoned. Could these embryos, created for other purposes, be donated for research or therapy without devaluing human life? Many people—about 60 per cent in most countries—would agree to using these embryos for research, with about 30 per cent opposed. [66]

The Ethics Committee of the American Society for Reproductive Medicine has recommended that discarded or abandoned embryos be used for research but with prior consent from the donors.[67] This would make the donation of stem cells akin to parents donating the organs of a child who dies suddenly; they turn their tragedy into meaning by donation of their offspring's organs or tissue for the benefit of others.

Respect for things human

As has been noted earlier in this book, Immanuel Kant believed in the intrinsic value of each individual's life. He argued that human beings should never be treated merely as a means to obtain some supposed "greater good" because this renders them mere "stepping-stones" to someone else's welfare or happiness.[68]

By the lights of the Kantian view, parents ought never to see their offspring as mere extensions of themselves and their own needs. Is the Kantian view of offspring too precious, though? After all, parents have children for all kinds of emotional, economic, and cultural reasons, but our culture does not privilege one set of reasons. There is no moral litmus test prospective parents must pass—we do not question why they want a new child. So, why not, then, produce an offspring, a so-called "saviour child," to rescue the life of an imperiled one? Moreover, it is sometimes argued, the early embryo is not a person with rights, so why the concern about its fate, as compared with the fate of a real imperilled person?

DISCUSSION OF CASE 10.5

Although not undertaken to serve the health interests of the donor child, there would be little reason to hesitate with sibling-to-sibling donation if the suitable donor child already exists, even if that child is unable to consent. Presuming the risks to be undertaken by the healthy sibling are small and the psychological benefits to the family (including to the donor child) evident were the ill child to survive, then donation could take place. (Similar reasoning—a broadened sense of "best interests" —authorizes bone marrow donation from an incapable adult patient to another family member.[69])

Is it more unacceptable for the parents to conceive a new child to save the life of their imperiled child? If doing so is acceptable to them and easy to do (for example, they want another child anyway, they are young, and can afford it), should someone stand in their way? But, if the couple simply wants an embryo for its stem cells in order to save the life of their three-year-old child, would it be wrong to help them? Is destroying an embryo which could save the life of a child more unacceptable than letting a child die? Common sense should dictate that the harm caused by the loss of an actual life is greater than the harm done by the loss of a potential life.

Other people would refuse to trade one human life (the embryo's) for that of another (the child's)—this is similar to the Kantian view of human life. One worry is that embryo use, even for a valid therapeutic purpose, might open the floodgates to raising and harvesting embryos to serve as tissue or organ factories. This worry might be countered if ART were to be strictly regulated and offered only by accredited facilities, not an easy task.[70]

Optimists put faith in technology and our ability to control it; pessimists are not as sanguine about human rationality and hanker for a simpler world. I tend to the eternal-optimism view, recognizing that the path forward is rarely controversy-free. Many of these rather Byzantine ethical and legal conundrums may disappear with the advance of the science that induced them.

Conclusion

Modern medicine has made pregnancy and its termination safe and reliable options. Reproduction can now be a matter of choice and not destiny for women and men. There will remain moral differences over these choices that ought to be explored and understood by clinicians in order to foster and enable authentic choice. Once a child is born alive, however, the situation changes almost entirely—there is priority of the interests of the child, as opposed to the wishes of the mother or the parents, as was considered in Chapter 7.

We will now go from life's beginning to life's end. In the next chapter, we examine some of the most recurring and disturbing issues in modern ethics, the issues connected with the care of the dying, the lost, and the dead. If life's beginning is about possibility and promise, then life's end may be more about destiny and purpose.

Cases For Discussion

CASE 1: A REPRODUCTIVE DILEMMA

You work as a healthcare professional in a clinic evaluating individuals and couples as to their suitability for IVF services. A young heterosexual couple, Mr and Ms J, with a history of infertility, linked to male and female factors, come for assessment. Both are deaf due to congenital hearing loss. Neither has a cochlear implant, but converse in sign language. They request help with getting pregnant and assistance as well with ensuring, by using PGD, (Preimplantation Genetic Diagnosis) that their child will be, like them, congenitally deaf. If pregnancy is successful, they intend to raise the child within the Deaf community and express their intention not to allow him or her to receive a cochlear implant.

Questions For Discussion

1. Should PGD or other forms of antenatal testing be used to screen for conditions that satisfy parental wishes as regards future offspring?
2. What if both parents were high-functioning Down's adults and wanted help with reproduction?

CASE 2: JUDGMENT OF SOLOMON

A 23-year old healthy female, Ms N, has decided to donate a few of her oocytes to a fertility centre and also act as a gestational mother for a upper middle-class couple seeking reproductive assistance. She is unemployed and will find the money from the oocyte harvesting ($5,000 per oocyte) quite helpful to pay her bills. She's unattached at the time of the donation and has never been pregnant. Her oocytes are successfully conjoined *in vitro* with male gametes and two are implanted in case one fails. Both are successful in achieving viability and she will deliver twins. The contracting parents are delighted. Ms N receives a handsome monthly retainer fee to offset the cost and inconvenience of pregnancy.

During her pregnancy, Ms N reads a magazine article arguing against surrogacy. It posits that surrogacy, such as she has undertaken, exploits poor women and treats offspring as chattel to be bought and sold, like calves at an auction. As her pregnancy progresses, she develops an increasing attachment to her embryonic duo and begins to consider keeping the babies. She then meets a partner who is willing to help her raise the children but is not able to support her financially. Ms N feels some twinges of guilt towards the contracting couple; she and her partner decide to offer one of the children to them at birth.

Questions For Discussion

1. Should there be a law preventing such arrangements? Why or why not?
2. Is dividing the twins between the two couples a fair compromise?
3. Who are the parents here? Does the answer change if the male gametes come from the ordering husband?

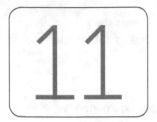

11

A Dark Wood
End-of-Life Decisions

The life of man, solitary, poor, nasty, brutish, and short.
Thomas Hobbes, 1651[1]

We are born in open field and die in a dark wood.
Russian proverb, n.d.

This Russian proverb reflects the pessimism with which, for most of human history, death has been viewed. Although religion can provide the promise of paradise in the afterlife, dying is something over which people have had little control and much to fear. The act and process of dying tends to be viewed (and indeed experienced) as "solitary, nasty, brutish" and, contrary to Hobbes' statement, is all too often anything but short, at least in modern times. In this chapter we look at how precedents in law and ethics have changed the process of dying in modern medicine. Although these precedents do not yet take death out of the woods, they do shed light on how patients, families, and healthcare providers may proceed to make dying a less forlorn journey.

I. Allowing Death: Refusals by the Patient

The option to forego treatment has by now become so well established in North American healthcare that to write about it now seems like reciting ancient history. Circumstances surrounding end-of-life decisions have changed considerably in medicine in the past 30 years.

Nancy B, a 25-year-old woman from Quebec, was hospitalized in 1988 with an unusual and extremely severe form of Guillain-Barré syndrome (an inflammatory nerve condition that usually resolves on its own with supportive care). In Ms B's case, the condition had resulted in an irreversible and almost complete decay of her respiratory motor nerves, so much that she could not breathe without the aid of a ventilator. Bedridden and hooked up to the ventilator every hour of every day, she was considered incurable but not "terminal" (she could be kept alive by technology indefinitely).

Nancy B expressed a firm and fixed wish in 1991 to be removed from the ventilator and be allowed to die—"life was no longer livable" for her. Could the hospital comply? it was asked.

Her request to be removed from respiratory support was seen as novel in the early 1990s. (In fact it wasn't; there were many similar cases from other jurisdictions such as the US.) Her care providers worried they might be charged with negligence or assisted suicide if they acquiesced to Ms B's request. This was not an unfounded concern. Section 215c of Canada's *Criminal Code* requires care providers to provide the "necessaries of life" to a person under their charge "if that person (i) is unable, by reason of detention, age, illness, mental disorder or other cause, to withdraw himself from that charge, and (ii) is unable to provide himself with necessaries of life."[2] Moreover, section 217 concerns "the duty of persons undertaking acts": "Every one who undertakes to do an act is under a legal duty to do it if an omission to do the act is or may be dangerous to life."[3]

Together these sections suggest treatment cannot be stopped if doing so might constitute a threat to the life of a patient who is dependent on others for care. If so, how do these provisions in law square with the liberty and privacy rights of competent persons to be free from unwanted interventions? The answer is not very well at all (aspects of the *Criminal Code* as they pertain to assisted suicide would indeed be found unconstitutional in 2012 for these very reasons—this will be discussed later in this chapter).

The Quebec Superior Court ruled that stopping Ms B's ventilator would not be culpable negligence but a reasonable treatment option and therefore should be allowed: "What Nancy B is seeking, relying on the principle of autonomy and her right of self-determination, is that the respiratory support treatment being given her cease so that nature may take its course; that she be freed from slavery to a machine as her life depends on it." This, the Court recognized, would require the assistance of another person—her doctor—to remove the ventilator. This, too, the Court allowed, as it was not considered suicide or assisted suicide but merely allowing "the disease [to] take its natural course."[4]

BOX 11.1

"The duty of the State to preserve life must encompass a recognition of an individual's right to avoid circumstances in which the individual himself would feel that efforts to sustain life demean or degrade his humanity."[5]

The bottom line: Nancy B's life was unacceptable to *her*. Core aspects of her life—her extreme disability, dependence on others, loss of privacy, loss of dignity—could not be "palliated." It is respecting the patient's point of view, the value of treatment as she sees it, which is the key to doing the right thing.

Little legal risk

Once the right to refuse life-sustaining care was clarified at a national level in Canada, it allowed end-of-life decisions to usually be made *consensually* by a competent patient, his or her doctor, and the family (or substitute decision-maker). Section 216 of the *Criminal Code* expects clinicians, in the exercise of their due skill, to act with "reasonable knowledge, skill and care."[6] Objectionable acts, ones open to criminal prosecution for criminal negligence, would be those done with "wanton or reckless disregard for the lives or safety of other persons" (section 219).[7] Healthcare professionals can stop life-sustaining treatment, *providing* they do so carefully and exercise the "standard of care." (As we shall see, however, the definition of a standard of care for end-of-life decisions is a contested notion.)

"Almost everything else physicians do (or do not do) puts them at greater risk of legal liability than withdrawing or withholding treatment in appropriate cases."[8] The courts invariably find that the laws governing suicide or homicide do not apply to such treatment decisions when made "in good faith" and by the patient's informed choice.[9] That the patient does not initiate the underlying death-inducing condition distinguishes such treatment decisions from suicide (and so the actions of professionals in such instances would not be considered "assisted suicide") (see Box 11.2).

BOX 11.2

"Refusing medical intervention merely allows the disease to take its natural course; if death were eventually to occur, it would be the result, primarily, of the underlying disease, and not the result of a self-inflicted injury."[10]

In some cases the patient's wishes are less clear and so have to be surmised by those who know the patient best. This has sometimes been referred to as "substituted judgment," a poor term in that it suggests someone else's judgment takes the place of the patient's. This is, of course, not the idea—instead, the decision-maker is obligated to make the decision the patient would have made in the circumstances if capable.

CASE 11.1 A DEATH NOT FORETOLD

Mr G, a 76-year-old male patient, handsome still, a true "gentleman" of the old school, is found unresponsive in his house by his granddaughter. Brought to the ER, he is put on a ventilator because his respiratory status is declining. Over the next day, no cause for his deterioration is found. His brain CT is normal, toxic screen negative, septic workup unrevealing, and the rest of his blood work unremarkable. On the second day, Mr G's 51-year-old daughter requests cessation of the ventilator, saying her father would never have wanted to be kept alive by machines.

Should the care providers abide by her wish?

DISCUSSION OF CASE 11.1

This real-life case was hard because Mr G had previously been well and the cause for his sudden decline was a mystery. In uncertainty, it is unwise to "give up" on a patient, so the health professionals explored the rationale for removing life support.

The patient's family physician and psychiatrist were contacted. Was the patient depressed? Yes, but not suicidal. Would he have wanted to be rescued in this circumstance? Not likely, although no living will could be produced. Mr G had suffered a number of losses—a sister to cancer, a wife to dementia—but he had also made a recent trip to the "old country" where he had reconciled with a long-estranged offspring. He had subsequently told his family doctor he had achieved a sense of resolution and was prepared to die. The doctor at the time put little stock in those words but it was only a month later that Mr G was found in a comatose state. Did he cause it? No one could answer that question but all who knew him were aware he would not thank them for saving him even if they could do so. That fact, plus his ongoing decline, was sufficient to tip the decision in favour of the daughter's request. It was not a happy decision but seemed right in the circumstances. The patient was removed from the ventilator and died peacefully within minutes.

The refusal of life-sustaining treatment by a patient (or a family) should not always be accepted at face value as an "autonomous" choice. The prudent and caring professional must always consider distracting features of the patient's life, such as disabilities, alcoholism, or psychiatric illness, that may undermine unbiased decision-making. Sometimes treatment refusals are precipitated by problems such as unhealthy family relationships, poor communication, or a lack of empathy or caring. Patients who feel uncared for may seek "negative" ways (by appearing resistant, by harming themselves) in order to get *more* care and attention, not less.

The values driving medical decision-making here, as elsewhere, should be the patient's values and not the values of others or the "values of technology." We can try to ensure this by understanding the patient's situation (see Box 11.3).[11, 12]

BOX 11.3

Conditions for the "proper" cessation of treatment include the following:

- the request is made by a competent informed patient;
- the request is consistent with the patient's beliefs, values and attitudes;
- the decision is freely made neither with coercion nor under circumstances such as severe depression, drug use, etc.;
- alternative forms of treatment and support have been explored and offer no further help to the patient;
- the patient's condition or illness would be considered by a neutral observer to be reasonable grounds for the wish to stop treatment.

As Case 11.1 suggests, care must be taken when the patient cannot participate in the decision-making process. The following is one such case where the team may have bent too far backwards to accommodate a family's wishes.

CASE 11.2 A SHOCKING SHOT

Mr V, an active 80-year-old man with coronary artery disease, is admitted with a large and serious, but quite survivable, self-inflicted gunshot wound to the side of his face. He had become despondent as the primary caregiver for his spouse with advanced dementia but had never been treated for a psychiatric disorder. Neither suicide note nor advance directive is found. At the time of admission to the ICU Mr V appears neurologically intact but is heavily sedated and intubated to protect his airway. A plastic surgeon seeks consent for the surgical repair of his facial injury from the appropriate substitute decision-makers, Mr V's two grown children.

Surprising to staff, they refuse consent on the grounds that he has "suffered enough" and that, at his age, further intensive treatment would not work. They request all treatment be withdrawn and their father be allowed to die.

What should be the response to the children's refusal of consent?

DISCUSSION OF CASE 11.2

Mr V's children have doubts regarding the helpfulness of treating their father's depression. "Who wouldn't want to die at his age with his problems?" they seem to say. However, depression in an 80-year-old can be just as amenable to treatment as depression in a younger person. (See also the discussion of suicide notes in Case 7.6.)

Discussion with the children should be continued and vigorously pursued to enable the necessary immediate clinical interventions, such as surgery, to be undertaken for Mr V. Later, more definitive assessment and management of his mental status and home situation should be initiated.

FOLLOW-UP TO CASE 11.2

After much cajoling and discussion, the children finally assent to the needed plastic surgery for their father. Surgery is long but successful in closing the wound. Unfortunately, on day 1 postoperatively, Mr V's bowel is accidentally punctured when a feeding tube is inserted. He quickly becomes very ill with peritonitis. As the patient is still obtunded, consent is sought from the children who, once again, refuse surgery, saying they "never should have agreed in the first place."

Lacking consent from the children, a consultant gastro-intestinal (GI) surgeon refuses to intervene. ("They're the next of kin. What can I do?") The plastic surgeon quarrels with the GI surgeon. An ethicist who is called in tries to mediate this discussion by asking the disputing surgeons: "What would you do if it were *your* father?"

The plastic surgeon immediately replies he would of course perform the operation. The GI surgeon, surprisingly, expresses reluctance to get involved, not on account of ageism *per se*, but because she feels this patient is on a relentless downward spiral. Surgery is not performed and so, not surprisingly, the patient expires several days later, never regaining consciousness.

DISCUSSION OF THE FOLLOW-UP TO CASE 11.2

Was Mr V's demise inevitable? (The relative ease, it seems, with which his problem could have been fixed is one distinguishing feature as compared with the situation in the previous case.) This question is hard to answer—judgments about "downward spirals" are often complex clinical judgments. Expense or resource shortfall (for example, availability of personnel or operating room time) was not an issue, so in one sense the case's resolution was not unjust. But the outcome could still be unjust if consideration of age alone was used to deny the patient potentially beneficial care. If the team felt the best interests of the patient were being thwarted by the children's refusal, counsel could have been obtained to have their status as decision-makers for Mr V evaluated in court or a regional tribunal.

Inappropriate requests to stop treatment

We have seen, throughout this book, cases where requests to stop potentially helpful treatment and life support have been made for various less than optimal reasons—negative transference (Case 1.4), misunderstood capacity (Case 6.8, p, 137), and misguided autonomy (Case 2.6). Such requests may be inappropriate if they fail to explore alternatives or too readily agree to treatment limitations—sometimes for the "wrong" reasons.[13]

Health professionals who experience patients in a negative way may collude in a patient's resistance to treatment by seeing the patient as "deserving" of death. "Negative transferences" are the hostile or futile reactions or "projections" from health professionals towards the resistant, severely disabled, or "unlikable" patient.[14] These reactions can manifest themselves as a too ready acceptance of death of patients with severe disabilities by clinicians and by patients themselves. Negative attitudes towards the so-called hopeless case must be thoroughly explored before treatment cessation decisions are made.

CASE 11.3 NO CRAP VERSUS NO CPR

A 58-year-old homeless man, Mr X, with no known relatives, is admitted in respiratory distress with resistant tuberculosis. Emaciated and disheveled, he looks 20 years older than his stated age. His verbal communication is minimal. Confined to a ward, he undergoes various procedures including bronchoscopy and urinary catheterization. Although he does not specifically verbalize a refusal to the procedures, he is resistant and difficult. He yells at the staff, spills his food tray ("I can get better food on the street!"), and repeatedly pulls out his tubes ("What is all this crap for? Get it off me!").

At one point during his hospitalization, Mr X is approached about the issue of cardio-pulmonary resuscitation (CPR). If his heart stops, would he want them to try to restart it? "What?" he said. "What kind of crap is this? I don't want any more crap!" He turns away from the staff and refuses any further discussion. The staff takes this as meaning he does not want CPR. They do not return to discuss the No CPR order that is entered on his chart. He arrests three weeks later and dies. CPR is not performed.

Why is there cause for concern in Mr X's care?

DISCUSSION OF CASE 11.3

Although anyone has the right to refuse potentially life-saving treatment, refusals should be properly explored. Saying one wants "no more crap" seems a bit different than saying one does not want CPR.

Mr X had several "red flags" for less than optimal management— he was homeless, impoverished, and difficult medically and personally; he had previously refused treatment and looked as if he was at the end of his life. Maybe he was, but his care providers could have been a little more diligent about assessing his wishes. (Of course, one can question the whole matter: should they have raised CPR with him in the first place? Would he have benefitted from it? A more appropriate discussion might have focused on how sick he was and on his likely imminent demise.)[15] On the face of things, it is not clear what he wanted. The decision about CPR did not appear to take place as part of an overall treatment plan. Mr X's refusal of "crap" may have been less a refusal of care than an acerbic observation on the state of his care. That being said, some patients are difficult to assess and a patient who has spent a lifetime refusing assistance— Mr X's true self may be seen in his past consistent behaviour to avoid medical care—may, finally, get his wishes met.

End-of-life studies

Care that concedes the inevitability of death and focuses on the prospect of a "natural death" is increasingly recognized as appropriate. Any kind of care, be it feeding or artificial breathing, be it considered "ordinary" or "extraordinary," may be stopped or withheld. Stopping dialysis is, for example, the second leading cause of death in patients with End Stage Renal Disease (ESRD) in Canada and the third in the United States.[16] In 2002 it was reported that 28 per cent of patient deaths with ESRD in New England followed treatment cessation.[17]

Other forms of life-sustaining treatment including cardio-pulmonary resuscitation, intravenous fluids, antibiotics, and artificial feeding are not infrequently stopped for patients with irreversible multi-organ failure, terminal malignancies, advanced cognitive impairment, coma, and other end-stage conditions. In fact, the majority of all ICU deaths, up to 85 per cent, are preceded by a decision to forego life support on the basis of either being incompatible with the patient's wishes or no longer being helpful.[18]

II. Advance Directives

Clinicians vary widely in end-of-life decisions in different countries.[19] One way to address this disparity and make decision-making more patient-responsive is through the completion of a "living will." Living wills were originally advocated by "right to die" groups in the 1970s, and included vague directives refusing "extraordinary treatment" if the person was "irreversibly ill."[20] In the US, under the *Patient Self-Determination Act*, hospitals must ask patients on admission if they have such documents.

Living wills are also known as "advance (not advanced!) directives." They may state in writing what sort of treatment the person would accept or reject if ill (an "instruction directive") and/or may name others, the "substitute decision-maker(s)," prepared to make medical decisions for the person in case of his or her incapacity (in some places, this is a "power of attorney" [POA] for personal care). The more precise the advance instructions, the easier it may be for families to let their ailing relative die "naturally," without technological encumbrances.[21]

Not having spelled out in advance the limits of care, irreversibly critically ill patients may be overtreated, resulting in, for example, unwanted burdensome care[22] and unnecessary trips to the hospital.[23] This may contribute to large, unwanted, and avoidable expenditures prior to death.[24] Although living wills may exaggerate the patient's ability to predict or control his or her future medical care and state of life,[25] well-crafted advance directives can better align treatment with the patient's preferences and will increasingly be used to direct care.[26] (See below, "Life, Hope, and the ICU.")

On the other hand, an advance directive can create a barrier to the true communication of a patient's intent if others take an overly rigid approach to it.[27] In addition, many patients do not always want their directives strictly followed and are willing to give surrogates the right to override their wishes.[28]

Then there is the question as to whether one can or should follow all prior wishes.[29]

Consider the case of a man who, when younger and well, shunned pills and analgesics, putting up with root canals without anaesthetic. Now incapacitated by dementia and suffering from a fractured hip, is he to be denied drugs for pain relief despite howling in pain? Even if he had gone so far as to write that into an advance directive, are we obliged to abide by it?

III. Who Is the Patient?

"The past," Karl Marx wrote, "weighs like a nightmare on the brain of the living."[30] Indeed it can, especially for those brains transfixed by the past. The influence of the past on the present is all too often the new contested territory between families and healthcare professionals. The battle to refuse care having been won, the struggle has now become, for some, one of obtaining whatever care the patient wants or, purportedly, would have wanted. Many of us are re-born as we age—or at least we come to lead lives we could not have predicted. It is our families who often have the hardest time adapting to the "new self" and accepting "natural" limits to care. Not surprising, sick patients[31, 32] and their surrogates[33] may misinterpret their condition and their future, seeing them in a rosier fashion than they actually are. This may impair realistic assessments of the usefulness of aggressive care.

In 1998 Mr Sawatsky was a 79-year-old resident of a nursing home with advanced Parkinson's disease and multiple other co-morbidities including previous strokes. These had resulted in severe cognitive impairment, limited communication, and difficulty swallowing. Despite having a tracheostomy to protect his airway, he experienced repeated episodes of pneumonia. After one such bout, the treating physician decided Mr Sawatsky's condition was deteriorating such that he would not benefit from "calling a code."[34] Previous attempts to write a No CPR order had been met with resistance from Mrs Sawatsky who some clinicians felt had an unrealistic understanding of her husband's capabilities and limitations. The physician wrote the order in Mr Sawatsky's chart but did not discuss it with his wife.

Several months earlier, Mrs Sawatsky had refused consent for the tracheostomy which led to the public trustee taking over as the substitute decision-maker for her husband. The public trustee was contacted by the physician about the No CPR order but declined to be involved, seeing this as having to do with "non-treatment" rather than active treatment. When Mrs Sawatsky eventually discovered such an order had been written, she sought and received a court ruling to block this.[35]

With the aid of a retrospectoscope, there are aspects of this case's management that may have predicted the trip to court. First, there was a communication problem that was not resolved before the No CPR order was written. Second, why did the doctor think Mr Sawatsky could benefit from a tracheostomy then and *not* from CPR now? Did Mrs Sawatsky appreciate that the tracheostomy tube could prevent problems and maintain comfort whereas performing CPR would do neither? Third, it appears the No CPR order was written without input from other clinicians. Fourth, the order was not communicated to Mrs Sawatsky in a respectful way—she found out only after the fact, a circumstance that may have made the order appear untrustworthy. Had these issues been addressed, it is *possible* this trip to court could have been avoided (see Box 11.4). But there would have to be agreement that the question as to "*who* should make the decision?" should be replaced by "*how* will the decision be made?" This would require efforts on both sides to "talk it out."[36]

As it turned out, Mr Sawatsky was transferred to another institution where, presumably, his wife's wishes were accommodated.

BOX 11.4

A decision not to resuscitate should "be, as well be seen to be, well thought out. The reasoning and criteria applied by the physician should be sufficiently clear so any decision can be supported should it be questioned later."[37]

No CPR orders

A cardiac arrest can be a devastating situation; even if CPR is "successful"—and success, even in the best case scenarios, is far from certain—patients or their SDMs need to be made aware of the risks of multi-organ failure (in particular the risk of neurological injury) and the very likely (except in rare cases) necessity of life support. This is, however, a state in evolution.[38]

The problem is how to limit the use of CPR to patients for whom it would be beneficial.[39] To this end, by a consensus of opinion from a variety of healthcare authorities, a "basic national guideline for use by all those involved in the care of the terminally ill," was released in 1994[40] and is still considered the standard of care in Canada in this area.[41]

This document delineates three groups of patients: (1) those for whom CPR is likely to be successful or for whom CPR is of uncertain help (CPR will be done unless they object), (2) those for whom CPR, even if "successful," is not likely to return them to their pre-arrest state (CPR will only be done if requested), and (3) those for for whom survival is unprecedented or who are "permanently unable to experience any benefit" (CPR should not be offered as an option).

The legal reliability of these guidelines has not been often tested but, until recently, opinion would likely have been that professionals who follow them in offering or not offering CPR to patients would be seen as taking "due care." Communication with the patient and family early in the hospital stay is critical for getting the intensity of care just right.[42, 43]

In a Manitoba case, the Court of Appeal was asked to rule on the refusal by two parents to consent to a No CPR order on their 13-month-old who was in a persistent vegetative state. The Court found that parental consent for a No CPR order was not required and physicians had the exclusive authority to withhold this treatment. The Court held that:

> Whether or not such a direction [No CPR] should be issued is a judgment call for the doctor to make having regard to the patient's history and condition and the doctor's evaluation of the hopelessness of the case. The wishes of the patient's family or guardians should be taken into account but neither their consent nor the approval of a court is required.[44]

Life, hope and the ICU

In Ontario, a different ruling occurred.[45] Here the Superior Court of Justice refused to uphold a lower tribunal's ruling that two daughters were acting inappropriately for their mother, an 81-year-old patient hospitalized with end-stage dementia (for whom treatment abatement and a No CPR order had been recommended by critical care providers).[46] Despite their mother being bed-bound, unaware of her surroundings, and suffering, her daughters had refused to consider any diminution in her treatment (they refused, for example, the suggestion that she not be re-admitted to the ICU) because she had said, some years previously, "Where there's life, there's hope."

This statement, one that many may say in an offhand way, was taken in two entirely different ways. Her daughters interpreted this as meaning that health professionals should stop at nothing to keep her alive. The healthcare team (and the lower tribunal) considered it to be virtually devoid of meaning and too vague to direct care in *any* way. Lacking a patient wish applicable to the circumstances, the team wanted to treat her according to the "standard of care" which does not require the provision of non-beneficial care. (The lower tribunal—the Consent and Capacity Board—had agreed with that.)

Her daughters, by contrast, saw their mother's statement in a very uncompromising way: they could not imagine *any* circumstance of life in which their mother would not want to be kept alive. The Court ruled that the team (and the tribunal) should *not* have dismissed the patient's vaguely expressed statement and so overruled the ruling of the tribunal that had replaced the daughters as her decision-makers. The patient's vague statement ought to play a role, the Court ruled.

Persons making grand statements about end-of-life care—whether in writing or in the spoken word ("I want everything . . . ") should be careful who may be listening. They might get more than they bargained for: yoked to a Procrustean bed of technology at life's end because some relative or court takes such statements too literally. Of course, on any reasonable understanding of advance directives, patients should be able to ask only for medical options within the standard of care. Such statements should not be interpreted as a legal means to torture patients with the exquisite and extravagant technologies of "life support." The courts have ruled, as in the *Malette v. Shulman* case, that deeply held objections to treatment should not be held to the "transitory" standards of reasonableness of the day. Although that might be fine for *refusals* of treatment, what about requests *for* treatment? Refusals of treatment are easier as they involve *not* doing something, but requests for treatment involve an obligation on the part of someone to *provide* that care. How far do such obligations extend?

IV. Lost Souls

One area where values can seem to clash is in the debate over those who are "almost dead," but not dead yet—especially those patients in a "persistent" or "permanent" vegetative state (PVS).[47] Obviously, without the miracles of modern medicine, such patients would never survive. With these "miracles," such patients can survive for a long, long time.

The legal and moral acceptability of withdrawing life support from PVS patients has been recognized. In 1976, the New Jersey Supreme Court ruled that Karen Ann Quinlan, a young woman in a PVS for almost a year, had a constitutional "right to privacy" to forego treatment, specifically the ventilator, given her poor quality of life ("no reasonable possibility of the patient returning to a cognitive, sapient state"). This right could be exercised on her behalf by her parents.[48]

Since the *Quinlan* ruling, courts and jurisdictions across North America have recognized a broad right of relatives or the courts to stop treatment in PVS patients.[49, 50] Similar precedents have been set in Ireland and the UK.[51]

Nonetheless, one dilemma is that PVS patients are not yet dead and sometimes seem to recover some level of awareness. The latter indicates the difficulty of distinguishing true PVS from the "minimally aware/conscious" state. Even if a PVS patient "lightens" a little in terms of unconsciousness, he or she will almost certainly remain profoundly neurologically impaired and never regain true awareness. There is some evidence that some patients in deep comatose-like states—up to 19 per cent in one study—indicate an ability to respond to verbal stimulus by exciting the same areas of their cortex as do uninjured persons.[52] What this means is unknown, with doubts having been cast on the validity of the methods in these studies.[53]

CASE 11.4 THE LONGEST GOODBYE

Hassan Rasouli was a patient in his late 50s admitted to a large teaching hospital in Toronto in 2010 for removal of a benign brain tumour. Unfortunately, he declined into a PVS after developing meningitis post-operatively. He has since been diagnosed as being in a minimally conscious state. Neither of these states are states of death *per se*, as some part of the brain, likely a very rudimentary part, is still functioning. Yet neither state is compatible with sentience or personhood. Patients such as Mr Rasouli require 24-hour complete care, tube feeding, and, sometimes, artificial respiratory support.

At issue in this case was whether aggressive medical care (admission to the ICU, ventilation) was of benefit to Mr Rasouli and who should make the decision as to what treatment was beneficial.

It was the consensus of the critical care team that the burdensomeness of ICU care for Mr Rasouli was not balanced by any benefit to him. Mr Rasouli's wife disagreed with this assessment and wanted his life-support continued indefinitely. By contrast, the clinicians predicted that his very minimal neurological state would never change and so intensive care was only prolonging his suffering. His physicians sought relief in court from the duty to provide life-sustaining care and asked for permission to remove it without family consent, (*and* without judicial review), arguing such care was non-beneficial (and, as such, not the "standard of care"). In doing so, they were following established end-of-life care guidelines, such as the ones regarding CPR. Ultimately, at trial, this argument did not help the clinicians. The Ontario Court of Appeal directed the physicians to carry on treating Mr Rasouli aggressively, as opposed to palliatively.[54] It opined that consent by the family for non-treatment was required since, in order to abate treatment (e.g., remove the ventilator), palliative care then needed to be offered. This in turn would necessitate the administration of a *positive* treatment. For example, patients are normally sedated with drugs while being removed from a ventilator.

One could not, from the Court's perspective, separate out the withdrawal of care from the provision of palliative measures and so, as the family was refusing the latter, life-sustaining treatment could not be withdrawn. The Court's finding of a duty to seek consent for non-treatment—deemed a "Rasouli consent"—by one observer[55]—seemed odd. By this ruling, you could be found guilty of battery for *failing* to touch someone if consent for non-treatment was not obtained. The argument can be made, however, that ceasing treatment is active treatment as it does involve touching the patient, e.g., in removing the patient from a ventilator.

So, how should treatment decisions be made in such cases?

Trouble with families

Intractable disagreements with families deserve careful ethical analysis before going the legal route. What are the particular issues families have with their relative's care? Are the family's requests based on the patient's autonomous wishes and/or the patient's best interests? Or, do they arise out of family issues, for example, not being able to let go, unresolved guilt feelings that are then projected onto medical professionals, or something as venal as financial considerations? In such difficult situations with families, healthcare professionals must step back and initiate and continue conversations.[56] Exploration of how the family is feeling and learning about the family dynamics rather than getting into an adversarial relationship is important, but not always possible.

BOX 11.5

When working with families:[57]

- assess understanding: Ask: "What have you been told about your [relative]'s condition?"
- assess feelings: Say: "It must be very hard to see your [relative] like this."
- assess cultural factors: What are their fundamental beliefs? What are their views about suffering? The nature of death? The role of technology?
- assess for guilt or fears: Listen for statements such as: "I can't live without [relative]."
- allow for information handling: Suggest, "You may have more questions later. Write them down and we'll discuss them." State a definite time and be there.
- avoid using jargon and value-laden words and phrases that can mislead or appear to denigrate the patient, for example, "vegetable" (demeaning); "doing everything" (not possible); "restart his or her heart" (rarely that easy); "brain dead" (such a patient is simply dead).
- avoid asking the family to shoulder too much of the burden of decision-making, for example, asking families, "Do you want to keep [your relative] alive?"

One-sided decisions?

At issue is what has been called "unilateral decision-making" by physicians: may physicians withhold life-sustaining care such as CPR without family consent when they think it will not be of benefit? Or is benefit something only families can decide? The College of Physicians and Surgeons of Manitoba in 2008 adopted end-of-life guidelines allowing physicians in limited circumstances to end life-support to patients without requiring family consent. Treatment is not necessary if it cannot achieve "the maintenance of or recovery to a level of cerebral function that enable patients to: achieve awareness of self; achieve awareness of existence; and experience his or her own environment." Moreover, a "physician cannot be compelled by a patient, proxy, representative or member of the patient's family to provide treatment that is not in accordance with the current standard of care."[58]

This is generally the law of the land: where treatment is offered or not by a clinician, so long as "usual care" is followed, the courts are unlikely to question it . . . usually, anyway.

DISCUSSION OF CASE 11.4

The Rasouli case was reviewed by the Supreme Court of Canada (SCC) in 2013.[59] Its ruling was not surprising: where the dispute with families concerns end-of-life care, clinicians must make use of the available dispute mechanisms—such as the Consent and Capacity Review Board in Ontario. This does not mean that families have an unfettered right to whatever care they want, no matter how inappropriate that might be or that healthcare professionals must defer to unprofessional requests for treatment made by patients and/or their families. (As we have seen in earlier chapters, healthcare professionals make decisions every day about what treatment options are and are not to be offered to patients.) But it does mean that, in some circumstances, a tribunal may disagree with a physician's judgment that the continuing life support is not appropriate. "A physician's duty of care may require that treatment not be withdrawn despite the physician's ethical objections to its administration."[60] Clinicians have the option of seeking higher judicial review of disputed cases or seeking transfer of the patient to another facility.

A limit to choice?

The SCC in Rasouli puts great faith in judicial tribunals for performing independent and unbiased reviews of contentious decisions. While this provides an administrative way of "resolving" a problem, it does not address the deeper moral issues at stake. Hopelessly "minimally conscious" states could be ones of utter hell. The indefinite support requested by some families for patients in a PVS, with the hope that the person who the patient once was will be "found," seems uncompromising and unrealistic as regards the return of sapient life.

When persons are lost at sea or in the wilderness, rescue efforts are appropriate but do not, and *cannot*, go on forever. It is assumed—after reasonable search and rescue efforts—that the persons are irrecoverably lost and presumed dead. After a period of time, even the search for world celebrities, such as Amelia Earhart, is called off. (In Earhart's case the search lasted three weeks in 1937 at a cost at the time of several million US dollars.) This may seem unfair or ungenerous—and indeed stories of miraculous rescues do occur—but it is a social decision that only so many resources can be expended on the rescue of one lost soul. Patients in a PVS state are truly lost souls—the overwhelming majority are irrecoverably lost—with their higher brain functions, their cerebrum, damaged to such an extent that the persons they once were will never be again. (They would fail to meet the Manitoba College's "minimal state" required to authorize treatment.) They survive only because their brainstem may be intact and their vital functions supported artificially.

Would it not be more dignified to "call off the search and rescue" operations after a "reasonable" period of time? What would be a reasonable time is a contentious issue as the thorny issues of futility and of the expensive costs of providing "futile" care inevitably come up. (The best metaphor for futility is the notion of trying to carry water in a sieve—in Greek mythology the daughters of Danaus were sentenced to an eternity of trying to fill a huge urn using only sieves—an impossible task.) That intensive care is very expensive cannot be ignored. Patients are due "reasonable care"— care that follows reasonable guidelines and makes reasonable attempts at rescue. When rescue goes awry or is very unlikely to succeed, then continued efforts become harder to justify. Exactly when a rescue attempt should be aborted will vary with the circumstances of each case, but end it must. The more the costs escalate, the more careful must be one's rationale for the ongoing rescue attempts. One must consider all the others who may be affected by excessive efforts at rescue. As we saw in the chapter on justice, prioritizing one patient means posteriorizing others. "Shared goals of care" (see Chapter 9) is the route to look for from the very beginning.

Where the costs of continued rescue arise, discussions should not take place behind closed doors but at or near the patient's bedside. (I say that as I think "local" decision-making is better than turning to the courts or tribunals and helps avoid the perception that healthcare providers are doing something secretly and illicitly.) The potentially diverging views of life, death, and suffering should be explored. Obviously, such discussions with families can be very difficult. By listening more and talking less we may better understand a family's concerns over the clinical course of the patient—especially if that course is a downward one toward death—and help them cope with the death of their loved one.[61] The right words and tone can help.[62] ("We left no stone unturned in trying to help your loved one from this deeply comatose state. All the evidence points to an irrecoverable loss of consciousness and of self. It's time we talked about letting him go . . . ") "Clinicians must be willing and able to have difficult discussions with patients and their loved ones . . . and craft recommendations for care that are evidence based yet framed by the patient's values."[63] This requires clinicians to be aware of, sensitive to, and try to incorporate, if possible, the patient's cultural values.

V. Physician-Accelerated Death (PAD)

Medical care that allows an underlying condition to result in death, through withdrawal or withholding of treatment, and that eases a patient's passing, through "palliative care," should be distinguished from "physician-accelerated death" (PAD). In the latter, the clinician, typically a physician, plays an active role in the death of the patient, either by "euthanasia" (EU) or "assisted suicide" (AS). Although palliative care "assists" patients in the dying process, it does not typically *aim* to shorten the patient's life.[64]

In physician-assisted suicide (PAS) the clinician knowingly provides the means of inducing death (such as prescribing a lethal dose of medication), but the final act inducing death is performed by the patient. Although suicide has been legalized in Canada, helping another do so is not (see Box 11.6). More controversial than PAS is EU where the professional is responsible for actually carrying out the final death-inducing action.

BOX 11.6 THE *CRIMINAL CODE* OF CANADA

Everyone who

(a) counsels a person to commit suicide, or
(b) aids or abets a person to commit suicide,

whether suicide ensues or not, is guilty of an indictable offence and liable to imprisonment for a term not exceeding 14 years.[65]

"Euthanasia" is defined in the *Oxford English Dictionary* as "bringing about a gentle and easy death, especially in the case of incurable and painful disease." Although this sounds innocuous enough, it has been considered an unacceptable task for physicians since Hippocrates ("I will give no deadly drug . . . "). In the controversial form of EU the healthcare professional intentionally causes a patient's death through direct means, such as injecting a lethal drug. Since in many jurisdictions, Canada included, there is no legal entity such as "compassionate homicide," deliberately ending the life of another by EU could be considered murder, irrespective of the patient's condition, consent, or compliance.

Palliative care may need to use escalating doses of drugs such as narcotics for pain control but there is little evidence, if used "properly," that this causes an earlier death of the patient.[66] While death *will* almost certainly take place with "advanced" palliation such as continuous deep sedation, the distinction from PAD should be obvious. The patient's death is not the purpose of treatment, unlike PAD. When death occurs in palliative care, it is accepted as an unavoidable consequence of easing the patient's dying process. This is known as the doctrine of "double-effect": an unwanted outcome is morally acceptable if there is no other way of achieving the good effect.

Sue R's plea

Sue Rodriguez was a 42-year-old Canadian woman in the advanced stages of amyotrophic lateral sclerosis (ALS). When life became intolerable, she hoped to be able to obtain help from a physician to end her life if she could not do so on her own. This wish conflicted with section 241(b) of the *Criminal Code* prohibiting assisted suicide, so Ms R went to the courts to challenge the law.[67]

As suicide itself has been decriminalized in Canada since 1972, the SCC was asked to consider whether this prohibition on assisted suicide interfered with the Charter rights of personal autonomy and security of the person (section 7) as well as equality (section 15) of a person so disabled she could not commit suicide on her own.

The Supremes decide

In 1993 by a 5-to-4 margin, the Court voted to uphold the prohibition against assisted suicide.[68] According to the majority, "the respect for human dignity, while one of the underlying principles upon which our society is based, is not a principle of fundamental justice within the meaning of s. 7." The majority expressed concern there would be no safeguards to distinguish more legitimate cases of assisted suicide from illegitimate cases of involuntary euthanasia. This, in turn, could open the floodgates to the wholesale murder of vulnerable disabled persons.

The opposing judges by contrast were more swayed by the argument that the desire of patients to control their dying was "an integral part of living." Chief Justice Lamer recommended a constitutional exemption for Ms R if certain conditions were met:

- she would have to be certified competent by two physicians;
- her request for assisted suicide would have to be freely made;
- a physician would have to be present at the assisted suicide;
- the act causing death could only be performed by her alone.

The judgment and its surrounding arguments made no difference to Ms R. She committed suicide with someone's assistance in 1994. No one was ever charged.

Assisted suicide (AS) redux

The illegality of assisted suicide in Canada was challenged in 2011 before the BC Supreme Court (BCSC) by, among others, a 63-year-old BC woman, Gloria Taylor. Like Sue Rodriguez, she suffered from ALS. Ms Taylor wanted to preserve her dignity and face death on her own terms by having the option of AS when her suffering became too great. The presiding judge ruled that to deny a disabled person assistance at death was to deny that individual an option available to a non-disabled person (suicide not being a criminal act), and therefore discriminatory in an unjust way. Unlike the SCC, the BCSC viewed dignity as a fundamental construct. Distinguishing the case of *Rodriguez*, Justice Smith concluded that the law is overbroad and "the legislative response—an absolute prohibition—is grossly disproportionate to the objectives it is meant to accomplish."[69] In her 2012 ruling, the justice gave the federal government one year to fix the law and granted Ms Taylor a constitutional exemption from the law. Ms Taylor never exercised this option as she died of an acute illness in July 2012. In 2013 the BC Court of Appeal, in a 2–1 decision, upheld the law prohibiting AS, ruling against the BCSC.[70]

Public and professional views: a house divided

In 2012, a UK Commission on Assisted Dying recommended decriminalizing AS[71] as did two new Canadian reports, one from the Collège des Médecins du Quebec in 2009[72] and the other from the Royal Society. The 2011 Royal Society report by well-known authorities provides perhaps the most comprehensive overview of the arguments and evidence concerning this topic.[73]

Public opinion polls since at least the early 1990s in Canada and the US have revealed widespread public support for some form of physician-accelerated death, but the public remains divided.[74, 75] Opinions among healthcare professionals are also divided although many are sympathetic to patient requests for some form of PAD, with PAS being the most common. In a 1993 Alberta survey, 44 per cent of physicians supported active euthanasia and 51 per cent felt it should be legalized. If legalized, 28 per cent were prepared to practise it.[76] In a 1998 study, about one-quarter of US healthcare professionals surveyed expressed support of "physician-assisted death" (meaning something more than palliative care) although few were prepared to practise it.[77] Similarly in 2000 a minority of oncologists supported PAS and even fewer supported euthanasia.[78] The figures from a 2003 study of family physicians showed 39 per cent in favour of PAS, with 44 per cent opposed; even if legalized, 58 per cent said they would not practise it.[79]

In 2013, Donald Low, a highly respected Infectious Disease specialist in Toronto, died of a brain stem tumour. Eight days before death he made an impassioned video decrying the absence of compassionate PAD in Canada.[80] It would be surprising if events such as this dampened support in the community for some form of AD. For many, Dr Low's video is an indictment of the limits of care at life's end.

Legalizing suicide with drugs dispensed by physicians—PAS, in effect—passed by popular vote in Oregon in 1994 and has since been reaffirmed.[81] PAS is legal in the states of Montana and Washington, being seriously considered in the province of Quebec, and allowed under the law, along with euthanasia, in various European countries such as the Netherlands, Luxembourg, Belgium, and Switzerland.[82]

Let us consider some of the more common positions for and against PAD.

Reasons for professionals to oppose PAD

Implications for public policy
There may be serious risks in allowing aid in dying, namely, that others might be injured by such practices for two broad reasons:

1. The challenge of how to "draw the line": should anyone be able to access PAD or just the terminally ill? How does one define who is terminally ill?
2. The dilemma of the "slippery slope": what would prevent abuse? In a permissive milieu, those who cannot consent, such as the cognitively disabled and the very sick, or those who are vulnerable, such as the depressed, the disabled, and the aged, might be coerced into accepting death.

Contrary to medical training
Ending someone's life prematurely, hastening their death, would be contrary to health professional training (which is to save lives), would erode public confidence in the profession, and might cause clinicians to expend

less effort in saving lives. According to this view, it should be condemned as being akin to medical assistance at capital punishment, widely regarded as unethical, even if it is legal in some jurisdictions. The solution to the problem of barbaric state executions is not to train "experts in execution."[83]

Over-reliance on autonomy

Acceding to requests of patients for PAD suggests to some that autonomy is always the trump principle in ethics and minimizes the ethos of the beneficent-physician-guided decision-making. Healthcare professionals become, in this view, a mere "means" for their patients. [84]

Cost to professionals

As reported by Emanuel, several studies have shown 12 to 19 per cent of physicians who participated in PAD were uncomfortable afterwards, with feelings of guilt or sadness unrelated to fear of prosecution. [85]

Lack of necessity if palliative care is done properly

This may be stated in a strong version (all pain and suffering can be relieved by good palliative care) or in a weak version (much suffering can be relieved). Superb palliative care makes requests for aid in dying unusual.[86]

Reasons for professionals to support PAD

No different than accepted practice

Some of the reasons given for opposing PAD also serve as arguments against letting patients *refuse* life-sustaining care. Removing someone from life-support and "allowing" death to come can be just as contentious as providing a patient with the means to hasten his or her death. Morally, however, there is no difference if the end result is the same: the death of the patient. How sure can we be, for example, that someone has authentically consented to forego care? Uncertainties about foregoing care do not suggest that we end the practice, only that we exercise it carefully.

In addition, "palliative sedation" and voluntary cessation of oral intake ("palliative care options of last resort") have been largely accepted by the medical community. The stopping of eating will result in death in days to weeks and can be a comfortable process with good care. In palliative sedation, a patient with intractable suffering is sedated to unconsciousness and maintained there with sedatives, without feeding, until death occurs.[87] The clinician participation needed for these accepted palliative practices is little different than the processes required where PAD is legal.

Obligation is to the patient first

Many arguments against PAD consider the implications for others. But the idea that permitting it in *some* circumstances makes the principle of autonomy *always* the "trump card" does not follow. This underestimates the ability of clinicians to individually evaluate patient requests and would undermine shared decision-making.

Moreover, adequate palliation for every patient is *not* always possible, especially as seen through the patient's eyes. Psychological misery—from loss of dignity and loss of autonomy—resists easy palliation.

Should be a matter of conscience

Quill provided a moving defence of assisted suicide in describing his decision to give a prescription for a lethal dose of barbiturates to a woman with leukemia who had decided to forego treatment.[88] After discussing her views with her over time, he decided to grant her request: "I . . . felt strongly that I was setting her free to get the most out of the time she had left, and to maintain dignity and control on her own terms until her death." Giving dying patients a sense of control over an undignified and autonomy-undermining illness is important to many patients and their families.[89] One author, well known for her opposition to all forms of PAD had a change of heart when it was her own dying father who requested her assistance at accelerating his imminent demise.[90]

Oregon's Death with Dignity Act

Only in Oregon and Washington has AS been legalized on account of a popular vote. If certain conditions are met, patients are eligible for a lethal prescription of drugs from a physician (see Box 11.7).

BOX 11.7

Under the Oregon's *Death With Dignity Act*,[91] patients requesting assisted suicide must

- be adult (more than 17 years old) state residents;
- be suffering from an incurable disease (life expectancy less than six months);
- have their diagnosis confirmed by two independent physicians;
- make a verbal request and sign a written request for the prescription in the presence of two witnesses attesting that the patient is competent and acting voluntarily; and
- wait for a minimum of 15 days.

A report on the first six years of this law noted that PAS was the cause of death of one eighth of 1 per cent of the deaths in Oregon.[92] There are few reports of failures of AS (that might, some feared, turn it into euthanasia). The use of palliative care has increased (suggesting this law does not undermine good end-of-life care). Any inappropriate use of AS by patients not fitting the inclusion criteria (such as psychological suffering or incapable patients) has not been reported. Patients who had chosen AS had issues that were less easily addressed by palliative care—loss of autonomy and a desire to control the way in which they die.[93] Physicians grant about one in six requests for lethal medication. Some patients change their minds after better attention is paid to their palliative care needs.[94] A 13-year audit reveals its use by 30–50 patients per year (even fewer may actually use the prescription); these numbers have stabilized.[95] A 10-year review of EU and AS practices showed "transparent practices" and indicated they accounted for 2.8 per cent of all deaths in the Netherlands. This is a relatively stable proportion over that time, despite the law legalizing such practices being enacted only in 2002.[96] (This suggests, as many realize, that aid in dying, including "advanced" palliative care practices, was and is practised even in the absence of judicial sanction and that judicial sanction need not open the floodgates to abuse.)

These are moderated results. Judging by these outcomes, it seems possible to devise guidelines that will be followed by patients and professionals. It may be that, having received support from the electorate twice, the law is well known and, Oregon being a relatively small jurisdiction, compliance easier to monitor.

Conclusion

One UK judge, sympathetic to an active form of physician aid in dying, has commented: How can it be lawful to allow a patient to die slowly, though painlessly, over a period of weeks from a lack of food but unlawful to produce his immediate death by a lethal injection, thereby saving his family from yet another ordeal to add to the tragedy that has struck them? I find it difficult to find a moral answer to that question.[97]

This judge's concerns, widely held, can *almost* be met under current law and practice. Death after the withdrawal of food and fluids usually occurs in less than eight days (but may take longer). The patient can be kept comfortable by sedation, good oral care, and pain medications. A lethal injection is rarely needed, should never be given for the family's sake anyway, and may deprive the patient of experiencing the process of dying.

The great twentieth-century Austrian-English philosopher Wittgenstein said we can never experience the moment of our death.[98] Maybe so, but all the moments before that ultimate one, being our last ones, may be of great import for the person dying. We interfere with this process at our peril. Do we really want all deaths to be quiet and quick? Perhaps we are all really trying to escape from *thanatos*.[99] Professionals and the public need to learn of comforts beyond technology and pills and learn to be *with* individuals as they die.[100]

Cases For Discussion

CASE 1: NIGHT TERRORS

Ms Y has had a troubled life. She has been estranged from her parents since leaving home as a teen. Since finishing high school, she has done a variety of jobs but has been unable to hold any of them very long due to emotional issues and substance abuse (cocaine, crystal meth). Ms Y can be very charming but also very manipulative. Having engaged in unsafe sexual practices, she has been diagnosed with HIV and Hepatitis C. Nonetheless, her physical status is quite stable and her immune system reconstituted, with no active viremia. Ms Y, now 35, hates her life—she is often depressed, anxious, and has chronic insomnia with disturbing nightmares.

She comes to see you one day and asks you for something stronger for sleep. "I need something really strong," she says, "Those benzodiazepines don't help at all. My brain is too wired! If only I could get a good night's rest, I'm sure I'd feel better. Can you please prescribe something that will work?!"

Questions For Discussion

1. You happen to know that barbiturates would help her sleep. In overdose they pose a risk of death. If the patient asked you for these, would you provide them?
2. What if she told you she might want to use them, if things got intolerable for her, to end her life? Would you still prescribe them?

CASE 2: A PAINFUL DECISION

Ms W, a feisty patient of 91, comes to hospital with severe back pain and difficulty breathing of a week's duration. Thought to have pneumonia, she turns out to have an unusual spinal malignancy that has spread to her ribs. Treatment options are limited—surgery is out of the question but radiotherapy might help her pain. She has a large family and many friends have come to visit. Bright as a pin, her social interactions are "well-preserved." She had agreed to a No CPR order on admission to the ward, but otherwise has not completed an advance directive.

By accident, two days after admission, she is given 10 times the prescribed dose of long-acting morphine and quickly lapses into a comatose state with very shallow breathing. She is in danger of acute respiratory failure and cardiac arrest. A family member in the room pleads for you to do something.

Questions For Discussion

1. Should CPR be performed on this patient despite the No CPR order, given that the cause of her sudden deterioration is due to an error in her care?
2. Would you act any differently if she were 45?

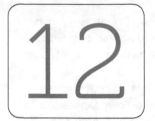

Questions of Culture, Genetics, and Science

"[C]ultures differ from one another, sometimes radically. The nagging question remains: What, if anything, follows from the facts of cultural relativity?"

Ruth Macklin, 1999[1]

"Everyone ought to follow the principles whose being universal laws would make things go best . . . "

Derek Parfit, 2011[2]

Medicine is a practical enterprise. Based in part on science, it is also rooted in culture and society. Healthcare is at the interface of culture and science—not quite applied science but certainly not just another form of social life. Modern medicine has been able to contribute to the advancement of humankind because its findings do not apply to just one group. Medicine is both governed by deontological (universal) principles and by a utilitarian ("striving for best outcomes") ethos. Its findings are meant to be universal but how medicine's findings are actualized and made effective in the real world is the rub. We need to be sensitive to local cultural matters but not forget that the attitudes of care and respect cross cultural boundaries.

I. Cultural Connections

"Culture matters. The question is: how does culture matter?"[3] Culture can mean many things: we speak of the culture of ignorance, of science, of medicine, of religion, of devotion, of consumerism, and of sacrifice. We also speak of Deaf culture, Gay culture, macho culture, Western culture, Islamic culture, and so on. Shared norms, values, beliefs, practices, and attitudes characterize a culture—they may be explicitly held and defended or they may be found and defined by sociologists or anthropologists. Cultures may be as big as a society or religion or as small as the aging person who lives next door.

CASE 12.1 A CLASH OF GENERATIONS

Jacqui W is a determined medical student. Nose to the grindstone, she had studied chemistry, physics, and biology for a university degree, receiving a 98 per cent average. Now she is in her first year of medicine and happily memorizing the intricate details of human anatomy and histology.

This week is more challenging for her and her fellow students (who, like Jacqui, also excelled in science). They are sent out, as a part of a new course on illness and health in the community, to interview a patient, Ms E (from Case 7.5, "No Fools Allowed"). A widow in her 80s, Ms E is cantankerous and somewhat rude. She complains bitterly about her family being unavailable, getting older, and how little good help she can get at home. Unsure how to respond, Jacqui suggests, "Have you consider moving into a home for the aged? We recently visited a very nice one. It was clean and people there were so friendly!" This is not advice Ms E wishes to hear—she doesn't consider herself like other "aged" folks and certainly is not going to leave her home ("except in a pine box," she always said). Ms E sends the students away.

What went wrong here?

DISCUSSION OF CASE 12.1

This may be just a clash of generations—but "cultures" are involved as well. There is the culture of science, purportedly objective and rational, and then there is the culture of patients, subjective and not always "rational." Ms E feels Jacqui is being condescending. Jacqui, by contrast, is merely trying to be helpful—she thinks if she were Ms E she would not want to live like that, all alone, with no family. Perhaps Jacqui and her colleagues are a little too eager to help Ms E. Or maybe they have had too little preparation for the real world of medicine—the social and personal aspects of care. Concentrating on one aspect of medicine—the culture of science, they may fail to consider what may be just as important: the unpredictable culture of patients.

The only ethical issue raised by Case 12.1 is whether healthcare trainees will get the kind of education they need to learn to be sensitive to the values and beliefs of others—whether they share your culture or not. Box 12.1 lists some of the understandings and attitudes a "culturally competent" practitioner requires.

BOX 12.1

To be "culturally competent" means having the knowledge, attitudes, and skills to be able to

- avoid bias and stereotyping of patients;
- avoid presumption of a patient's allegiance to his or her identified group;
- appreciate the diversity within the relevant groups;
- accommodate patient/family "culture-dependent" views;
- ask about patient/family experience of illness and what matters to them;
- appreciate the need to negotiate resolutions.[4]

Although one would rarely fulfill or address all these considerations in one interview with one patient, they are some of the prerequisites permitting and facilitating the process of communication. We have seen already how cultural norms can affect conceptions of autonomy (Case 2.6), privacy (Case 3.2), truthtelling (Case 4.6), consent (Case 5.4), and personhood (Case 11.4). Not all of these situations were resolved to the satisfaction of each side, but that may be inevitable when it comes to making reasonable compromise. Success may require accepting less than perfect results.

Culture as "bricolage"

Cultures not only vary tremendously, they also overlap: one can simultaneously be part of a consumerist culture, a scientific culture, and a transgendered culture. Differing cultures also overlap like Venn diagrams, sharing some things, rejecting others. In other respects a culture is not a fully integrated whole but a "bricolage," a term used by the anthropologist Claude Lévi-Strauss to denote an activity combined of various and not always consistent elements.[5] People and cultures are, as Sen has written, "diversely different."[6] As individuals, we are characterized by a multiplicity of allegiances and beliefs which may not be consistent but give meaning to, and help make sense of, different aspects of one's life.

Worlds apart?

One of the best and most popular books about the influence of culture on medical practice is *The Spirit Catches You and You Fall Down: A Hmong Child, her American Doctors, and the Collision of Cultures* by Anne Fadiman.[7] It concerns a Laotian refugee family in California during the 1980s. They speak little English, have next to no understanding of American medicine, but do have very strong beliefs about why illness strikes some people and not others. When one of the family's young children develops a serious seizure disorder, the family's views about it are never explored. As a result, the child does not receive proper and timely treatment, her parents suffer legal consequences for failing to provide her with necessary care and, in the end, the child dies. This tragic tale is characterized by misunderstandings, a failure to communicate across a cultural divide, and a total breakdown in trust.

The lesson is deceptively simple: trying to better understand another culture may result in treatment choices being more inclusive and so more likely to be accepted.[8] But mutual understanding can be difficult when protagonists don't share common ground. Healthcare professionals do not have to reject input into a patient's care from other cultural perspectives. Asking the following questions can help better appreciate the "explanatory model" of a patient/family from a different culture.

BOX 12.2

Some questions to ask a patient or family across a cultural gap are

- What do you think the problem/sickness is?
- What do you think caused the problem?
- Why do you think it started when it did?
- What other problems/difficulties has the sickness caused?
- How severe is the sickness?
- What do you fear most about the problem?
- What kind of treatment do you think should be used?
- How will you know the treatment is working?
- Who else would you wish to be involved in the healing process?[9]

Some questions in Box 12.2 will be more pertinent than others. It depends on how new and different a patient's culture is from your own. Many of the questions, quite frankly, should be asked of *every* patient and/or family in order to get a sense of a patient's/family's experience, priorities, and beliefs concerning the problem or illness. For example, one person may fear loss of autonomy, another loss of beauty; one family may be concerned about their ability to care for the ill relative, another may feel guilt that something they neglected to do may have created the problem.

I do not think the message from Fadiman's book is that we cannot communicate across cultures and language—we can, it can just be hard to do. The message is there are deep cultural differences which must be recognized by healthcare professionals, not simply dismissed as superstition or dogma, but instead treated in a respectful way. Mutual understanding can still be found since cultures and languages are never entirely consistent wholes; they always provide some inconsistency, some shared piece of turf to be used as to permit communication. For this, one needs an interest and a good translator not just of language but of the ideas behind the language.

CASE 12.2 A NATURAL CURE

Ms A is an 18-year-old college student who had chemotherapy for Hodgkin's lymphoma at 16. You are her primary care provider. Unfortunately, it has recurred and she is very reluctant to undergo another round of chemotherapy. She found the first round to be very unpleasant—nausea, weight loss, hair loss, and extreme fatigue. Ms A is skeptical about the lymphoma's recurrence given she feels better. She is convinced chemo will only weaken her. Instead she and her parents have found a clinic in Mexico that provides an alternative "traditional" cure involving non-toxic plants and roots.

Is there an ethical problem here and, if so, how might it be managed?

DISCUSSION OF CASE 12.2

Given the high success rate in treating even recurrent Hodgkin's lymphoma in a young adult, this case does seem to pit autonomy against beneficence. Many people are entranced by the idea of traditional medicines that are supposedly effective and also without side effects.

For Ms A and her family the notion of beneficence appears to exclude the use of modern therapeutics. With a good bit of persuasion—trying to understand their understanding of the disease and how it can be cured—your best hope is to convince Ms A to integrate what modern medicine has to offer with what an alternative medical practice might utilize. Perhaps you could seek a local naturopath who can develop an alternative course of therapy that is compatible with modern medicine. If she and her family are adamant about their intended course all you can do is promise you will try to help her when the "treatment" in Mexico fails—as it inevitably will.

Local matters matter

Ethnography, the study of "local" behaviours and mores, it is claimed, can illuminate the cultural complexity behind the everyday world of medical practice.[10] Clinicians are not expected to be anthropologists or ethnographers, just as they need not be lawyers or philosophers. Ethnography is a helpful reminder that what is at stake may sometimes depend on unique, contextual "local" factors. But it cannot replace bioethics or solve all medicine's moral dilemmas. In the clinical encounter the clinician attempts to integrate the universal aspects of medicine with the unique views of the patient and his or her cultural background. This is the model of concordance or shared decision-making discussed in earlier chapters. It is not mission impossible but does take interest and some time.

Transcending culture

For every cultural perspective, there are "facts," or circumstances, that transcend the culture. These may involve circumstances of commerce or exploration, scientific knowledge or works of philosophy or literature. Any of these can be used as a "lever" by people to get out of their culture and/or to work with and understand what other cultures have to offer. In past times such items were not always reliable or accepted. Today there may be more room for mutual respect among differing cultures. Accepting this can encourage dialogue and create a safe harbour, an "ethical space," for co-operative action and learning.[11]

Yet one has to be careful as to how closely one takes into account cultural factors. To be sensitive to another's culture does not mean one must relinquish one's own local culture.

CASE 12.3 FAR FROM HOME

A 36-year-old single Aboriginal man, Mr M, is flown in from his Reserve to a large tertiary care hospital following a severe MVA. His car having struck a moose, he was launched through the window and is now quadriplegic secondary to transection of his upper cervical spinal cord. Mr M is now in the ICU, intubated and heavily sedated. Whether he can breathe on his own will not be known until next week.

A few days later, Mr M's mother and brother arrive from the Reserve where they all reside. They insist all treatment be stopped and he be allowed to die. "He's a fisherman and a trapper," his mother exclaims. "His whole life is the outdoors. I can't see him ever coming home. There's no place for anybody in a wheelchair, there aren't really sidewalks on the Reserve." He would not want, she declares, to be kept alive in this state. "He told us, after watching a TV show one time, that he wouldn't want medical treatment if he were ever to become paralyzed. Nope, I don't think he'd like this at all."

The intensivist, Dr D, is reluctant to withdraw treatment as she does not yet fully know Mr M's prognosis given his very recent arrival in the ICU. He might be able to breathe on his own, for example. She is doubtful he will regain much, if any, use of his limbs but, who knows, he might be grateful to be alive. Told this, the family's anger increases. "It's not just about him, you know. This affects the whole community. We don't think this decision is yours or his to make!"

What is the major ethical dilemma in this case?

DISCUSSION OF CASE 12.3

This case challenges us as to how we think ethical issues should be resolved. One component of the ethics decision procedure is to involve the right people. Surely Mr M's family members are the right people. They are, but that does not mean the decision is theirs alone to make. A professional assessment must be made as to their ability to act as SDMs. Are they acting out of self-interest as they don't want the burden of looking after Mr M? Or do they actually have a better appreciation of the dependent patient's true wishes and that to which he and his community can accommodate? They seem to be saying the profession ought to respect Mr M's prior wishes and the views of his community. It is not clear how those views would be elicited. The finality of the family's choice—Mr M's imminent death—is not one the team wants to concur with *now* as, in a few days, he will likely be able to make his own decision about his care.

Many people with traumatic quadriplegia get over the initial shock and distress and accept what life they have left. Some patients recover some limb mobility, so the outlook for Mr M is not entirely bleak. As important as it is to provide culturally sensitive care, one should not forget the advances in care for the severely injured achieved by modern medicine. An altered life may be a life of permanent and severe disability; that does not mean it is not a life worth saving. This discussion is attempted with the family, but to no avail; they angrily leave the hospital.

The next week, Mr M brightens up neurologically and is successfully extubated. He expresses unhappiness with his condition but says he is happy to be alive. "Better a quadriplegic than to be dead," he says. As for his future on the Reserve, he states he'll figure that out later. "They've got lots of money, they [the Reserve] can support me for a while!"

Knowing a culture

So it all turns for the best, then? Culture must adapt to the individual? In retrospect, the ethicist involved with the critical care team feels he did not provide very good input. He didn't know much at all about the indigenous culture to which Mr M belonged. He knew little about how flexible this culture was and how resilient Mr M could be. He could, and should, have found out more—perhaps inviting the family to return with tribal elders or others from the community to help make a consensual decision. As it was, the family was faced with a unilateral decision by the healthcare team. When the ethicist ponders this later, he realizes he didn't really consider (or follow) Mr M's future. What kind of life *could* he have? What kind of life *did* he have? Unfortunately, he never found out.

The upshot of this case is

- throwaway statements by people should not be taken as wishes carved in stone;
- even a state of extreme disability can be a life worth living;
- working with different cultures does not mean reflexively following their mores;
- individual patients are unique and their preferences not always those predicted by their family/group/culture; but you should be well informed about another's culture before riding roughshod over it.

However, the medical interests of the patient and the medical limitations of what is possible must, at times, take precedence over cultural mores or family concerns.

Limits to cultural compromise

Attention to and acknowledgment of cultural diversity will result in such issues arising more frequently. Certain cultural convictions can seem at odds with humane and dignified care. The question here is: is it more appropriate and culturally sensitive to allow a family to set the tone for end-of-life care or should the clinicians play a more leading role? There is no one right answer but, where the stakes are high, principled and respectful negotiation should be sought.

CASE 12.4 A DISPUTE OVER DEATH

A 44-year-old man, Mr N, with a large extended family is admitted to the ICU with raised intracranial pressure from an untreatable cerebral malignancy. Despite various measures, he has continued to decline and is now on a ventilator. It is obvious to the ICU staff that the patient's brain is too compressed to respond to any treatment. On no sedatives, he has been in a deep coma for several days, completely unresponsive to any stimulation. His Glasgow Coma Scale is 3—as low as you can get—and there is complete absence of any brainstem reflex activity on two assessments.

Mr N's strongly religious family feels everything possible must be done to extend his life, arguing: "If God wanted him to die, he wouldn't have allowed mankind to invent ventilators."

As is standard practice, an "apnea test" to establish brain death is arranged.[12] This entails temporarily removing the patient's attachment to the ventilator. In response to rising carbon dioxide levels in the body, an individual who is brain-dead will fail to initiate respiration as would normally occur. As the ICU resident and attending neurologist are about to perform the test on the patient, a family member exclaims, "Don't touch him! If you remove him from the breathing machine, we'll sue you!" According to the family's (and the patient's) religion, where there is breathing, there is life and so one may not stop an artificial breathing apparatus.

What should the response of the ICU staff be?

"Reasonable accommodation"

The idea that death may be defined or defied by modern medicine seems to be a widely held view and may be the cause of cross-cultural conflict in the ICU. In many jurisdictions, however, religious objections to brain death are not acceptable. Even where they are accepted, such as in New Jersey and New York states, it is expected only that clinicians offer families "reasonable accommodation."[13, 14] A "brain-dead" person is dead, full stop, and only remains in an ICU for exceptional reasons (for a coroner's/medical examiner's inquiry or while awaiting organ retrieval[15]). Out of respect for a family's wishes, one may delay transfers to the morgue, allowing time for grieving and/or any religious rites to be performed.

The inevitability of complete somatic collapse following entire brain death (within seven days even with cardiovascular support) used to limit how long a body could be kept perfused after death.[16] In some cases, this limit can now be extended much longer with maximal ICU support.[17] This means increasingly one cannot wait for "nature to take its course" and assume time will solve all ethical problems. Clinicians should play a more active role in directing the resolution of such cases—especially as such care is so expensive (see Chapter 11 for this thorny issue).

DISCUSSION OF CASE 12.4

This case seems to pit religion against science. A "reasonable" accommodation to a cultural or religious objection to death (as defined by standard neurological criteria) should be, at most, 24–48 hours; in some jurisdictions, any further continuance of critical care maintenance of somatic function, if allowed at all, would be at the family's expense.[18] However, the idea that one might be able to "buy" a bed in the ICU to provide somatic support for a dead person seems repugnant and suggests a questionable commercialism. It is also a poor use of a scarce resource.

Cultural objections to death cannot be grounds for preventing measures to determine death.

There may be a limit as to how far any society can accommodate cultural preferences. Where serious harm to patients or overuse of scarce resources may result from cultural adherence, one may have some responsibility and allowance to examine and challenge cultural assumptions.

With the advent of genomic medicine there will be challenges to many cultural assumptions about life. If culture suggests diversity, genetics suggests predisposition and a physical limit on human variability. However, this is far from the case, as we shall now see.

II. All in the Genome?

"Genome" is a neologism from an amalgam of "gene" and "chromosome." The genome, be it of a cell, an individual, a group, or a species, refers to all of the hereditary material of the individual, not simply one's "genotype" but one's nuclear DNA and mitochondrial DNA (mtDNA). The exception to Sen's claim that we are all "diversely different" is here. Genomes, it is true, vary from species to species. But the genetic overlaps are striking. Humans show just 1 per cent divergence in their nuclear genomes from chimps and gorillas. Different humans show less than 0.1 per cent sequence divergence in their mtDNA genomes. Clones and identical twins have virtually the same genome: they are truly identically identical.[19]

While we are far from being determined by our genome, there is a very complex relationship between one's inherited genetic profile and the illnesses to which one might be susceptible as well as the treatments which might work and those which might not. This is the advent of the era of truly "personalized medicine" that may take some of the guesswork out of diagnostics and therapeutics in medicine.[20] The new genetic-oriented medicine has had its biggest impact on testing for diseases or for inherited susceptibilities to diseases in oneself or one's offspring.

CASE 12.5 ALL IN THE FAMILY?

You are a primary care provider looking after a 24-year-old man, Mr P, who develops ataxia and paranoid ideation. Noticing unusual copper-tinged rings in his pupils, you make a diagnosis of Wilson's disease (a serious illness with protean manifestations that has genetic markers and is amenable to treatment).[21] After the diagnosis is confirmed through further serological and genetic testing, the patient is started on effective treatment.

Mr P has two siblings also in your practice. You advise him to disclose his diagnosis to his siblings, recognizing they each have a one in four risk of also having the disease. This, the patient refuses to do, saying he has never gotten along with his siblings and they can "rot in hell" as far as he's concerned.[22]

What would you do in this case?

DISCUSSION OF CASE 12.5

There exists tension in this case between confidentiality due to the patient and beneficence owed to others. The patient's wishes are clear but the possible harms to his siblings are also evident. In general, in a conflict between the prevention of serious harm to others and the preservation of privacy, beneficence should prevail. It is unconscionable to allow serious, preventable harm to another person take place simply on the basis of a blanket principle to protect a "right to privacy" (see Chapter 3).

A good clinician—genetics advisor, nurse, social worker, or doctor—would spend time with the patient in an attempt to understand his decision in context. Is his desire to allow potential harm to befall his siblings a manifestation of his paranoid illness? Or is it an extension of bad feelings he has harboured for years?

The right thing is for someone to warn the patient's siblings—it would be best if this took place with the patient's consent and indeed if he told them himself. Their awareness of their risk of the illness could be heightened if you, as their clinician, had a relationship with them. You would certainly be within your professional duty to bring the siblings in for a routine examination and look for evidence of Wilson's disease. You could carefully question them regarding symptoms and signs of the illness. Sowing seeds of suspicion in this way would be allowable but seems a bit morally suspect.

Preventative ethics

This ethical dilemma could have been avoided if the informed consent requested prior to genetic testing were more assiduous. The patient could have been warned in advance that those also potentially affected must, ethically, be informed if testing revealed a serious inherited disease. This is especially true now that interventions can be undertaken for genetic conditions, such as for those carrying genes increasing susceptibility to breast cancer, familial non-polyposis or long QT syndrome. Where practitioners are uncertain about what to advise the identified individual regarding his or her relatives, help should be sought from more experienced consultants. Some have suggested that, although the information is derived from an individual, that information is not his or hers alone; rather it is part of a familial "joint account" that ought to be shared.[23] This seems reasonable enough as long as there are protections from scrutiny by those outside the family's circle such as employers or insurance companies. International bodies have suggested certain rules be followed in studying the human genome.

BOX 12.3

Persons who undergo genetic testing must be provided full information on the procedure and that they freely give their informed consent. Patients also have the right to be informed of the results or, if they so desire, the right not to be informed of them.[24]

International Declaration on Human Genetic Data (2003) and the Universal Declaration on Bioethics and Human Rights (2005).

Seemingly straightforward genetically-induced disease is not so straightforward for most of the host's conditions of wellness or ill-health. The "causes" behind the latter states usually involve multiple, sometimes hundreds, of genes.[25] Whole genome sequencing (WGS) can reveal unique individualized data such as alterations in a person's abilities to metabolize a drug (resulting in increased susceptibility to adverse drug reactions) or mutations in the genome of malignancies making them more susceptible to anti-neoplastic drugs. Genomic sequencing has already had an impact on drug therapy for breast cancer, allowing affected women the opportunity to avoid having to start and then stop therapy because of side effects. The genome of the tumour also plays a central role in a patient's response to anti-cancer agents. This has become so well established that genetic testing is routinely done looking for biomarkers of a tumour's likely susceptibility to a specific drug.[26]

> ## BOX 12.4
>
> "Genomic studies do not raise wholly new ethical issues, but they cast these issues [of biomedical research] in a fresh light."[27]

In the era of genomic medicine, it should be remembered that large "anonymized" genomic data banks can be used to uniquely identify individuals if they have a distinct genetic aberration or variant.[28] Hence, non-traceability may be a relic of the era of non-personalized medicine. As well, whole groups of people or communities may be identifiable by linkages established through genetic predispositions and genomic associations, so one must be sensitive to local mores and local jurisprudence in this area. In many parts of the world there are few, if any laws, protecting privacy of genetic data. That should not give researchers free rein over such data.[29]

Indigenous objection

In 2010 a settlement of $700,000 US was levied against an American university for having allowed its researchers to study blood samples from a native tribe for genetic purposes to which they had not consented.[30] Assuming their samples were being used for the study of diabetes, tribe members did not realize their samples were (and did not consent to their samples) also being used to study schizophrenia and "inbreeding."

The outcome of this case should be a reminder that some communities/cultures with increased prevalence of diseases may have a unique interest in research conducted on them. This may be due to the increased burdens of those ill-understood diseases and the wish not to be stigmatized on account of disease association. Aboriginal communities have been long used (and abused) by researchers and are now looking to benefit more directly from the results of research. Guidelines recommend they are owed a role in "shaping the conduct of research that affects [them]."[31]

It is not surprising, then, to find indigenous peoples creating guidelines for ethical research involving their communities. Researchers dropping into a community, conducting whatever research interests them and then promptly leaving, is no longer a viable option. Instead, such behaviour is considered exploitation of indigenous people and a legacy of colonialism. "Aboriginal ownership, control, access, and possession of research process and products" (OCAP) guidelines, developed by indigenous scholars, promote the interests of local populations and allows them to help set the agenda and reap some of the benefits of research.[32]

To avoid such disputes, it is important to clarify to what research participants are agreeing—some participants and communities will have particular needs to control information concerning them. However, too strict controls by donors over genomic information gathered from thousands of individuals might seriously hamper accurate genome-wide research and thereby unduly slow down medical progress.[33] Too loose consent, on the other hand, provides donors with little or no control over how their genetic material is used and by whom. Likely most individuals would not object to the scientific use of their specimens if they were confident that researchers were using them for benign purposes of health. But discomfort is raised by the spectre of their ill-use (e.g., personal identification by the state or by insurers or employers), and their purely commercial use (e.g., cloning, "Frankenstein" creations by mad scientists).

While genetic knowledge can be beneficial to patients, clinicians, and researchers alike, it also creates new professional responsibilities—not only to protect that information but as well to ensure that information is used to best advantage. Genetically-based risk assessments are complex and as yet fraught with uncertainty. It is also true that the only way to resolve such uncertainties is to conduct more genomic-wide studies on larger populations.[34]

We shall now look at some other critical considerations for the ethics of medical research.

III. Ethical Regulation of Research

The Nuremburg trials of Nazi doctors following World War Two implicated physicians in the most deliberately heinous forms of research on humans, resulting in a sacrosanct standard for any human research: *all* research involving humans must occur *only* with the *voluntary* consent of participants. Despite this inviolable standard, Beecher in the US and Pappworth in the UK, in the early to mid-1960s, laid bare the ongoing conduct of numerous unethical research trials in each country.[35] Patients were enrolled in risky protocols without their knowledge. Vulnerable subjects such as children and the mentally ill were the subjects of experimentation without substitute consent or knowledge. While these exposés took a professional toll on both men, their writings helped launch the explicit ethical regulation of research since then. Yet unethical research did not end there. The most infamous was the Tuskegee "experiment" (poor, black farm labourers were not told for decades they had, nor were they treated for, syphilis) which was halted only in 1972 when it came to public attention.

The culture of science increasingly pervades medicine; effective care would not be possible without it. Nevertheless, abuses of patients for the purposes of "science" have resulted in the proliferation of rules and regulations to guide research involving humans. (For a very simple, but actually quite demanding, set of requirements from the Council for International Organizations and Medical Sciences, see Box 12.5.)

BOX 12.5

CIOMS Requirements for Consent to Research

- Participants must have the capacity to consent.
- Consent must be voluntary.
- Patients must have received sufficient information for choice.[36]

The most pertinent feature of research is that it is not meant to be primarily, therapeutic for the participants. The impetus for research is to contribute to the fund of knowledge by testing a hypothesis. By contrast, clinical practice is meant to help the patient based on best medical guidelines.

Equipoise

Clinical trials are most appropriate when there is genuine controversy— some call it "equipoise," a term coined by Benjamin Freedman—in the medical community as to effectiveness of a treatment. Lacking convincing evidence regarding one option over another provides good grounds for a clinical trial to try to resolve the uncertainty.[37]

This is not as straightforward as it might seem, however: what and where is the "standard of care"? Does it reside with the researcher's immediate colleagues? In the hospital? Across the country? In the most advanced hospitals in the world? The trouble is there may not be agreement as to the evidence required for a trial's results to *resolve* the state of equipoise. When would it be unethical to propose a trial? When should a trial be stopped? The answers depend on the risk of harms versus the chance of benefits of trial participants as compared with risks faced by similarly situated patients not in the trial. Well conducted studies should have clear rules set in advance for stopping the trial on grounds of harm, efficacy, or futility. Adherence to these rules is ensured by a "data safety monitoring board" (DSMB), a group of independent experts in biostatistics and trial conduct with the authority to monitor and halt a trial. DSMBs should be part of the oversight and monitoring of any significant clinical trial—such as drug trials that test the efficacy of one drug against another and that involve some risk of serious harm.

Consent for research

Much emphasis in research ethics is put on informed choice and the Informed Consent Form (ICF). The rigour and completeness these forms are meant to embody sometimes outweigh their helpfulness to would-be participants trying to decide if they should take part in a trial. (See Box 12.6)

BOX 12.6

The requirements for research consent are as follows:

- explain why the subject is being asked to take part;
- explain the voluntary nature of participation and the right to withdraw;
- explain in simple terms the trial's rationale and the study design (randomization, placebo arm, safety measures);
- explain what is expected of participants (e.g., duration of the trial, requirements as regards extra testing, what will happen to donated specimens, if any);
- explain clearly the possible risks and benefits. Include information as to the availability of the test substance at the conclusion of the trial and how participants will be informed about any new and relevant findings;
- explain alternatives to participation and reasons a trial might be halted;
- disclose investigator remuneration, if any, to participants;
- disclose any conflicts of interest the investigator may have;
- ensure the subject knows what to do in an emergency (what to look for, who to call);
- explain privacy protections and who may receive what aspects of patient data;
- disclose compensation for research-related injury;
- provide names of whom to contact, including the researcher and the reviewing ethics board.[38]

Even the best-written consent form cannot make up for a morally dubious trial.

CASE 12.6 POLES APART

It is suggested that a new drug, Invidia, is superior to lithium, the standard of care for maintenance therapy of bipolar disorder. A study is proposed whereby 100 patients with bipolar disorder stable on lithium will be enrolled in a randomized controlled trial (RCT). Patients will be randomized to three groups: one to remain on lithium, another to be switched to Invidia, and a third group to receive a placebo pill. Would-be participants are told about the randomization but neither the researcher nor the patient will know to which group they are assigned.

Are there ethical concerns about this trial?

DISCUSSION OF CASE 12.6

Lithium is a known efficacious therapy for prevention of relapse in bipolar disorder. However, it does not work for everyone, can cause intolerable side effects for some, and has the potential for serious side effects. Hence, there is certainly a rationale for the study of a new drug with possible equal efficacy but fewer adverse effects. The moral acceptability of the trial depends on the science behind the study: how good is the evidence behind the new substance? Without a solid scientific rationale, a study ought not to be mounted. Another concern would be patient safety. How well monitored will study participants be? Is it safe to allow some patients to be without a maintenance medication? Who is the best judge of the acceptability of the hazards a trial might pose to participants? (Although the usual answer is a research review board, some argue this is too paternalistic, instead recommending patient input into all aspects of a trial from planning to execution.[39]) If these kinds of questions are properly addressed, the research trial could be mounted.

Research trials and placebos

In general, RCTs are most acceptable if all participants receive known effective treatment. RCTs have more than one "arm"—each arm is a group of patients, each group comparable in number and composition. Study participants are randomly assigned to one of the arms. One arm gets the test substance while those in the other receive a placebo look-alike, both on top of the standard of care. In other RCTs, more controversially, one arm gets the test substance while the other gets *only* a look-alike placebo. The first type of study will look at whether the test substance is as good as or better than standard treatment while the second will tell you only if the test substance is better than nothing. This latter type of RCT is considered acceptable only if there is no standard effective treatment for the studied condition or if the standard of care is poorly tolerated.

Researchers often claim placebo arms without the standard of care are necessary to prove to drug regulators that their new drug is better and safer than taking nothing. The studies that use placebo-only arms also allow trials to be conducted with *fewer* participants. Demonstrating the efficacy of a new agent can be more easily accomplished by comparing it to "no active drug" (the placebo arm) than comparing it to the standard of care medication (which presumably is somewhat efficacious). But in practice, however, clinicians are most interested in its comparison with the latter. Does the new test substance perform *better* and is it *safer* than what is used already? Has it a better side effect profile? This can be determined only if each group receives the standard of care. Currently, researchers may carry out studies that deny some participants an effective standard of care if they can show that those not receiving it will not be harmed, there is a guarantee of close clinical vigilance of all participants in the trial, and participants give their informed consent to the trial.

For RCTs, therapeutic benefits cannot be guaranteed for participants because of the possibility they may assigned to the placebo arm or because the test substance (the "active arm") may not end up working. Despite this, patients may enter a trial for the *chance* of benefit, with the hope they will not be randomized to the placebo arm. They may be motivated to do so because the existing standard of care for their condition may not be sufficiently efficacious or is associated with adverse effects they prefer to avoid.

The tissue issue

Patients can contribute to science unsuspectingly. It is common, for example, for donors of blood or tissue samples to be uninformed about how their samples will be used.

In her gripping and wonderfully written book, *The Immortal Life of Henrietta Lacks*, Rebecca Skloot documents the sad tale of an impoverished woman who died of cervical cancer in the early 1950s but not before her doctors had kept part of her tumour, eventually and for the first time, creating an "immortal" cell line from her all-too lethal yet fecund cancer cells.[40] The "HeLa" cells, as they are called, have been widely used for research on a variety of topics including immunization, genetics, and cancers of all types. The saddest part of this story is that while many researchers and multitudes of patients benefitted from this cell line, neither Ms Lacks nor her family reaped any advantages; for many years, they were even without basic health insurance. It took decades for her family to obtain any recognition for her contribution to medical science. This book is a reminder of the human cost of some modern medical advances and lack of respect given to some patients and study participants.

Does the use of patient tissue excised during surgery require patient consent? It depends. Assuming proper consent was obtained for the surgery, the question is whether the tissue sample was obtained for clinical purposes or removed for research purposes only. Clinically-garnered tissue is removed with prior patient consent and, akin to medical information, can be subsequently used for research, educational, and epidemiological purposes if so authorized by the patient and/or a research ethics board.[41] (In the case of Ms Lacks, although the tissue was removed for clinical reasons, consent for its research use was never obtained—and probably never even considered.) Tissue removed for research purposes alone requires patient consent as does, in general, the use of personally identifiable material (as in the Lacks case). Non-identifiable material may not require patient consent as it cannot be linked to specific individuals. But it may then be problematic as to whether one can, or should attempt to, re-contact a population or individuals (to warn them of, for example, incidental findings that may affect their well-being) who may have unknowingly "donated" the blood or tissue.

CASE 12.7 AN UNEXPECTED ASSOCIATION

A 27-year-old woman, Ms T, has responded well to treatment for T-cell leukemia and has been disease-free for three years. As part of the treatment for her condition, she participated in a clinical trial of a new anti-leukemic agent which she tolerated well. She also donated samples of her blood that were to be "anonymized" and used for future research "purposes connected with her condition." Since that trial, new genome-wide studies have revealed that the first-degree relatives of patients who responded well to the drug were at increased risk for a hormonally-dependent breast cancer due to unexpected genetic associations. The researchers involved in the newer trials seek to de-anonymize the code for the trial in which Ms T was enrolled in order to study the health and genomes of her relatives.

Should the institutional ethics board charged with overseeing the trial allow them to "break the code" and warn the families of participants?

DISCUSSION OF CASE 12.7

In the case of Ms T, this is really a question of research ethics. We do not know precisely to what she had consented. Was it her understanding that her stored blood could be retained indefinitely and potentially used for any "legitimate" research purposes? Or did she think her samples would be used only for leukemia-related research and destroyed within a fixed period of time? Was she told she might be re-contacted or did she assume, once anonymized, that any future contact with her by the researchers was verboten? The broader the consent obtained, the less restrictive is the use of a participant's study samples and the more open the door for any further research on it and future re-contact. This is advantageous in many ways—for society, for future patients—but does infringe upon the right to privacy and the right to be left alone. It also opens the door more widely for the use of that information for commercial purposes never considered by the original researchers or the participants.

Whose tissue is it?

The US courts have been consistent in finding that research participants do not have a right to ownership over donated samples—they are considered "gifts" to the institution (e.g., the university, the hospital, the biobank) that harbours them. They belong neither to the patient nor to the researcher. In one well-known 2007 US court hearing,[42] a bank of thousands of prostate tissue samples collected by a physician over many years was considered the property of the university where he worked. It was felt that giving over rights of ownership to him or his patients carried the risk of rampant commercialization. In the judge's opinion,

> If left unregulated and to the whims of [donors], these highly prized biological materials would become nothing more than chattel going to the highest bidder . . . Selling excised tissue or DNA on e-Bay would become as commonplace as selling your old television on e-Bay.[43]

This may be a legitimate concern, but it goes both ways. A less charitable interpretation is that the original sponsoring institution had a strong pecuniary interest in retaining the samples for its own commercial purposes and wished to use them no matter what the participants were told or expected.

Obtaining, in advance of any deposition of tissues or blood, what has been called "tiered consent" from patients or research participants is one solution to these complexities (see Box 12.7, next page).

> **BOX 12.7**
>
> A tiered consent should include language such as the following:
>
> - "With your permission we would like to store your blood/tissue from this study for future research. You do not have to agree to this to participate in the study, but it is important for us to know how we might use your samples."
> - "Regarding my blood/tissue collected for my illness in this study, I request that this (please choose one of the following options):
>   a. only be used for research concerning the illness I have.
>   b. may be used for research concerning any health problems.
>   c. may be used in future only if I am contacted.
>   d. may not be used at all beyond this study."[44]

In trust

Even with these provisos, whether patients will truly understand to what they are consenting—and whether the courts will recognize their attempt to corral the use of their samples and personal information—is another matter. Do they truly wish to bind researchers' hands in what is already a complicated area of study? Would patients prefer a "use-unless-opt-out" option? Should there be some form of local community control over how this information is to be used and by whom? Some authors have suggested more community involvement, especially in less well-developed regions, by the creation of tissue databanks to be held "in trust" for those contributing to it. This would help ensure local control over genomic studies on the tissue. Tissues held in trust would enable public, even world, benefit without exploiting individuals or their cultures.[45]

IV. Some Questions and Answers Regarding Research

In this section I will address a few common questions regarding medical research involving humans.

Must all research receive ethics review?

In all cases an independent research ethics board is required to review and approve any research before it is undertaken. Community involvement in such a board is essential for maintaining transparency and helping lay people understand the rationale behind the research. Good and comprehensive ethics review may help prevent bad science.[46]

Is consent always necessary?

The answer is generally yes, but there are exceptions. Consent is not needed for non-interventional research such as retrospective chart reviews or research involving the secondary manipulation of large anonymized data sets, so long as privacy is protected and the collected data not sensitive.

Consent may also be waived or deferred for research conducted on patients in emergency settings. While this type of research strictly goes against the Nuremberg consent requirement, it is considered acceptable, if certain conditions are met:

- time must be of the essence, i.e., there is a narrow window of opportunity;
- the patient is incapable and cannot give consent or cannot do so in the window of time;
- the standard of care is of very limited efficacy;
- the trial can be reasonably supposed to help or address the patient's condition;
- the trial is not considered to be more harmful than the standard of care.

This is the rationale underlying studies of CPR in ambulatory settings and of the use of thrombolytic and neuroprotective drugs in the setting of acute stroke. If the test substance is unlikely to make would-be participants worse off and, if seeking consent would undermine the possibility of demonstrating the intervention's effectiveness, the normal consent process can be waived. Trial subjects and their families, needless to say, should be told of the trial as soon as feasible.

May children or incapable patients participate in research?

The answer would seem to be yes, but again there is the issue of consent. How can young children be expected to be capable of consenting to participate in a study? Because children cannot consent, the risks must be assessed as no more than minimal and, obviously, parental consent is generally required. *Adults may assume risks for the benefit of others, children are unable to do so.*[47] Patients with reduced capacity are considered a "vulnerable" group if they cannot consent to the particulars of a trial and ought never to be enrolled for reasons of convenience (e.g., by virtue of living in a residential or long-term care facility) or because they may not be able to dissent from a trial. Nevertheless, in research on conditions affecting the incapable it may be quite appropriate to include such patients (with SDM consent), otherwise it may be impossible to generalize the results from other trials that enroll only well or less afflicted subjects.

Must researchers caution participants about unanticipated findings during a study?

The answer is generally yes—especially if the findings are relevant to a participant's well-being (e.g., an unanticipated finding on a study X-ray) or if they concern the safety or usefulness of an ongoing trial. If a reasonable person would want to know such new information in order to continue enrolment in that trial, for example, new side effects are discovered or results from competing studies make the trial's completion irrelevant, that information should be promptly conveyed to participants (and the trial halted or the patients "re-consented").

May a researcher accept recompense from the trial sponsor?

Yes, but the value of such recompense must be disclosed to the reviewing ethics board and in the ICF. Payment should be only for work done and not so excessive as to be seen to sway a researcher's judgment. Any involvement of the researcher with the sponsor of a trial outside the context of the trial, for example, as an advisor to or investor in the sponsor, must be disclosed to the appropriate review board as it may place or be seen to place the researcher in a conflict of interest.

How can participant privacy be assured?

This concern is especially important given the capacity of modern medicine to capture and manipulate huge banks of information.

CASE 12.8 ARE YOU COMING HOME SOON, DAD?

A medical researcher is running a study looking at the possible benefits of a new type of medication for diabetes. Because his wife and young children have repeatedly expressed resentment of his staying at the hospital after hours to analyze this data, he has agreed to work on this at home after the children have been put to bed. The information from the study is put onto his laptop. The data includes patient names, their dates of birth, diagnoses, and test results. One day, he stops off at the grocery store on the way home to buy some bread and milk. When he returns to the car, he discovers that his laptop has been stolen from the back seat.

What should the researcher do?

DISCUSSION OF CASE 12.8

The right thing for the researcher to do is to inform the appropriate authorities in his hospital about the loss of patient data. Depending on the particular jurisdiction, there may also be an obligation to inform the research subjects of this incident (in some jurisdictions, such as Ontario, such notification is mandatory). There are several ways to ensure privacy of research data, including separating out identifiable information from study data, using only randomly generated study identification numbers for event reporting, avoiding inclusion of unique patient identifiers such as initials or birthdates, ensuring no research files leaving the office contain identifiable personal information, and using encryption and password protection protocols.

Quite frankly, privacy in research cannot ever be entirely guaranteed. Once health information leaves the institution of origin—especially if sent to another country—attempts at limiting the information's use and disclosure will be lost. One sometimes can only hope that the receiving country will have good information privacy protections. In case it does not, any information to be transmitted elsewhere should only be in the form of anonymized, not personalized, health information. All information must be encrypted and stored on a secure server. Anyone working with personalized data must be trained in privacy practices and held to strictly enforced oaths of confidentiality.

What about quality improvement (QI) studies?

Quality improvement (QI) "research" does not usually require ethics review, especially if the risks are zero or minimal, there is no participant randomization or hypothesis testing, and any data is de-identified. For example, the retrospective evaluation of the success of a new program of diabetes education would not require research review. It would require ethics review if the QI project had compared two different educational interventions. Requiring board review of every QI study is overly onerous and might hinder patient safety efforts.[48] However, as the line between research and QI is not always clear, it is prudent, when uncertain, to seek the opinion of the local research review board as to whether review is needed.

Must a research review board review all research with the same depth?

Not necessarily, but research review ought to be proportionate to the risks involved. There must be careful scrutiny of, for example, research involving vulnerable subjects, research undertaken in emergencies, research that involves risks of surgery or sham surgery, novel test substances with uncertain side-effect profiles, and "first in human" trials (trials that test a new drug or device in humans for the first time).

Must research be carried out throughout the world according to the same standards?

CASE 12.9 AN UNFAIR TRIAL

Radha, a 3-year-old girl in a poor country, is playing at home when she suddenly suffers a seizure. Her parents rush her to the hospital in the nearest town where she is stabilized. The doctor explains she most likely has a seizure disorder, but that further testing, including a CAT of her brain, is needed to rule out other causes. When her parents tell the doctor they cannot afford the tests, he asks if they would consent to enrolling Radha in a pharmaceutical company-sponsored study comparing two types of anti-seizure drugs. If so, the study sponsors will pay for her hospitalization, the investigations, and the drugs as well. She will be required to come to the hospital every month but the study will pay for transport.

Radha's parents readily agree. She does well in the trial. At study end 18 months later, her parents are informed they will no longer receive free medicines. The local clinic does not carry either of the test medications. One week later Radha suffers another seizure.

What was wrong with this trial?

International standards

No matter what the milieu or culture, the same standards of research must hold. There are ICH-GCP ("International Conference on Harmonization of technical requirements for registration of pharmaceuticals for human use"—"Good Clinical Practice") guidelines that set out international standards for human research.[49] Burdensome as they may sometimes be,[50] the standards of research review boards exist to prevent the abuses of human rights identified by Beecher and Pappworth over 50 years ago. Clearly, some standards, such as free and informed consent, are harder to implement in regions of impoverishment, illiteracy, and paternalism or authoritarianism. Where research appears to be conducted for the benefit of others, there must be genuine social value, participants must be fairly selected, and the risks ought to be minimized. "Mutual aid" is an important principle that can be applied to clinical research and justify participation in research that may not directly help individual participants.[51] One could say that, absent such altruism, much medical research would not occur. Unfortunately, this altruism by participants may not be matched by the ethics of a trial's sponsor.

DISCUSSION OF CASE 12.9

Just about everything was wrong with this trial. It typifies the problems of conducting research in the developing world.[52] The parents' decision to join the trial was motivated by financial factors—not at all unusual in poor regions—but the researchers did not inform the parents how limited the free ride would be and failed to plan for the trial's end. This is not unusual almost anywhere; research participants are used to "try out" medications they will not be able to obtain at the trial's completion, no matter how beneficial the test substances might be. This seems unjust as participants risk their well-being for the benefit of others but, even if lucky enough to benefit in the short-term, fail to reap benefits in the long run.

Impoverished participants may be less used to asking questions of researchers and may be happy with whatever assistance they can get. They cannot be blamed for that; it is the researcher's responsibility to protect the rights and welfare of participants wherever the research is conducted. The ICH-GCP guidelines are known in India and throughout the world.[53] Failure to follow them may stem from lack of effective local oversight. As more research is transferred to developing countries, it will be crucial to ensure this is not because of lower local ethical standards.[54]

Conclusion

In this chapter, we have briefly touched on complicated areas involving cross-cultural care, genetics and the human genome, and the ethics of medical research. All areas are under constant evolution and deserve deeper examination than an introductory text can plumb. Medical ethics is itself in evolution as more areas of medicine and social life undergo ethical review and moralization. Progress in healthcare has been made possible not only by our advances in the basic sciences but also through improved understanding of the social determinates of health and illness and the role of culture in the provision of appropriate care. Ethics is a small part of that process of improvement but is, I hope you would agree, a vital and enduring component.

Cases For Discussion

CASE 1: A FORM OF PROTEST?

You are a primary care provider working in an inner city clinic with a large number of immigrant patients, not all of whom are legal, most speaking little English. Many are ordered returned to their country of origin when their cases are heard before the immigration board. A small group of families awaiting deportation has taken refuge in a church in your clinic's catchment area. The local media report the group has gone on a "hunger strike" in protest—children are among them, the youngest being 5 years old.

One very articulate 8-year-old boy states he is fasting of his own free will, wants to help his parents, and does not want to go back to the awful living conditions in his home country. "It's much nicer here. I can have fun," he declares.

Questions For Discussion

1. Is this child abuse?
2. What are your obligations, if any, towards the children involved in this protest?

CASE 2: THE NEW DRUG ON THE BLOCK

A research study proposes to use a new drug, Superbia, for the maintenance of positive symptom regression in schizophrenia. There are already two drugs used for this purpose. It is thought that Superbia will have a better patient tolerability profile and possibly be safer as there appears to be less risk of agranulocytosis, a serious side effect of one of the accepted drugs. In this 48-week study, one third of the 200 patients to be enrolled at 30 sites will be randomized to either stay on their current regimen, one third will be randomized to Superbia, and one third to placebo.

All participants will be seen every 2 weeks initially, then every 4–6 weeks, with some visits conducted by telephone. Blood tests will be done throughout the study to look for evidence of reduced white cells, liver inflammation, and kidney damage.

Other side effects noted with Superbia, akin to other maintenance drugs, include high blood pressure, dizziness, headaches, fatigue, dry mouth, nausea, rashes, numbness in the body, a fuzzy feeling in the head, and diarrhea. Additional side effects, previously unidentified, may also occur.

Doses 15 times as high as used in this study resulted in weight loss, inflammation of the gastrointestinal tract, and red swollen gums in rats and dogs. No deaths have been reported to date with Superbia. Patients who deteriorate during this study will be withdrawn from the study and offered "rescue" antipsychotics.

Questions For Discussion

1. What concerns might you have about this trial?
2. Discuss what improvements could be made in the trial to make it more appropriate.

Conclusion
Going from Here

Since this book's first edition there has been continued and deepening interest in medical ethics. Newspapers, journals, social media sites, bloggers, and the Internet all carry stories and issues of ethical import. Throughout the world, people are disappointed in the cynical and often self-serving attitudes and practices of leaders in various areas of public life. Bioethics has become more sophisticated, and ethicists—"experts" (better, "consultants in ethics")—populate hospitals and other institutions. Fortunately, hospitals, despite significant budget deficits, seem to have found ways, albeit often meager, to continue to support bioethics. No doubt this is due to the useful role it can play in hard decision-making.

Some, however, still see such support for ethics in a less benign light and predict the demise of bioethics, suggesting it will be eaten for breakfast by the quotidian unethical realities of modern healthcare. According to these critics, bioethics, hemmed in by bottom-line thinking and priority setting, will either become a lapdog of administrators or wither on the vine. So it is with some institutions—for them, ethics is mere window dressing; for others, ethicists are "bullies." I'm not *that* skeptical or scared of all bioethics and ethicists. Much good work is going on, and will continue to go on, in the field. Certainly, progress in human affairs and ethics in particular should never be taken for granted.[1] The advantaged do not hand the disenfranchised their due rewards on a silver platter.

Patient rights and patient-based care are among the hard-won achievements that, I believe, will be difficult, if not impossible, to reverse. Like democratic rights and freedoms generally, once citizens have a taste of them and see their tangible benefits, they won't readily let them go. As such, the room for ethical debate will widen, not contract.

The professions of healthcare and their institutions—hospitals, universities, colleges, examining and credentialing bodies—are slowly mutating away from paternalism and hierarchies into more morally positive directions. These achievements, moral (as well as political and social) advances, are buttressed by the courts, the regulatory authorities, professional associations, academies, in charters, and conferences, and by the millions of people who have experienced and benefited from the modern "advantage-reducing" impact of ethics (see Chapter 1).

Hard lessons have been learned by the healthcare professions out of their past failures to meet the expectations of their patients and society. Out of these disappointments a new professionalism has arisen that is all about ethics and quality patient care: the centrality of the autonomous patient, the importance of evidence-based care as opposed to clinical pragmatism, teamwork and collaboration as opposed to "flying solo," transparency as opposed to secrecy, and a commitment to quality improvement over repeating the mistakes of the past.[2] I have stressed many of these themes throughout this book.

Ethics may ultimately be a private affair ("What am *I* to do? How can I do this? How should I live?"), but professional ethics is also about the attitudes, beliefs, values, and practices of healthcare professionals that can best protect and promote the welfare and wishes of patients. Seen in this way, an ethos for all the healthcare professions gives unity to the human race riven by credo, violence, and intolerance.

Lacking a commitment to such an ethics—an ethics for everyone— we are in danger, in hard times, of falling back into a Hobbesian state of nature where every man is at war with all others and no one is secure. Hardly a pleasurable prospect. The modern healthcare professional, by doing the hard work that progress in ethics and in social affairs requires, can help ameliorate the old ways of doing things, the intolerances, the thoughtlessness, and uncaring attitudes that have plagued humankind.

Ethics may seem an unlikely foundation for stability and reliability but not if you believe in ethical progress in human affairs. The world is an immeasurably (and measurably!) better place on account of the abolition of slavery, the advent of the eight-hour workday, the decline in racism, the liberation of women, the acknowledgement of the rights of children, the acceptance of interracial marriage and the rights of people of any sexual orientation, the extirpation of smallpox, the expectation of veracity of healthcare professionals by patients, and the recognition of the rights of research participants. These are but a few of the hard won moral advances societies have made, admittedly incompletely so in many places.

The central tasks of medicine—to prevent disease and premature death, to alleviate suffering and ameliorate illness—correspond to the duty of beneficence in medicine. What differs from one culture to the next is the social and political landscape that may be inhospitable to, or more fertile for, the practice of medicine. So ethics *does* vary, you might say. It does to some degree, but so does illness: how common is severe anorexia nervosa in societies where starvation is prevalent? Or dementia in regions where the average lifespan is under 50 years of age? If in a society 90 per cent of the population lacks running water and most children die of preventable infectious diarrhea, what place is there for transplant medicine? Patient choice may at times necessarily take a back seat to a population-based best interests standard. This is a loss for individuals, but it does not have to be a permanent one. The ethical tools for analysis are the same everywhere, the conditions for their use and priority varies.

This book may be the beginning of a journey for you or a refresher for those of you already on the road. If you've slogged your way through it, you have some powerful tools for ethical analysis and practice, tools that can be used for good or ill but hopefully for the good of patients and the profession of medicine. Ethics is a core curricular activity and an examinable subject, along with communication skills, necessary for entry into practice. As a healthcare professional you will be scrutinized every day for your ethical acumen by your patients and your peers. Trainees who do well in these areas exhibit better patient care attitudes and are less likely to be the subject of professional complaints.[3] Extra searching and reading are always advisable in order to keep up.

There are so many outstanding books on ethics that I can only list a few. The classic text in philosophical bioethics is Tom Beauchamp and James Childress's *Principles of Biomedical Ethics*.[4] Another helpful book is *Clinical Ethics* by Albert Jonsen, Mark Siegler, and William Winslade.[5] *Principles of Health Care Ethics* is an excellent collection covering an almost encyclopedic variety of topics.[6] *The Cambridge Textbook of Bioethics* provides a fine overview of the field with a clinical persepective.[7] The most comprehensive reference book for bioethics can be found in the five-volume *Encyclopedia of Bioethics*, now in its third edition.[8] The Office of the Surgeon General of the United States Army has produced an interesting two-volume opus, *Military Medical Ethics*, that can be recommended as a comprehensive coverage of medical ethics with, obviously, special attention to the ethics of wartime and ethics under extreme conditions.[9] The British Medical Association has provided a very practical set of well-thought-out recommendations for physicians in *Medical Ethics Today*, now in its third edition.[10]

Sugarman and Sulmasy's *Methods in Medical Ethics* is an excellent review of the different approaches, theoretical and empirical, to ethics.[11] Two books by the contemporary UK philosopher Simon Blackburn are highly recommended: *Think: A Compelling Introduction to Philosophy* and *Being Good: A Short Introduction to Ethics*.[12] Their titles are self-explanatory. The musings on ethics by the contemporary US philosopher Harry Frankfurt—*The Reasons of Love* and *The Importance of What We Care About*—are stimulating and accessible as well, if a little challenging.[13]

For practical advice on research ethics, consider Amdur and Bankert's *Institutional Review Board: Management and Function*.[14]

The following have been particularly helpful to me in writing this book: John Rawls' *Justice as Fairness: A Restatement*, although hard-going, is an elegant exploration of justice from the twentieth-century's foremost theorist of that topic;[15] Martha Nussbaum's *The Frontiers of Justice* provides a readable and cogent argument for the "opportunities" approach to justice;[16] Norman Daniels' *Just Health*, is an excellent up-to-date presentation of his arguments for fairness and reasoning in distributive justice;[17] and Amartya Sen's *Identity and Violence* which counters the "culturist" tendencies in the "post-modern" world.[18]

There are some very good compendiums of ethics cases. I will mention only two here: *Complex Ethics Consultations* by Ford and Dudzinski[19] and Lavery et al.'s *Ethical Issues in International Biomedical Research*.[20]

Almost a Revolution: Mental Health Law and the Limits of Change by Paul Appelbaum, from which I adapted the title to Chapter 2 of this book, is still an outstanding discussion of the interaction between modern health law and the practice of psychiatry.[21] Quasi-ethical and intensely interesting reflections on medicine may be found in Michael Balint's *The Doctor, His Patient and the Illness*,[22] John Berger's *A Fortunate Man: The Story of a Country Doctor*,[23] and the acerbically written *Hippocratic Oaths: Medicine and its Discontents* by a geriatrician, Raymond Tallis.[24]

Narration is an important perspective; there are many books by physicians in this field, such as Orfi's *Medicine in Translation*.[25] Books by Gawande,[26] Groopman,[27] and Sacks[28] are always worth reading for their reflections on medicine and life. In this regard, the journal, *Ars Medica*, which bridges the gap between the humanities and medicine, is highly recommended.

A well-written and comprehensive view on disability and difference may be found in Andrew Solomon's book, *Far From the Tree*; not a work in ethics, it nevertheless has important insights into the lives and experiences of those who fall "far from the family's tree" and have been, historically, poorly treated by medicine and society.[29] Mediation skills to help overcome distance and difference are critical to anyone involved in ethics consultations and for this purpose Dubler and Liebman's *Bioethics Mediation* is a very useful guide.[30] *I Shall Not Hate* by Abuelaish is a cry, in the wake of irrecoverable losses, for tolerance across cultures and cycles of violence and despair.[31] Rebecca Skloot's *The Immortal Life of Henrietta Lacks* gives eloquent voice to those used by and excluded from medical science.[32] The future of medicine and the seemingly infinite capacities of digital technology to capture and utilize complex informational fields, such as genomics, making truly personalized medicine possible, are well presented in Eric Topol's book, *The Creative Destruction of Medicine*.[33]

Want to read more? Go no further than your favourite medical journals. From the *Lancet* to the *British Medical Journal*, the *Canadian Medical Association Journal*, the *New England Journal of Medicine*, the *Annals of Internal Medicine*, and the *Journal of the American Medical Association*, all medical publications carry articles on contemporary ethical and jurisprudential issues regularly, as the footnotes throughout this book attest. The

Annals also regularly publishes poems and brief, but often riveting, stories from the lives of doctors and patients.

Many journals, of course, specialize in ethics (*Ethics, Cambridge Quarterly of Healthcare Ethics, Journal of Medical Ethics,* and *Journal of Medicine and Philosophy,* to name just a few); it is worth consulting them for guidance in vexing cases and for in-depth discussions of contemporary issues. Other journals, such as *Alberta Law Review, The Journal of Legal Medicine,* and *Law, Medicine and Health Care,* cover the more strictly legal aspect of medicine.

Finally, many websites and blogs are devoted to ethics. One only has to web-search any ethics topic to discover hundreds, if not thousands, of sites and articles. They will be of varying reliability, and seekers will not want to rely on one source of information alone.

Professional ethics is not just about individual right or wrong. It's about how we—as members of the public and members of civil societies, as patients and as healthcare professionals—should make decisions, some pedestrian, some momentous. The public and patients are involved more and perhaps, at times, even respected more, as the tides turn in favour of patient safety and public trust. These are key components of our evolving healthcare systems in fragile societies facing economically and politically challenging times.

Progress in professional ethics in a world characterized by value and moral divides is possible but will be made not by one profession or one nation alone, but by the combined efforts of many. Medicine's greatest historian, Roy Porter, explains, "Medicine's finest hour is the dawn of its dilemmas." But there is hope. "Many of these quandaries," he writes, "can be resolved with common decency, goodwill, and a sensible ethics committee."[34]

To this I can only say: *"Hear, hear."*

Notes

Preface

1. G. Annas, Doctors, patients, and lawyers: two centuries of health law, *N Engl J Med* 367 (2012): 445–50.
2. E. Gellner, *Thought and Change* (Chicago: University of Chicago Press, 1964. Midway Reprint, 1974), 59.
3. A. Montagu, *On Being Human* (New York: Henry Schuman, 1951).
4. E. Ostrum, *Governing the Commons: The Evolution of Institutions for Collective Action* (Cambridge UK: Cambridge University Press, 2008).
5. P. Gourevitch, D. Lake and J. Gross Stein, *The Credibility of Transnational NGOs: When Virtue is not Enough* (Cambridge UK: Cambridge University Press, 2012).

Introduction

1. C. Dickens, *Hard Times* (London: Chapman & Hall, 1854), 1.
2. S. Harris, *The Moral Landscape: How Science can determine Human Values* (Toronto: Free Press, 2010), 2.
3. For example, the new curriculum for UK medicine "focuses on the development of more generic professional competences such as communication, working in multi-professional teams, encouraging self-care, increasing shared decision-making between patients and healthcare professionals, and the ability to assure and improve the quality of care." Academy of Medical Royal Colleges, *The Foundation Programme: Curriculum* (June 2007), 4.
4. Similar efforts to expand and clarify the physician's role in society may be found in other places, too. See: J.R. Frank, (ed), *The CanMEDS 2005 Physician Competency Framework. Better standards, Better physicians, Better care* (Ottawa: The Royal College of Physicians and Surgeons of Canada, 2005).
5. T. Ferguson, *E-Patients: How They Can Help Us Heal Healthcare* (San Francisco: Creative Commons, 2007). Available at: http://www.e-patients.net.
6. See the journal *Ars Medica: A Journal of Medicine, the Arts, and Humanities* which, as its title suggests, grapples with the altogether human experience of healthcare.
7. Narrative medicine which allows us to better stand in the shoes of others has been particularly helpful in this regard. Narrative medicine generates an ethics of its own.
8. K. Popper, *Conjectures and Refutations: The Growth of Scientific Knowledge* (New York: Harper & Row, 1968), 322–24.
9. A. MacIntyre, *A Short History of Ethics: A History of Moral Philosophy from the Homeric Age to the 20th Century,* 2nd edn. (Notre Dame, Indiana: Notre Dame U Press, 2008), xvi: "Each fundamental moral philosophy . . . has its own set of first principles."
10. D. Macrae, The Council for International Organizations and Medical Sciences (CIOMS) Guidelines on ethics of clinical trials, *Proc Am Thorac Society,* 4 (2007): 176–79.
11. S. Hoffman, Ending medical complicity in state-sponsored torture, *Lancet* 378 (2011): 1535–7.
12. R. Goodman and M.J. Roseman, eds. *Interrogations, Forced Feedings, and the Role of Health Care Professionals* (Cambridge, MA: Human Rights Program at Harvard Law School, 2009).
13. C. Elliott, *White Coat, Black Hat: Adventures on the Dark Side of Medicine* (Boston: Beacon Press, 2010).
14. S. Sherwin, Whither Bioethics? How feminism can help reorient bioethics, *Int J of Feminist Approaches to Bioethics,* 1 (2008): 7–27; R.Edgman-Levitan, "[People] have wildly unrealistic views about what can be improved how quickly." Quoted in D. Malina, Performance anxiety—What can health care reform learn from K-12 education? *N Engl J Med,* 369 (2013): 1270.
15. T. Nagel, Moral epistemology, in R. Bulger, E. Bobby, and H. Fineberg (eds.), *Society's Choices: Social and Ethical Decision Making in Biomedicine* (Washington, DC: National Academy Press, 1995), 202.

16. D. Parfit, *On What Matters*, Vol. 1 (New York: Oxford University Press, 2011), 35.

17. See, for example, H. Frankfurt, *The Reasons of Love* (Princeton NJ: Princeton University Press, 2004), 6: "Morality is less pertinent to the shaping of our preferences and to the guidance of our conduct . . . than is commonly presumed . . . it does not necessarily have the last word."

18. B. Egman-Levitan, Shared decision-making—The pinnacle of patient-centered care, *N Engl J Med*, 366 (2012): 780–1.

19. J.S. Mill, *On Liberty* [1859] (New York: Appleton-Century Crofts, 1947), 10–11.

20. A. Sen and B. Williams, eds. *Utilitarianism and Beyond* (Cambridge MA: Cambridge University Press, 1981).

21. I. Kant, *The Metaphysical Principles of Virtue* [1797] (New York: The Bobbs-Merrill Company, Inc., 1964), 23, 25.

22. J. Rawls, *A Theory of Justice* (Cambridge MA: Harvard University Press, 1981).

23. G.A. Cohen, *Rescuing Justice and Equality* (Cambridge, MA: Harvard University Press, 2008).

24. Parfit, *op. cit.*

25. G. Harman, *The Nature of Morality: An Introduction to Ethics* (New York: Oxford University Press, 1977), 162.

26. E. Pellegrino and D. Thomasma, *The Virtues in Medical Practice*. (Oxford: Oxford University Press, 1993).

27. R. Charon, Narrative and medicine, *N Engl J Med*, 350, (2004): 862–4.

28. M. Divinsky, Stories for life, *Can Fam Physician*, 53, (2007): 203–5.

29. A. MacIntyre, *After Virtue*. 2nd ed., (Notre Dame, Indiana: University of Notre Dame Press, 1984), 216.

30. R. Garland-Thomson, Integrating disability, transforming feminist theory, *NWSA J Feminist Disability Studies*, 14 (2002): 1–32.

31. A. Donchin, Converging concerns: Feminist bioethics, development theory, and human rights, *Signs*, 34 (2004), 299–324.

32. H. Meekosha, The complex balancing act of choice, autonomy, valued life, and rights: Bringing a feminist disability perspective to bioethics, *Int J of Feminist Approaches to Bioethics*, 3 (2010): 1–8.

33. A. Jonsen and S. Toulmin, *The Abuse of Casuistry: A History of Moral Reasoning* (Berkeley: University of California Press, 1988), 265.

34. K. De Ville, What does the law say? Law, ethics, and medical decision making, *West J Med*, 160 (1994): 478–80.

35. H. MacDonald, Irish abortion laws to blame for woman's death, say parents, *The Guardian*, (Nov. 15, 2012). Accessed at www.guardian.co.uk/world/2012/nov/15/irish-abortion-law-death.

36. M.G. Bloche, The Supreme Court and the purposes of medicine, *N Engl J Med*, 354 (2006): 993–5.

37. C. Wilson, *Moral Animals: Ideals and Constraints in Moral Theory* (Oxford: Clarendon Press, 2007): 9–10.

38. J.A.M. Gray, *The Resourceful Patient* (Oxford: eRosetta Press, 2002).

39. J. McKinlay and L. Marceau, When there is no doctor: Reasons for the disappearance of primary care physicians in the US during the early 21st century, *Social Science & Medicine*, 67 (2008): 1481–91.

40. R. Desjarlais and A. Kleinman, Violence and demoralization in the new world order, *Anthropology Today*, 10 (1994): 9–12.

41. L. Dyrbye, M. Thomas, S. Massie, D. Power, et al., Burnout and suicidal ideation among US medical students. *Ann Intern Med*, 149 (2008): 334–41.

42. R. Macklin, *Enemies of Patients: How Doctors Are Losing Their Power and Patients Are Losing Their Rights* (New York: Oxford University Press, 1993).

43. A. Zuger, Dissatisfaction with medical practice, *N Engl J Med*, 350 (2004): 69–75.

44. N. Edwards, M.J. Kornacki, and J. Silversin, Unhappy doctors: What are the causes and what can be done? *BMJ*, 324 (2002): 835–8.

45. J. Adams, et al., *Healthcare 2015: Win-win or Lose-lose: A Portrait and a Path to Successful Transformation*. IBM Global Business Services. NY USA 2006, 3: 'Today value in healthcare is hard to see . . ."

46. "While it has been frequently suggested that the aim of professionalism and ethics preparation is not to midwife virtue or to assure sound moral character, medical students and residents themselves believe it may confer positive qualities and preservation of compassion." L.W. Roberts, K.A. Green Hammond, C.M.A. Geppert, and T.D. Warner, The positive role of professionalism and ethics training in medical education:

A comparison of medical student and resident perspectives, *Acad Psychiatry*, 28 (2004): 170–82.

47. C. LeBlanc and J. Heyworth, Emergency physicians: "burned out" or "fired up"? *CJEM*, 9/2 (2007): 121–3.

48. S. Schulz, B. Woestmann, B. Huenges, C. Schweikardt, and T. Schäfer. How important is medical ethics and history of medicine teaching in the medical curriculum? An empirical approach towards students' views. *GMS Z Med Ausbild*, 29 (2012): Doc 8. Available online at: < 10 3205/zma000778 >

49. C. Horowitz, A. Suchman, W. Branch, and R. Frankel, What do doctors find meaningful about their work? *Annals of Int Med*, 138 (2003): 772–75.

50. R. Porter, *The Greatest Benefit to Mankind: A Medical History of Humanity* (New York: W.W. Norton & Co., 1997).

Chapter 1

1. J.S. Mill, *On Liberty* [1859] (New York: Appleton-Century Crofts, 1947), 58.

2. S. Blackburn, *Being Good: A Short Introduction to Ethics* (London: Oxford University Press, 2001), 132–3.

3. "In view of the casual attitude towards antibiotics that prevails, it is hardly surprising that resistance has increased worldwide over the past few decades." J. Carlet, P. Collignon, D. Goldmann, et al., Society's failure to protect a precious resource: antibiotics, *Lancet*, 378 (2011): 369–71.

4. H. Frankfurt, *The Reasons of Love* (Princeton, NJ: Princeton University Press, 2004).

5. K. Margittai, R. Moscarello, and M. Rossi, Medical students' perception of abuse, *Annals RCPSC*, 27 (1994): 199–204.

6. G. Cohen, *What's Wrong with Hospitals?* (Middlesex, UK: Penguin Books, 1964).

7. R. Srivastava, Speaking up: When doctors navigate medical hierarchy, *N Engl J Med*, 368 (2013): 302–5.

8. H. Silver and A. Glicken, Medical student abuse: Incidence, severity, and significance, *JAMA*, 263 (1990): 527–32.

9. L. Hicks, Y. Lin, D. Robertson, D. Robinson, and S. Woodrow, Understanding the clinical dilemmas that shape medical students' ethical development: Questionnaire survey and focus group study, *BMJ*, 322 (2001): 709–10.

10. S. Rennie and J. Crosby, Are "tomorrow's doctors" honest? *BMJ*, 322 (2001): 274–5.

11. "[N]eophytes cannot perform high-stakes procedures at an acceptable level of proficiency . . . [We must] develop approaches to skills training that do not put our patients at risk in service to education." M. Cook, D. Irby, W. Sullivan, and K. Ludmerer, American medical education 100 years after the Flexner Report, *N Engl J Med*, 355 (2006): 1339–44.

12. D. Parfit, *On What Matters*, Vol. 1 (Oxford: Oxford University Press, 2011): 375.

13. Aristotle, *Nicomachean Ethics*, Book II, 1103a-b. (New York: Bobbs-Merrill, 1962): 33–5.

14. D. Lyons, *Ethics and the Rule of Law* (Cambridge, UK: Cambridge University Press, 1987), 7–35.

15. D. Sontag, Deported in coma, saved back in US, *New York Times*, (Nov 9, 2008): s.A, 1, 34.

16. R. Perkin, Lecture Notes "Medical Ethics," Period III Curriculum, (Toronto: University of Toronto, unpublished,1967). Personal communication to the author (2013).

17. Adapted from: A. Peterkin, Practical strategies for practising narrative-based medicine, *Can Fam Physician*, 58 (2012): 63–64.

18. T. Beauchamp and J. Childress, *Principles of Biomedical Ethics*, 5th edn. (New York: Oxford University Press, 2000).

19. A. Jonsen and S. Toulmin, *The Abuse of Casuistry: A History of Moral Reasoning* (Berkeley: University of California Press, 1988).

20. Oath of Hippocrates, in W. Reich (ed.), *Encyclopedia of Bioethics*, rev. edn., vol. 5 (Toronto: Simon & Schuster Macmillan, 1995), 2632.

21. N. Rohrhoff, Becoming a physician. What life is like, *N Engl J Med*, 366 (2012): 683–85.

22. T. Brewin, *Primum non nocere? Lancet*, 344 (1994): 1487–8.

23. Such was Ivan Illich's criticism of modern healthcare: "The medical establishment has become a major threat to health." I. Illich, *Medical Nemesis:The Expropriation of Health* (Toronto: McClelland & Stewart, 1975), 11.

24. A. Esmail, Physician as serial killer: The Shipman case, *N Engl J Med*, 352 (2005): 1843–4.

25. R. Brook, Quality of care: do we care? *Ann Intern Med*, 115 (1991): 486–90.

26. C. von Gunten, Discussing Do-Not-Resuscitate status, *J Clin Oncol*, 19 (2001): 1576–81.

27. E. Pellegrino and D. Thomasma, *The Virtues in Medical Practice* (New York: Oxford University Press, 1993), 80–1.

28. B. Lo, *Resolving Ethical Dilemmas: A Guide for Clinicians*, 2nd edn. (Philadelphia: Lippincott, Williams & Wilkins, 2000); T. Thomasma, Training in medical ethics: An ethical workup, *Forums on Medicine* (Dec. 1978): 33–6; M. Siegler, Decision-making strategy for clinical-ethical problems in medicine, *Arch Intern Med*, 142 (1982): 2178–9; L. McCullough, Addressing ethical dilemmas: An ethics work-up, *The New Physician*, 33 (Oct. 1984): 34–5.

29. Thanks to Mary Rose MacDonald for emphasizing this.

30. A. Sen, *Identity and Violence: The Illusion of Destiny* (New York: Norton & Co, 2007), 13.

31. W. Styron, *Sophie's Choice* (New York: Vintage Books, 1992).

32. S. Callahan, The role of emotion in ethical decision making, *Hastings Cent Rep*, 18 (June/July 1988): 9–14.

33. J. Sevulescu, Conscientious objection in medicine, *BMJ*, 332 (2006): 294–7.

34. A.C. Grayling, *Meditations for the Humanist: Ethics for a Secular Age* (Oxford: Oxford University Press, 2002), 38.

35. G.E.R. Lloyd, *Aristotle: The Growth and Structure of his Thought* (London: Cambridge University Press, 1968), 244.

36. "Forcible feeding is never ethically acceptable." J. Welsh, Responding to food refusal. In R. Goodman and M.J. Roseman, *Interrogations, Forced Feedings, and the Role of Health Professionals*, (Cambridge, MA: Human Rights Program at Harvard Law School, 2009), 154.

37. E. Attia, Eating disorders, *Annals of Intern Med*, 156 (3 April 2012): ITC1-14.

38. A. Robb, T. Silber, J. Orrell-Valente, A. Valadez-Meltzer, N. Ellis, M.J. Dadson, and I. Chatoor, Supplemental nocturnal nasogastric refeeding for better short-term outcome in hospitalized adolescent girls with anorexia nervosa, *Am J Psychiatry*, 159 (2002): 1347–53.

39. V. Levy-Barzilai, Death wish: Does an anorexic whose life is in danger have a right to starve herself to death? *Ha'aretz*, 17 Aug. 2001.

40. M. Christodoulou, Pro-anorexia websites pose a public health challenge, *Lancet*, 379 (2012): 110.

41. "The 'psychiatric patient' is a person who fails, or refuses, to assume a legitimate social role." T. Szasz, *Ideology and Insanity: Essays on the Psychiatric Dehumanization of Man* (New York: Anchor Books, 1970), 210.

42. H. Bruch, *The Golden Cage: The Enigma of Anorexia Nervosa* (Cambridge, MA: Harvard University Press, 1982).

43. E.L. Langston, Ethical treatment of military detainees, *Lancet*, 370 (2007): 1999.

44. G. Annas, Hunger strikes at Guantanamo: Medical ethics and human rights in a "legal black hole," *N Engl J Med*, 355 (2006): 1377–82.

45. L. Schneiderman, K. Faber-Langendoen, and N. Jecker, Beyond futility to an ethic of care, *Am J Med*, 96 (1994): 110–14.

46. S. Strauss, Death: one, Medicine: no score, *CMAJ*, 177 (2007): 903–4.

47. P.C. Hébert and M. Weingarten, The ethics of forced feeding in anorexia nervosa, *CMAJ*, 144 (1991): 141–4.

48. R. Palmer, Death in anorexia nervosa, *Lancet*, 361 (2003): 1490.

49. D. Hume, *A Treatise of Human Nature*, in H. Aiken, (ed.), *Hume: Moral and Political Philosophy* (New York: Hafner Press, 1975), 43. Hume was pessimistic about the role of rationality in disputes over ethics: "reason alone can never be a motive to any action of the will . . . and . . . it can never oppose passion in the direction of the will" (*ibid.*, 23).

50. D. Hume, in L. Selby-Bigge, (ed.,) *A Treatise of Human Nature* (London: Oxford University Press, 1967), "The rules of morality, therefore, are not conclusions of our reason" (*ibid.*, 457). Nevertheless Hume would write, "The interest, on which justice is founded, is the greatest imaginable, and extends to all times and places" (*ibid.*, 620).

51. "What people disagree about is what is true, and not merely what is true for

them. If there is no such thing as truth in a certain area people cannot disagree." R. Trigg, *Reason and Commitment* (London: Cambridge University Press, 1974), 152.

Chapter 2

1. H. Cockerham, *The English Dictionarie* (1623), accessed in *Oxford English Dictionary* [CD-ROM], 2nd edn., Version 3.0 (Oxford: Oxford University Press, 2002).
2. *Schloendorff v. Society of New York Hospital*, 1914, 105 N.E. 92, (N.Y.C.A.).
3. A. Sen, *Identity and Violence: The Illusion of Destiny* (New York: Norton & Co, 2007): 120.
4. B. Venesy, A clinician's guide to decision making capacity and ethically sound medical decisions, *Am J Phys Med Rehab*, 73 (1994): 219–26.
5. A. Mol, *The Logic of Care: Health and the Problem of Patient Choice* (New York: Routledge, 2008).
6. D. Wolpaw, Seeing eye to eye, *N Engl J Med*, 365 (2011): 2052–53.
7. K. Pollock and J. Grime, Patients' perception of entitlement to time in general practice consultations for depression: qualitative study, *BMJ*, 325 (2002): 687.
8. L. Baker, D. O'Connell, and F. Platt, "What else?" Setting the agenda for the clinical interview, *Ann Intern Med*, 143 (2005): 766–70.
9. J. Coulehan, F. Platt, B. Egener, et al., "Let me see if I have this right . . ." Words that help build empathy, *Ann Intern Med*, 135 (2001): 221–7.
10. J. Walker, S. Leveille, L. Ngo, E. Vodicka, et al., Inviting patients to read their doctors' notes: Patients and doctors look ahead, *Ann Intern Med*, 155 (2011): 811–19.
11. "Autonomy is therefore the ground of the dignity of human nature and of every rational nature." I. Kant, *Groundwork of the Metaphysic of Morals* [1785] (New York: Harper & Row, 1956), 103.
12. W. Kaufmann, *Without Guilt and Justice: From Decidophobia to Autonomy* (New York: Dell Publishing, 1973).
13. "[T]he obligation to make all one's own decisions . . . states an unattainable and unwise standard." C. Schneider, *The Practice of Autonomy: Patients, Doctors, and Medical Decisions* (New York: Oxford University Press, 1998), 174.
14. "Autonomy is essentially a matter of whether we are active rather than passive in our motives and choices—whether, however we acquire them, they are the motives and choices that we really want and are therefore in no way alien to us." H. Frankfurt, *The Reasons of Love* (Princeton, NJ: Princeton University Press, 2004), 20.
15. W.W. Bartley III, *The Retreat to Commitment* (2nd ed) (Nashville: Open Court Publishers, 1984). Bartley was a committed rationalist but held that you could, rationally, relinquish one's rationalism.
16. R. Descartes, *Discourse on Method: Discourse 4* [1637] (Baltimore, MD: Penguin Books, 1968), 53.
17. S. Nadler, *A Book Forged in Hell: Spinoza's Scandalous Treatise and the Birth of the Secular Age* (Princeton, NJ: Princeton University Press, 2011).
18. W. Weston, J. Brown, and M. Stewart, patient-centred interviewing, *Can Fam Physician*, 35 (1989): 147–51.
19. R. Charon, Narrative medicine: A model for empathy, reflection, profession and trust, *JAMA*, 286 (2001): 1897–1902.
20. H. Carel and J. Macnaughton, "How do you feel?" Oscillating perspectives in the clinic. *Lancet*, 379 (2012): 2334–35.
21. R. Klitzman, *When Doctors become patients* (New York: Oxford University Press, 2008).
22. O. Sacks, *A Leg to Stand On*, (New York: Summit Books, 1984): 57, his emphasis.
23. *Malette v. Shulman* (1987), 63 O.R. (2d) 243 (H.C.J.).
24. *Ibid.*, 273.
25. *Malette v. Shulman* (1990), 72 O.R. (2d) 417 (C.A.).
26. *Ibid.*, 273.
27. P.A. Singer and F. Lowy, Refusal of life-sustaining treatment, the Malette case, and decision making under uncertainty, *Annals RCPSC*, 24 (1991): 401–3.
28. D. Sacks and R. Koppes, Caring for the female Jehovah's Witness: Balancing medicine, ethics, and the First Amendment, *Am J Obstet Gynecol*, 170 (1994): 452–5.
29. *Fleming v. Reid* (1991), 4 O.R. (3d) 86.
30. *Ibid.*, 75.

31. Tying the knot, *Maclean's*, 12 Nov. 2007, 51.

32. D. Reuben and M. Tinetti, Goal-oriented patient-care—An alternative health outcomes paradigm, *N Engl J Med*, 366 (2012): 777–9.

33. *Allen v. New Mt Sinai Hospital* (1980) 11 CCLT 299 (Ont HC) (1981) 19 CCLT 76 (CA).

34. D. Brock and S.Wartman, When competent patients make irrational choices, *N Engl J Med*, 322 (1990): 1595–9.

35. O.J. Bogunovic and S.F. Greenfield, Practical geriatrics: Use of benzodiazepines among elderly patients, *Psychiatr Serv*, 55 (2004): 233–5.

36. L. Farrell, The threat, *BMJ*, 332 (2006): 1399. "A prescription has many fathers, and physical intimidation is yet another"—on the difficulties of weaning patients from drugs.

37. A. J. Mitchell, O. Lord, and D. Malone, Differences in the prescribing of medication for physical disorders in individuals with v. without mental illness: meta-analysis, *Br J Psychiatry*; 201(2012): 435–43.

38. T. J. Heeren, P. Derksen, B. F. van Heycop Ten Ham, and P. P. van Gent, Treatment, outcome and predictors of response in elderly depressed in-patients, *Br J Psychiatry*, 170 (1997): 436–40.

39. M. Siegler, Critical illness: The limits of autonomy, *Hastings Cent Rep*, 7 (Oct. 1977): 12–15.

40. F. Ingelfinger, Arrogance, *N Engl J Med*, 303 (1980): 1507–11.

41. R. Hardy and C. Kell, Understanding and working with the concept of denial and its role as a coping strategy, *Nursing Times*, 105 (2009): 22–4.

42. J. Groves, Taking care of the hateful patient, *N Engl J Med*, 298 (1978): 883–7.

43. D. Bardes, Defining "patient-centered medicine", *N Engl J Med*, 366 (2012): 782–3.

44. C. Foster, Putting dignity to work, *Lancet*, 379 (2012): 2044–5.

45. R. Srivastava, Dealing with uncertainty in a time of plenty, *N Engl J Med*, 365 (2011): 2252–3.

46. N. Dubler and C. Liebman, *Bioethics Mediation: A Guide to Shaping Shared Solutions* (Nashville: Vanderbilt University Press, 2011).

47. Adapted with permission from J. Stutchbury, Who's meant to be teaching us? *Lancet*, 378 (2011): 2136–7.

Chapter 3

1. G. Lyttelton, *Personal Letters* LXXIX [1744], accessed from *Oxford English Dictionary* [CD-ROM], 2nd edn., Version 3.0 (Oxford: Oxford University Press, 2002).

2. W. Shakespeare, *Troilus and Cressida* [c. 1602], Act III, Scene iii, accessed from *Oxford English Dictionary* [CD-ROM], 2nd edn., Version 3.0 (Oxford: Oxford University Press, 2002).

3. P. Appelbaum, Privacy in psychiatric treatment: Threats and responses, *Am J Psychiatry*, 159 (2002): 1809–18.

4. S.D. Warren and L.D. Brandeis, The Right to Privacy, *Harv. L. Rev.*, 4 (1890): 193–220. Similarly, in 1988 the Supreme Court of Canada affirmed that "the liberty interest is rooted in the fundamental notions of human dignity, personal autonomy, privacy and choice in decisions regarding an individual's fundamental being." *R v. Morgentaler*, [1988] 1 S.C.R.

5. *McInerney v. MacDonald*, [1992] 2 S.C.R. 138.

6. Oath of Hippocrates, in W. Reich (ed.), *Encyclopedia of Bioethics*, rev. edn., vol. 5 (Toronto: Simon & Schuster Macmillan, 1995), 2632.

7. See *Kenny v. Lockwood* [1932] O.R. 141 (C.A.). Many thanks to Maria McDonald for this reference.

8. E. Gibson, Whither privacy of health information at the Supreme Court, in J. Downie and E. Gibson (eds.), *Health Law at the Supreme Court of Canada* (Toronto: Irwin Law, 2007).

9. *R v. Potvin* (1971), 16 C.R.N.S. 233 (Que. C.A.).

10. Canadian Nurses Association, *Code of Ethics for Registered Nurses* (Ottawa, 2008).

11. Supreme Court of Canada, *McInerney v. MacDonald* [1992] 2 S.C.R. 138.

12. Lü Yao-Huai, Privacy and Data Privacy Issues in Contemporary China, *Ethics and Information Technology*, 7 (2005): 7–15.

13. Privilege is especially important in psychotherapy whether conducted

by physicians, social workers or psychologists. "The psychotherapist privilege serves the public interest by facilitating the provision of appropriate treatment for individuals suffering the effects of a mental or emotional problem. The mental health of our citizenry, no less than its physical health, is a public good of transcendent importance." *Jaffee v. Redmond* (95–266), 518 U.S. 1 (1996)

14. M. Ross, Subpoenas: What to do, where to go, *CMPA Information Letter*, 10 (1995): 1–2.

15. Gibson, in J. Downie, *op. cit.*: 324.

16. Many thanks to Lori Luther for Boxes 3.1, 3.2 and 3.4.

17. E. Picard and G. Robertson, *Legal Liability of Doctors and Hospitals in Canada*, 3rd edn. (Toronto: Thomson Carswell, 1996), 21.

18. P. Beck, The confidentiality of psychiatric records and the patient's right to privacy, *Can J Psychiatry*, 46 (2001): No. 3, insert, CPA position statement. Available at: http://publications.cpa-apc.org/media.php?mid=121

19. J. Burnham, Secrets about patients, *N Engl J Med*, 324 (1991): 1130–3.

20. K.V. Rhodes, R.M. Frankel, N. Levinthal, E. Prenoveau, J. Bailey, and W. Levinson, "You're not a victim of domestic abuse, are you?" Provider–patient communication about domestic violence, *Ann Intern Med*, 147 (2007): 620–7.

21. J. Liebschutz and E. Rothman, Intimate-partner violence—what physicians can do, *N Engl J Med*, 367 (2012): 2071–3.

22. Note that the requirement of "imminence" is found in many Canadian privacy statutes (Personal Health and Information Acts) and Canadian case law (*Smith v. Jones*) but in Ontario privacy law (PHIPA, s. 40) refers to disclosure necessary to "eliminating or reducing a significant risk of bodily harm" without reference to imminence or emergency. How this actually translates is not entirely clear but it seems to suggest a slight broadening of the permission to disclose. Thanks to Lori Luther for this point.

23. J. Irvine, The physician's other duties: Good faith, loyalty and confidentiality, in B. Sneiderman, J. Irvine, and P. Osborne, *Canadian Medical Law: An Introduction for Physicians, Nurses and other Health Care Professionals*, 3rd edn. (Toronto: Thomson Carswell, 2003), 224.

24. *Criminal Code* (R.S.C., 1985, c. C-46).

25. M. Marshall and B. von Tigerstrom, Confidentiality and disclosure of health information, in J. Downie, and T. Caulfield (eds.), *Canadian Health Law and Policy* (Toronto: Butterworths Canada, 1999), 165–6.

26. *Medicine Act*, O. Reg. 856/93, s. 1(1)(10)

27. S. Vigod, C. Bell, and J. Bohnen, Privacy of patients' information in hospital lifts, *BMJ*, 327 (2003): 1024–5.

28. P. Ubel, M. Zell, D. Miller, G. Fischer, D. Peters-Stefani, and R. Arnold, Elevator talk: Observational study of inappropriate comments in a public space, *Am J Med*, 99 (1995): 190–4. One would hope that things have changed in the close to 20 years since this paper was published.

29. J. Campbell Rep. Cases King's Bench III. 81 [1814].

30. *Shulman v. CPSO* (1980), 29 O.R. (2d). 40 (Ont. Div. Ct.).

31. S. Solomon, Physician writer faces court martial over story, *Nat Rev of Med*, 4 (2007). Accessed at: http://www.nationalreviewofmedicine.com/issue/2007/08_30/4_patients_practice03_14.html

32. Accessed at: https://www.cpsbc.ca/files/u6/2009-10-annual-report.pdf

33. J. Irvine, The physician's other duties: Good faith, loyalty and confidentiality, in B. Sneiderman, J. Irvine, and P. Osborne, *op. cit.*, 212.

34. R. Neubauer, Paranoia over privacy, *Ann Intern Med*, 145 (2006): 228–9.

35. P. Collins, P. Slaughter, N. Roos, K. Weisbaum, M. Hirtle, J. Williams, et al., *Harmonizing Research & Privacy: Standards for a Collaborative Future*, Executive Summary: Privacy Best Practices for Secondary Data Use (SDU) (Ottawa: Canadian Institutes of Health Research, 2006).

36. "Where it is not feasible to use anonymous or anonymized data for research (and there are many reasons why data may need to be gathered and retained in an identifiable form), the ethical duty of confidentiality and the use of appropriate measures to safeguard information become paramount." Tri-Council Policy Statement, *Ethical*

Conduct for Research Involving Humans (Ottawa: TCPS 2, 2010): 56.

37. P. Collins, et al., *op. cit.*

38. D. Sittig and H. Singh, Rights and responsibilities of users of electronic health records, *CMAJ*, 184 (2012): 1479–83.

39. "[R]ules [regarding confidentiality] (i.e., the Quebec Charter of Human Rights and Freedoms, the Code of Civil Procedure, the *Medical Act*, and the Code of Professional Ethics for Physicians) are rules of protective public order." J. LeBel quoted in Gibson, Whither privacy, 336, see FN 8.

40. J. Duff quoted in *McInerney v. MacDonald* (1992) S.C.C. 12.

41. Failure to Report Communicable Disease is Negligence Per Se—*Derrick v. Ontario Community Hospital*, 47 Cal.App.3d 145, 120 Cal.Rptr. 566 (1975). By the *Health Protection and Promotion Act*: "26. A physician or registered nurse in the extended class who, while providing professional services to a person, forms the opinion that the person is or may be infected with an agent of a communicable disease shall, as soon as possible after forming the opinion, report thereon to the medical officer of health of the health unit in which the professional services are provided." R.S.O. 1990, c. H.7, s. 26; 2007, c. 10, Sched. F, s. 4.

42. See *US State Laws on Mandatory Reporters of Child Abuse and Neglect*. (Aug, 2012) https://www.childwelfare. gov/systemwide/laws_policies/statutes/ manda.cfm

43. S.K. Loo, N. Bala, M. Clarke, and J. Hornick, *Child Abuse: Reporting and Classification in Health Care Settings* (Ottawa: Health Canada, 1999) http://www.phac-aspc.gc.ca/cm-vee/ publicat/pdf/child_e.pdf. Accessed 28-03-2013.

44. M. Lachs and K. Pillemer, Abuse and neglect of elderly persons, *N Engl J Med*, 332 (1995): 437–43.

45. Many laws apply to elder abuse, but there is no "elder abuse" law in Canada. *A Practical Guide to Elder Abuse and Neglect Law in Canada* (Vancouver: Canadian Centre for Elder Law, University of BC, 2011). Accessed at: http://www.bcli. org/sites/default/files/Practical_Guide_ English_Rev_JULY_2011_0.pdf

46. *Toms v. Foster* (1994) OJ No. 1413 (CA).

47. D.A. Breen, D.P. Breen, J. Moore, P.A. Breen, and D. O'Neill, Driving and dementia, *BMJ*, 334 (2007): 1365–9.

48. *Assessing Fitness to Drive* (4th ed.) National Transport Commission (Sydney, Australia: March, 2012).

49. D. Redelmeier, V. Vinkatesh, and M. Stanbrook, Mandatory reporting by physicians of patients potentially unfit to drive, *Open Medicine*, 2/1(2008): E8–17.

50. D.A. Redelmeier, C. J. Yarnell, D. Thiruchelvam, and R. J. Tibshirani, Physicians' Warnings for Unfit Drivers and the Risk of Trauma from Road Crashes, *N Engl J Med*, 367 (2012): 1228–36.

51. *Determining Medical Fitness to Drive: A Guide for Physicians*, 8th edn. (Ottawa: Canadian Medical Association, 2012). Accessed at: http://www.cma.ca/ multimedia/CMA/pdf/CMA-Drivers- Guide-8th-edition-e.pdf

52. CANDRIVE is the Canadian research consortium looking at this issue, See: http://www.candrive.ca

53. s. 6.5 (1) *The Aeronautics Act.* http:// laws-lois.justice.gc.ca/eng/acts/A%2D2/ page-20.html#h-25

54. s. 35 (1) *The Railway Safety Act.* http:// laws-lois.justice.gc.ca/eng/acts/R-4.2/ page-21.html#h-30.

55. s. 27, 28 *Merchant Seamen Compensation Act* (R.S.C., 1985, c. M-6). http://laws.justice. gc.ca/eng/acts/M-6/page-7.html#h-7

56. Canadian Medical Protective Association quoted in *Newsletter of the Section on Occupational and Environmental Health* (Nov.) (Toronto: Ontario Medical Association, 1994).

57. Third Party Reports. CPSO Policy Statement #2-12, *Dialogue*. CPSO, Toronto Canada. Issue 2 (2012).

58. Mandatory Gunshot Wounds Reporting Act, 2005, S.O. 2005, c. 9. "ME/Cs have state statutory authority to investigate deaths that are sudden, suspicious, violent, unattended, or unexplained."

59. J.P. May, D. Hemenway, R. Oen, and KR Pitts, Medical care solicitation by criminals with gunshot wound injuries: a survey of Washington, DC, jail detainees, *J Trauma*, 48 (2000): 130–2.

60. J.P. May, D. Hemenway, and A. Hall, Do criminals go to the hospital when they are shot? *Inj Prev*, 8 (2002): 236–8.

61. D.L. Combs, R.G. Parrish, and R. Ing, *Death investigation in the United States and Canada*, 1995 (Atlanta: U.S. Department of Health and Human Services, CDC, 1995).

62. *Medical Examiner's and Coroner's Handbook on Death Registration and Fetal Death Reporting* (Hyattsville, Md, DHHS; 2003) Avialable at: http://www.cdc.gov/nchs/data/misc/hb_me.pdf

63. J. Bourke and S. Wessely, Confidentiality, *BMJ*, 336 (2008): 888–91.

64. J. Lenzer, Doctors outraged at Patriot Act's potential to seize medical records, *BMJ*, 332 (2006): 69.

65. *Smith v. Jones*, [1999] 1 S.C.R. 455.

66. Quoted in: M. Mills, G. Sullivan, and S. Eth, Protecting third parties: A decade after Tarasoff, *Am J Psychiatry*, 144 (1987): 70.

67. *V. Tarasoff et al. v. Regents of the University of California et al.* (1974), 329 Pacific Reporter (2d) 553–69.

68. *V. Tarasoff et al v. Regents of the University of California et al.* (1976), 17 Cal. 3d, 131 California Reporter 26 (S.C.C.).

69. Mills, Sullivan, and Eth, *op. cit.*, 68–74.

70. Box 3.9 is adapted from P. Appelbaum, *Almost a Revolution: Mental Health Law and the Limits of Change* (New York: Oxford University Press, 1994): 96.

71 P. Appelbaum, and T.G. Gutheil, *Clinical Handbook of Psychiatry and the Law*. 4th edn. (New York: Williams & Wilkins, 2007): 59-68.

72. *Fleming v. Reid by his litigation guardian, the Public Trustee; Fleming v. Gallagher*, etc. (1992), 4 O.R. (3d) 74–96 (C.A.).*Reid (Litigation Guardian)* (1991) 82 D.L.R. (4th) 298 (O.c.A.)

73. Mills, Sullivan, and Eth, *op. cit.*, 71.

74. S. Michalowski, *Medical Confidentiality and Crime* (London: Ashgate Books, 2003), 70.

75. *Ibid.* 69.

76. French psychiatrist sentenced after patient commits murder. Thomson Reuters, (18-12-2012). Accessed at: http://www.reuters.com/article/2012/12/18/us-france-murder-psychiatrist-idUSBRE8BH13X20121218

77. L. Ferris, H. Barkun, J. Carlisle, B. Hoffman, C. Katz, and M. Silverman, Defining the physician's duty to warn: Consensus statement of Ontario's Medical Expert Panel on Duty to Inform, *CMAJ*, 158 (1998): 1473–9.

78. T. Bailey and C. Jefferies, *Physicians with Health Conditions* (Edmonton; University of Alberta Health Law Institute, 2012). Available at: http://www.hli.ualberta.ca/en/ResearchandResearchPublications/~/media/hli/Physicians_with_Health_Conditions_Complete.pdf

79. The Bristol Royal Infirmary Inquiry, *The Inquiry into the Management of Care of Children Receiving Complex Heart Surgery at the Bristol Royal Infirmary*. July, 2001. Accessed at: http://www.bristol-inquiry.org.uk/final_report/rpt_print.htm

80. *Public Interest Disclosure Act* (1998) <www.opsi.gov.uk/acts/acts1998/ukpga_19980023_en_1>. Described at the time as the "most far-reaching whistle-blower act in the world," it makes it possible for employees, including doctors, and contract and agency staff, to raise concerns without endangering their own jobs or careers; C. Dyer, UK introduces far reaching whistleblower act, *BMJ*, 319 (1999): 7. See: https://www.gov.uk/whistleblowing/overview. Accessed 28-03-2013.

81. D. Greene and J. Cooper, Whistleblowers, *BMJ*, 305 (1992): 1343–4.

82. K. Lennane, Whistleblowing: A health issue, *BMJ*, 307 (1993): 667–70; Blowing the whistle on incompetence: One nurse's story, *Nursing* (July 1989): 46–50; The guidelines in Box 3.5 are adapted from A. Haddad and C. Dougherty, Whistleblowing in the OR, *Today's OR Nurse*, 13 (March 1991), 30–3.

83. A. Mostaghimi and B. Crotty, Professionalism in the digital age, *Ann Intern Med*, 154 (2011): 560–2.

84. E. Topol, *The Creative Destruction of Medicine: How the Digital Revolution Will Create Better Health Care* (New York: Basic Books, 2012).

85. Adapted from: S. Devi, Facebook friend request from a patient? *Lancet*, 377 (2011): 1141–2.

86. G. Gabbard, K. Kassaw, and G. Perez-Garcia, Professional boundaries in the era of the Internet, *Academic Psychiatry*, 35 (2011): 168–74.

87. H. Atherton and A. Majeed, Social networking and health, *Lancet*, 377 (2011): 2083.

88. M. Siegler, Confidentiality in medicine: A decrepit concept, *N Engl J Med*, 307 (1982): 1518–21.

Chapter 4

1. L. Durrell, *The Alexandria Quartet: Clea* (New York: E.P. Dutton & Co., 1961), 24.
2. *Oxford English Dictionary* [CD-ROM], 2nd edn., Version 3.0 (Oxford: Oxford University Press, 2002).
3. CJD is a degenerative untreatable neurological caused by "prions"—small fragments of genetic material of uncertain origin and transmission. It has been causatively linked to surgical instrument transmission. Death comes within months to a year after symptom onset.
4. I. Kant, *The Metaphysical Principles of Virtue* [1797] (New York: The Bobbs-Merrill Co., 1964), 90–1.
5. R. Fulford, Private secrets, public lies, *Queen's Quarterly*, 113 (Summer 2006): 187–96.
6. E. Gillian, K. Oakley, N. Connor, P. Hewitt, H.J.T. Ward, S.M.A. Zaman, Y. Chow, and T.M. Marteau, Impact of being placed at risk of Creutzfeldt-Jakob Disease: A qualitative study of blood donors to variant CJD Cases and patients potentially surgically exposed to CJD, *Neuroepidemiology*, 36 (2011): 274–81.
7. D. Craufurd, L. Kerzin-Storrar, A. Dodge, and R. Harris, Uptake of presymptomatic predictive testing for Huntington's disease, *Lancet*, 334 (1989): 603–5.
8. R. Lawrence and P. Appelbaum, Genetic testing in psychiatry: A review of attitudes and beliefs, *Psychiatry*, 74 (2011): 315–31.
9. L. Macdonald, D. Sackett, R. Haynes, and D. Taylor, Labelling in hypertension: A review of the behavioural and psychological consequences, *J Chronic Dis*, 37 (1984): 933–42.
10. V. Jenkins, L. Fallowfield, and J. Saul, Information needs of patients with cancer: results from a large study in UK cancer centres, *Br J Cancer*, 84/1 (2001): 48–51.
11. R. Sato, H. Beppu, N. Iba, and A. Sawada, The meaning of life prognosis disclosure for Japanese cancer patients: a qualitative study of patients' narratives, *Chronic Illness*, 8 (2012): 225–36.
12. M. Balint, *The Doctor, His Patient and the Illness*, rev. edn. (Madison, CT: International Universities Press, 1988), 215–29.
13. *Ibid.*: 240–42.
14. W.V.O. Quine, *The Roots of Reference* (LaSalle Ill: Open Court Books, 1974), 63–4.
15. H.M. Chochinov, D.J. Tataryn, K.G. Wilson, M. Ennis, and S. Lander, Prognostic awareness and the terminally ill, *Psychosomatics*; 4 (2000): 500–4. See: J. De Lima Thomas, When patients seem overly optimistic, *AMA Virtual mentor*, 14 (2012): 539–44. Available at: http://virtualmentor.ama-assn.org/2012/07/ecas2-1207.html
16. *Daniels v. Heskin* 1954 IR 73 at 86–7 (SC).
17. D. Nyberg, *The Varnished Truth* (Chicago: The University of Chicago Press, 1993).
18. T. Greenhalgh, Barriers to concordance with antidiabetic drugs: Cultural differences or human nature? *BMJ*, 330 (2005): 1250.
19. A. Bowling and S. Ebrahim, Measuring patients' preferences for treatment and perceptions of risk, *Qual Health Care*, 10/Suppl I (2001): i2–i8.
20. L. Egbert, G. Battit, C. Welch, and M. Bartlett, Reduction of postoperative pain by encouragement and instruction of patients—A study of doctor-patient rapport, *N Engl J Med*, 270 (1964): 825–7.
21. A. Luck, S. Pearson, G. Maddern, and P. Hewett, Effects of video information on precolonoscopy anxiety and knowledge: a randomized trial, *Lancet*, 354 (1999): 2032–5.
22. S. Woloshin, M. Schwartz, and H. Welch, The effectiveness of a primer to help people understand risk: two randomized trials in distinct populations, *Ann Intern Med*, 146 (2007): 256–65.
23. S. Kaplan, S. Greenfield, B. Gandek, W. Rogers, and J. Ware Jr, Characteristics of physicians with participatory decision-making styles, *Ann Intern Med*, 124 (1996): 497–504.
24. R. Logan and P. Scott, Uncertainty in clinical practice: implications for quality and costs of health care, *Lancet*, 347 (1996): 595–8.
25. H. Bursztajn, R. Feinbloom, R. Hamm, and A. Brodsky, *Medical Choices, Medical Chances: How Patients, Families, and Physicians Can Cope with Uncertainty* (New York: Dell Publishing, 1981).
26. E. Elkin, S. H. Kim, E. Caspar, D. Kissane, and D. Schrag, Desire for information and involvement in treatment decisions: elderly cancer patients' preferences and their physicians' perceptions, *J Clin Oncol* 25 (2007): 5275–80.

27. M. Elian and G. Dean, To tell or not to tell the diagnosis of multiple sclerosis, *Lancet*, 2 (1985): 28.

28. *Arndt v. Smith*, [1997] 2 S.C.R. 539.

29. L. Fallowfield, A. Hall, P. Maguire, M. Baum, and R. A'Hern, Psychological effects of being offered choice of surgery for breast cancer, *BMJ*, 309 (1994): 448.

30. Elian and Dean, *op. cit.*, 27–8. This is the situation, albeit encountered more rarely, with potential exposure to CJD. See reference 6 above. Disclosure of CJD risk did not cause any significant or longstanding emotional distress.

31. J. Groopman, *The Anatomy of Hope* (New York: Random House, 2005).

32. Anonymous, Once a dark secret [personal view], *BMJ*, 308 (1994): 542. See also: I.A. Hughes, J. Davies, T. Brunch, V. Pasterski, et al., Androgen insensitivity syndrome, *Lancet*, 380 (2012): 1419–28.

33. R.C. Cabot, The use of truth and falsehood in medicine: An experimental study, *Am Med*, 5 (1903): 344–9.

34. S. Bok, *Lying: Moral Choice in Public and Private Life* (Toronto: Random House of Canada, 1979), 247.

35. J. Davies and A. Bacon, When things go wrong, part II, *Anesth Rev*, 17(1990): 50–3.

36. *Chappel v. Hart* [1998] 195 CLR 232; *Rogers v. Whitaker* [1992] 175 CLR 479, 490.

37. *Canterbury v. Spence* [1972] 464 F 2d 772.

38. *Bolam v. Friern Hospital Management Committee* [1957] 1 WLR 582, 586.

39. L. Snyder and C. Leffler for the Ethics and Human Rights Committee, American College of Physicians, Ethics Manual, 6th edn., *Ann Intern Med*, 156 (2012): 73–104.

40. The British Medical Association, *Medical Ethics Today: The BMA's Handbook of Ethics and Law*, 2nd edn. (London: BMJ Publishing Group, 2004), 37–41.

41. Canadian Medical Association, CMA Code of Ethics, accessed on September 21, 2013 at www.cma.ca/code-of-ethics.

42. D. Oken, What to tell cancer patients: A study of medical attitudes, *JAMA*, 175 (1961): 1120–8.

43. D. Novack, R. Plumer, R.L. Smith, H. Ochitill, G.R. Morrow, and J.M. Bennett, Changes in physicians' attitudes toward telling the cancer patient, *JAMA*, 241 (1979): 897–900.

44. M. Delvecchio Good, B. Good, C. Schaffer, and S. Lind, American oncology and the discourse on hope, *Cult Med Psychiatry*, 14 (1990): 59–79.

45. O. Thomsen, H. Wulff, A. Martin, and P. Singer, What do gastroenterologists in Europe tell cancer patients? *Lancet*, 341 (1993): 473–6.

46. L. Iezzoni, S. Rao, C. DesRoches, C. Vogeli, and E. Campbell. Survey shows that at least some physicians are not always open or honest with patients, *Health Aff*, 31 (2012):383–91.

47. R. Samp and A. Curreri, Questionnaire survey on public cancer education obtained from cancer patients and their families, *Cancer*, 10 (1957): 382–4.

48. President's Commission for the Study of Ethical Problems in Medicine and Biomedical and Behavioral Research, *Making Health Care Decisions*, vol. 1 (Washington, DC: US Government Printing Office, 1982), 69–111.

49. P. Elson, Do older adults presenting with memory complaints wish to be told if later diagnosed with Alzheimer's disease? *Int J Geriatr Psych*, 21 (2006): 419–25.

50. M. Silverstein, C.B. Stocking, J.P. Antel, J. Beckwith, R.P. Roos, M. Siegler, et al., ALS and life-sustaining therapy: patients' desires for information, participation in decision making, and life-sustaining therapy, *Mayo Clin Proc*, 66 (1991): 906–13.

51. A. Ajaj, M.P. Singh, and A.J. Abdulla, Should elderly patients be told they have cancer? Questionnaire survey of older people, *BMJ*, 323 (2001): 1160.

52. L.J. Blackhall, S. Murphy, G. Frank, V. Michel, and S. Azen, Ethnicity and attitudes toward patient autonomy, *JAMA*, 274 (1995): 820–5.

53. E. Pucci, N. Belardinelli, G. Borsetti, and G.Giuliani, Relatives' attitudes towards informing patients about the diagnosis of Alzheimer's disease, *J Med Ethics*, 29 (2003): 51–4.

54. G. Ruhnke, S. Wilson, T. Akamatsu, T. Kinoue, Y. Takashima, M. Goldstein, et al., Ethical decision making and patient autonomy: a comparison of physicians and patients in Japan and the United States, *Chest*, 118 (2000): 1172–82.

55. A. Akabayashi, I. Kai, H. Takemura, and H. Okazaki, Truth telling in the case of a pessimistic diagnosis in Japan, *Lancet*, 354 (1999): 1263.

56. F. Fukuyama, *The Great Disruption: Human Nature and the Reconstruction of Social Order* (New York: Simon & Schuster, 2000).

57. A. Surbone, C. Ritossa, and A. Spagnolo, Evolution of truth-telling attitudes and practices in Italy. *Crit Rev Oncol Hematol,* 52 (2004): 165–72.

58. G. Sigman, J. Kraut, and J. La Puma, Disclosure of a diagnosis to children and adolescents when parents object, *Am J Dis Child,* 147 (1993): 764–8.

59. Anon, Delivering bad news, *BMJ,* 321 (2000): 1233.

60. U. Kreicbergs, U. Valdimarsdottir, E. Onelov, J.-I. Henter, and G. Steineck, Talking about death with children who have severe malignant disease, *N Engl J Med,* 351 (2004): 1175–86.

61. C. Atkins, *My Imaginary Illness: A Journey into Uncertainty and Prejudice in Medical Diagnosis* (Ithica: Cornell University Press, 2010).

62. A. Schattner, What do patients really want to know? *Q J Med,* 95 (2002): 135–6.

63. J. Brown, M. Boles, J. Mullooly, and W. Levinson, Effect of clinician communication skills training on patient satisfaction: A randomized, controlled trial, *Ann Intern Med,* 131 (1999): 822–9.

64. A. Mann, Factors affecting psychological state during one year on a hypertension trial, *Clin Invest Med,* 4 (1981): 197–200.

65. A. Jonsen, M. Siegler, and W. Winslade, *Clinical Ethics,* 5th edn. (New York: McGraw-Hill, 2002), 63.

66. M. Stewart, Effective physician–patient communication and health outcomes: A review, *CMAJ,* 152 (1995): 1423–33.

67. L. Fallowfield and V. Jenkins, Communicating sad, bad, and difficult news in medicine, *Lancet,* 363 (2004): 312–19.

68. *Stamos v. Davies* [1985] 52 OR (2d) 10 (H.C.).

69. R.C. Cabot, *op. cit.,* 344–9.

70. R. Buckman, *How to Break Bad News* (Toronto: University of Toronto Press, 1992).

71. This case is adapted from A. Burrows, The man who didn't know he had cancer, *JAMA,* 266 (1991): 2550.

72. C. Feudtner, D. Christakis, and N. Christakis, Do clinical clerks suffer ethical erosion? *Acad Med,* 69 (1994): 670–9.

73. F. Fang, K. Fall, M. Mittleman, et al., Suicide and cardiovascular death after a cancer diagnosis, *N Engl J Med,* 366 (2012): 1310–18.

Chapter 5

1. J.S. Mill, *On Liberty* [1859] (New York: Appleton-Century Crofts, 1947), 10.

2. *Canterbury v. Spence* 464 F.2d 772 at 784 (1972).

3. President's Commission for the Study of Ethical Problems in Medicine and Biomedical and Behavioral Research, *Making Health Care Decisions,* vol. 1 (Washington, DC: US Government Printing Office, 1982), 42–51.

4. Mill, *op. cit.,* 9.

5. M. Neuman and C. Bosk, What we talk about when we talk about risk: Refining surgery's hazards in medical thought, *Milbank Q,* 90 (2012): 135–59.

6. I. Health, A wolf in sheep's clothing: a critical look at the ethics of drug taking, *BMJ,* 327 (2003): 856–8.

7. A. Akkad, C. Jackson, S. Kenyon, M. Dixon-Woods, N. Taub, and M. Habiba, Patients' perceptions of written consent: questionnaire study, *BMJ,* 333 (2006): 528.

8. C.H. Braddock, K. Edwards, N. Hasenberg, T. Laidley, and W. Levinson, Informed decision making in outpatient practice: time to get back to basics, *JAMA,* 282 (1999): 2313–20.

9. S.J. Weiner, B. Barnet, T. Cheng, and T. Daaleman, Processes for effective communication in primary care, *Ann Intern Med,* 142 (2005): 709–14; S. Woolf, E. Chan, R. Harris, S. Sheridan, C. Braddock III, R. Kaplan, et al., Promoting informed choice: Transforming health care to dispense knowledge for decision making, *Ann Intern Med,* 143 (2005): 293–300.

10. C. Barry, C. Bradley, N. Britten, F. Stevenson, and N. Barber, Patients' unvoiced agendas in general practice consultations: qualitative study, *BMJ,* 320 (2000): 1246–50.

11. Box 5.2 is based on a quote from the College of Physicians and Surgeons of Ontario, *Consent to Medical Treatment Policy Statement #4-05* (Jan./Feb. 2006).

12. J. Kassirer, Incorporating patients' preferences into medical decisions, *N Engl J Med,* 330 (1994): 1895–6.

13. *Reibl v. Hughes* (1980), 16 O.R. (2d) 311–12.

14. College of Physicians and Surgeons of Ontario, *Report of Proceedings, Disciplinary Committee* (June 1992), 20.

15. D. Ziegler, M. Mosier, M. Buenaver, and K. Okuyemi, How much information about adverse effects of medication do patients want from physicians? *Arch Intern Med*, 161 (2001): 706–13.

16. S. Woloshin and L. Schwartz, Communicating data about the benefits and harms of treatment: A randomized trial, *Ann Intern Med*, 155 (2011): 87–96.

17. L. Schwartz, S. Woloshin, and H.G. Welch, Using a drug facts box to communicate drug benefits and harms: two randomized trials, *Ann Intern Med*, 150 (2009): 516–27.

18. J. Mitchell, A fundamental problem of consent, *BMJ*, 310 (1995): 43–6; M. Jones, Commentary: The legal position, *BMJ*, 310 (1995): 46; J. Lunn, Commentary: An anaesthetist's view, *BMJ*, 310 (1995): 47.

19. G. Ness and J. Menage [letters], *BMJ*, 310 (1995): 935.

20. *Marshall v. Curry* (1933), 3 D.L.R. 260: 275 (N.S.S.C.); *Murray v. McMurchy* (1949), 2 D.L.R. 442 (B.C.S.C.).

21. BMA Medical Ethics Department, *Advance decisions and proxy decision-making in medical treatment and research* (London: BMA Pub., June 2007). Accessed at: http://bma.org. uk/practical-support-at-work/ethics/ mental-capacity.

22. P. Angelos, D. DaRosa, D. Bentram, and H. Sherman, Residents seeking informed consent: Are they adequately knowledgeable? *Curr Surg*, 59 (2002): 115–18.

23. E. Picard, *Legal Liability of Doctors and Hospitals in Canada*, 2nd edn. (Toronto: Carswell, 1984), 91.

24. D. Studdert, M. Mello, A. Gawande, T. Gandhi, A Kachalia, et al., Claims, errors and compensation payments in medical malpractice litigation, *N Engl J Med*; 354 (2006): 2024–33.

25. M. Killoran and A. Moyer, Surgical treatment preferences in Chinese-American women with early-stage breast cancer, *Psychooncology*, 15 (2006): 969–84. See also: M. Morrow, J. Winograd, P. Freer, and J. Eichhorn,

Case 8-2013: A 48-year-old woman with carcinoma in situ of the breast, *N Engl J Med*, 368 (2013): 1046–53. The latter case is of a woman who wanted, and received, bilateral mastectomy, not the unilateral BCS that was initially offered.

26. K. Joseph, S. Vrouwe, A. Kamruzzaman, A. Balbaid, D. Fenton, R. Berendt, E Yu, and P. Tai, Outcome analysis of breast cancer patients who declined evidence-based treatment, *World Journal of Surgical Oncology*, 10 (2012): 118. See also: W. El-Charnoubi, J. Svendsen, U. Tange, and N. Kroman, Women with inoperable or locally advanced breast cancer—What characterizes them? A retrospective review of 157 cases, *Acta Oncol*, 51 (2012): 1081–5.

27. Based on R. Webb, A patient who changed my practice. The zero option, *BMJ*, 310 (1995): 1380.

28. *Kovacich v. St. Joseph's Hospital*, [2004] O.J. No. 4471 [2004] O.T.C. 942 (Ont. Sup. Ct); *Best v. Hoskins* [2006] ABQB 58.

29. The quotation in Box 5.7 is from G. Sharpe, *The Law and Medicine in Canada*, 2nd edn. (Toronto: Butterworths, 1987), 57.

30. *[I]n elective procedures even minimal or possible risks must be disclosed."* E. Picard and G. Robertson, *Legal Liability of Doctors and Hospitals in Canada*, 3rd edn. (Toronto: Carswell Thomson Canada, 1996), 26, FN 143.

31. CPSO *Disciplinary Decisions* (May 4, 2011). Available at: https://www.cpso.on.ca/ whatsnew/news/default.aspx?id=4972.

32. Somewhere, I believe, this quote originated from the CMPA—if so, I cannot now find where. It's a good rule of thumb for taking a personal approach to informed choice. See also K.G. Evans, *Consent: A Guide for Canadian Physicians*, 4th edn. (Ottawa: CMPA, 2006). Accessed 26-02-2013; available at: http://cmpa.org/cmpapd04/docs/ resource_files/ml_guides/consent_guide/ pdf/com_consent-e.pdf

33. M.K. Marvel, R. Epstein, K. Flowers, and H. Beckman, Soliciting the patient's agenda: have we improved? *JAMA*, 281 (1999): 283–7.

34. J. Stilgoe and F. Farook, *The Talking Cure: Why Conversation is the Future of Healthcare* (London UK: Demos Books, 2008).

35. R. Deyo, Tell it like it is: patients as partners in medical decision making, *J Gen Intern Med*, 15 (2000): 752–4.
36. A. Edwards, Communicating risk, *BMJ*, 327 (2003): 691–2.
37. C. Lavelle-Jones, D. Byrne, P. Rice, and A. Cuschieri, Factors affecting quality of informed consent, *BMJ*, 306 (1993): 885–90.
38. *Ciarlariello v. Schacter*, [1993] 2 S.C.R. 119.
39. *Nightingale v. Kaplovitch*, [1989] O.J. No. 585 (H.C.J.; unreported; 20 April 1989).
40. "13. Consent to medical care is not required in case of emergency if the life of the person is in danger or his integrity is threatened and his consent cannot be obtained in due time. It is required, however, where the care is unusual or has become useless or where its consequences could be intolerable for the person." *Civil Code of Québec*, S.Q., 1991, c. 64, s. 13. Authorized by Les Publications du Québec.
41. A. Back, R. Arnold, and T. Quill, Hope for the best, and prepare for the worst, *Ann Intern Med*, 138 (2003) 439–43.
42. *Ediger v. Johnston*, [2013] SCC 18.
43. D. Kerrigan, R. Thevasagayam, T. Woods, I. McWelch, W. Thomas, A. Shorthouse, et al., Who's afraid of informed consent? *BMJ*, 306 (1993): 298–300.
44. G. Lamb, S. Green, and J. Heron, Can physicians warn patients of potential side effects without fear of causing those side effects? *Arch Intern Med*, 154 (1994): 2753–6.
45. M. Gattellari, K. Voigt, P. Butow, and M. Tattersall, When the treatment goal is not cure: Are cancer patients equipped to make informed decisions? *J Clin Oncol*, 20 (2002): 503–13.
46. Thanks to Hannah Kaufman for this point.
47. Based on a short story by William Carlos Williams, The use of force. Available at: http://fiction.eserver.org/short/the_use_of_force.html.

Chapter 6

1. *Starson v. Swayze* [2003] S.C.J. No. 33, C.J.C. McLachlin, dissenting.
2. E. Saks, *Refusing Care: Forced Treatment and the Rights of the Mentally Ill* (Chicago: University of Chicago Press, 2002).
3. H. Bloom and M. Bay (eds.), *A Practical Guide to Mental Health, Capacity and Consent Law of Ontario* (Toronto: Carswell, 1996).
4. E. Cassell, A. Leon, and S. Kaufman, Preliminary evidence of impaired thinking in sick patients, *Ann Intern Med*, 134 (2001): 1120–3.
5. V. Raymont, W. Bingley, A. Buchanan, A. David, et al., Prevalence of mental incapacity in medical inpatients and associated risk factors: cross-sectional study, *Lancet*, 364 (2004): 1421–7. The authors of this study of hospitalized patients estimated at least 40 per cent lacked mental capacity, However, of 50 patients interviewed, only 24 per cent had been identified by their clinical team as lacking capacity.
6. L. Sessums, H. Zembrzuska, and J. Jackson, Does This Patient Have Medical Decision-Making Capacity? *JAMA*, 306 (2011): 420–7.
7. President's Commission for the Study of Ethical Problems in Medicine and Biomedical and Behavioral Research, *Making Health Care Decisions*, vol. 1: A Report on the Ethical and Legal Implications of Informed Consent in the Patient-Practitioner Relationship (Washington, DC: US Government Printing Office, 1982), 55, 171.
8. P. Applebaum, Assessment of patients' competence to consent to treatment, *N Engl J Med*, 357 (2007): 1834–40.
9. L. Roth, A. Meisel, and C. Lidz, Tests of competency to consent to treatment, *Am J Psychiatry*, 134 (1977): 279–84.
10. P. Appelbaum and T. Gutheil, *Clinical Handbook of Psychiatry and the Law*, 4th edn. (Philadelphia: Lippincott, Williams & Wilkins, 2007), 181-2.
11. The National Ethics Committee of the Veterans Health Administration, *Ten Myths About Decision-Making Capacity* (Washington, DC: National Center for Ethics in Health Care, Veterans Health Administration Department of Veterans Affairs, Sept. 2002).
12. *Consent to Treatment Act*, R.S.O. 1992, c. 31, S.G.
13. M. Farnsworth, Evaluation of mental competency, *Am Fam Physician*, 39 (1989): 182–90.
14. J. Kutner, J. Ruark, and T. Raffin, Defining patient competence for medical decision making, *Chest*, 100 (1991): 1404–9.

15. T. Grisso and P. Appelbaum, Comparison of standards for assessing patients' capacities to make treatment decisions, *Am J Psychiatry*, 152 (1995): 1033–7.

16. K. Byrick and B. Walker-Renshaw, *A Practical Guide to Mental Health and the Law in Ontario* (Toronto: Ontario Hospitals Association, 2012): 11, accessed at www.oha.com/KnowledgeCentre/Library/Toolkits/Documents/Final%20-%20Mental%20Health%20and%20the%20Law%20Toolkit.pdf.

17. P. Appelbaum and T. Gutheil, *Clinical Handbook of Psychiatry and the Law*, 4th edn. (Philadelphia: Lippincott, Williams & Wilkins, 2007): 194–200.

18. Adapted from Farnsworth, *op. cit.*: 186–8.

19. E. Etchells, P. Darzins, M. Silberfeld, et al., Assessment of Patient Capacity to Consent to Treatment, *J Gen Intern Med*, 14 (1999): 27–34.

20. J. Howell, Review: Several instruments are accurate for evaluating patient capacity for medical treatment decision-making, *Ann Intern Med*, 155 (2011): 1JC5-12.

21. The Québec *Civil Code* requires judicial involvement: "The authorization of the court is necessary where the person who may give consent to care required by the state of health of a minor or a person of full age who is incapable of giving his consent is prevented from doing so or, without justification, refuses to do so; it is also required where a person of full age who is incapable of giving his consent categorically refuses to receive care, except in the case of hygienic care or emergency. The authorization of the court is necessary, furthermore, to cause a minor 14 years of age or over to undergo care he refuses, except in the case of emergency if his life is in danger or his integrity threatened, in which case the consent of the person having parental authority or the tutor is sufficient." *Civil Code of Québec*, S.Q., 1991, c. 64, s. 16. Authorized by Les Publications du Québec.

22. *Consent to Treatment Act, 1992*, S.O. 1992, c. 31, s. 13, as amended.

23. *Substitute Decisions Act*, 1992, S.O. 1992, c. 30, s. 66, as amended.

24. The Quebec *Civil Code*, if less elaborate, is similar: "A person who gives his consent to or refuses care for another person is bound to act in the sole interest of that person, taking into account, as far as possible, any wishes the latter may have expressed. If he gives his consent, he shall ensure that the care is beneficial notwithstanding the gravity and permanence of certain of its effects, that it is advisable in the circumstances and that the risks incurred are not disproportionate to the anticipated benefit." *Civil Code of Québec*, S.Q., 1991, c. 64, s. 12. Authorized by Les Publications du Québec.

25. H. Venables, *A Guide to the Law Affecting Mental Health Patients* (Toronto: Butterworths, 1975), 75–6.

26. R. Pivec, A. Johnson, S. Mears, and M. Mont, Hip arthroplasty, *Lancet*, 380 (2012): 1768–77.

27. *Starson v. Swayze* [2003] 1 S.C.R. 772, 2003 SCC 32 at para 9.

28. *Fleming v. Reid (Litigation Guardian)* (1991), 82 D.L.R. (4th) 298 (O.c.A)

29. P. Appelbaum, *Almost a Revolution: Mental Health Law and the Limits of Change* (New York: Oxford University Press, 1994), 128.

30. *Starson v. Swayze* [2003] S.C.J. No. 33.

31. E. Saks, *op. cit.*: 190.

32. A .Williams and A. Caplan, Thomas Szasz: rebel with a questionable cause, *Lancet*, 380 (2012): 1379.

33. S. Wildeman, The Supreme Court of Canada at the limits of decisional capacity, in J. Downie and E. Gibson (eds.), *Health Law at the Supreme Court of Canada* (Toronto: Irwin Law, 2007), 290–2.

34. Appelbaum, *op. cit.*: 133–5.

35. *Ibid.*, 143.

36. P. Appelbaum, The right to refuse treatment with antipsychotic medications: retrospect and prospect, *Am J Psychiatry*, 145 (1988): 413–19.

37. N. Hewak, The ethical, medical and legal implications of the forcible treatment provisions of the Criminal Code, *Health Law Can*, 15/4 (1995): 107–16.

38. F. Orr, D. Watson, and A. King-Smith, Alberta's community treatment order legislation and implementation: the 1st 18 months in review, *Health Law Review*, 20 (Spring 2012): 5–12.

39. *Health Care Consent Act*, 1996, S.O. 1996, c. 2, Schedule A, Part III, Admission to Care Facilities, Crisis Admission: 47.(1).

40. M. Jones, A memorable patient: Caring for those who refuse help, *BMJ*, 328 (2004): 1546.

41. S. Harris, J. Hepburn, J. Gray, E. Murphy, and C. Carrie, What to do with a sick elderly woman who refuses to go to hospital, *BMJ*, 289 (1984): 1435–6.

42. T. Hope, J. Savulescu, and J. Hendrick, *Medical Ethics and Law*, 2nd edn. (London, UK: Churchill-Livingston, 2008): 84–5.

43. See P. Alderson, *Children's Consent to Surgery* (Buckingham, UK: Open University Press, 1993).

44. D. Coleman and P. Rosoff, The legal authority of mature minors to consent to general medical treatment, *Pediatrics*, 131(2013): 786–93.

45. *Gillick v. West Norfolk and Wisbech Area Health Authority* [1985] 3 All ER 402HL 31.

46. A. Elton, P. Honig, A. Bentovim, and J. Simons, Withholding consent to lifesaving treatment: three cases, *BMJ*, 310 (1995): 373–7.

47. *Region 2 Hosp Corp v. Walker* (1994), N.B.J. No. 242 (N.B.C.A.).

48. Re L.D.K.; *Children's Aid Society of Metropolitan Toronto v. K. and K.* (1985), 48 R.F.L. (2d) 164 (Ont. Prov. Ct.).

49. *Hughes (Estate of) v. Hughes*, 2006, ABQB 159.

50. Coleman and Rosoff, *op. cit.*

51. D.S. Diekema, Adolescent refusal of lifesaving treatment: are we asking the right questions? *Adolesc Med State Art Rev*, 22 (2011): 213–28.

52. The Quebec *Civil Code* distinguishes care that a minor may consent to and care which requires the involvement of his/her parents or "tutor." "A minor 14 years of age or over may give his consent alone to care not required by the state of his health; however, the consent of the person having parental authority or of the tutor is required if the care entails a serious risk for the health of the minor and may cause him grave and permanent effects." *Civil Code of Quebec*, S.Q., 1991, c. 64, s. 17. Authorized by Les Publications du Québec.

Chapter 7

1. Attributed to M. Balint by J. Norell, letter: The importance of the generalist, *Br J Gen Pract*, 42 (October, 1992): 443.

2. D. Hilfiker, *Not All of Us Are Saints* (Toronto: Hill and Wang, 1994), 198–9.

3. CMA Code of Ethics, accessed at cma.ca/code-of-ethics.

4. T. Brewin, *Primum non nocere? Lancet*, 344 (1994): 1487–8.

5. *Crits et al. v. Sylvester et al.* [1956] O.R. 132 (C.A.), aff'd [1956] S.C.R. 991: 143.

6. J. Smits, The Good Samaritan in European Private Law: On the Perils of Principles without a Programme and a Programme for the Future. Inaugural lecture, Maastricht University 19 May 2000 Available at: http://works.bepress.com/jan_smits/8.

7. *Egedebo v. Windermere District Hospital Association* [1991] BCJ No.2381 (QL) (SC), aff'd (1993) 78 BCLR (2d) 63 (CA).

8. *Woods v. Lowns* (1995), 36 NSWLR 344 (SC).

9. E.J. Emanuel, The Lessons of SARS, *Ann Intern Med*, 139 (2003): 589–91.

10. A. Caplan, Time to mandate influenza vaccination in health-care workers, *Lancet*, 378 (2011): 310–11.

11. *V.G.H. v. McDaniel* (1934) 4 D.L.R. 593 (P.C.) 597; *Wilson v. Swanson* (1956), 5 D.L.R. (2d) 113 (S.C.C.) 120. For a story of "overtreatment" see, H.J. Warraich, Opinion: The Cancer of Optimism, *New York Times*, May 5, 2013, SR9.

12. *Bolam v. Friern Hospital Management Committee* (1957), 2 All E.R. 118 (Q.B.D.) 122.

13. *Ter Neuzen v. Korn*, [1995] 3 SCR 674. *Per* La Forest, Sopinka, Gonthier, Cory, McLachlin and Iacobucci: "[T]here are certain situations where the standard practice itself may be found to be negligent. However, this will only be where the standard practice is *fraught with obvious risks (my italics)* such that anyone is capable of finding it negligent . . ."

14. J. Feinberg, The child's right to an open future, in J. Feinberg, *Freedom and Fulfillment: Philosophical Essays* (Princeton, NJ: Princeton University Press, 1992), 89.

15. D. Shaw and B. Elger, Evidence-based persuasion: An ethical imperative, *JAMA*, 309 (2013): 1689–90.

16. J. Wahl, K. Le Clair, and S. Himel, The geriatric patient, in H. Bloom and M. Bay (eds.), *A Practical Guide to Mental Health, Capacity, and Consent Law of Ontario* (Toronto: Carswell, 1996), 343–77.

17. L. Ferris, H, Barkun, J. Carlisle, B. Hoffman, C. Katz, and M. Silverman, Defining the physician's duty to warn: Consensus statement of Ontario's Medical Expert Panel on Duty to Inform, *CMAJ*, 158 (1998): 1473–9.

18. N. Hewak, The ethical, medical and legal implications of the forcible treatment provisions of the *Criminal Code, Health Law Can*, 15/4 (1995): 107–16.

19. F. Pochard, M. Robin, and S. Kannas [letter to the editor], *N Engl J Med*, 338 (1998): 261–2.

20. L. Ganzini and M. Lee, Psychiatry and assisted suicide in the United States, *N Engl J Med*, 336 (1997): 1824–6.

21. J. Grant, Liability in patient suicide, *Current Psych*, 3 (2004): 80–2.

22. D. Muzina, What physicians can do to prevent suicide, *Cleveland Clinic J Med*, 71 (2004): 242–50.

23. R. Gilbert, J. Fluke, M. O'Donnell, A. Gonzalez-Izquierdo, M. Brownell, P. Gulliver, et al., Child maltreatment: variation in trends and policies in six developed countries, *Lancet*, 379 (2012): 758–72.

24. L. Wissow, Child abuse and neglect, *N Engl J Med*, 332 (1995): 1425–31.

25. E. Picard, *Legal Liability of Doctors and Hospitals in Canada*, 2nd edn. (Toronto: Carswell, 1984): 47.

26. "Consent to medical care is not required in case of emergency if the life of the person is in danger or his integrity is threatened and his consent cannot be obtained in due time." *Civil Code of Québec*, S.Q., 1991, c. 64, s. 13. Authorized by Les Publications du Québec.

27. Quoted in P. Schroeder, Female genital mutilation – a form of child abuse, *N Engl J Med*, 331 (1994): 739–40.

28. *B.(R) v. CAS of Metropolitan Toronto* [1995] 1 S.C.R. 315, 176 N.R. 161, 26 C.R.R. (2d) 202, 78 O.A.C. 1, 122 D.L.R. (4th) 1.

29. *New York Times*, 6 Aug. 1990, 1.

30. *Superintendent of Family and Child Service v. RD and SD* (1983), 42 B.C.L.R. 173–87 (B.C.S.C.).

31. *Ibid.*, 187.

32. *Ibid.*, 177.

33. J. Carter quoted in Picard, *op. cit.*, 49.

34. S. Mukherjee. *The Emperor of All Maladies: A Biography of Cancer* (NY: Scribner Books, 2010).

35. *Minister of Social Services v. F & L Paulette* (1991), Saskatchewan Provincial Court, Sask. D. 1568–1605 (Prov. Ct.; unreported).

36. Picard, *op. cit.*, 50.

37. Canadian Physicians and Surgeons of Ontario, *Members' Dialogue*, 2/2 (1994): 31–2.

38. H. MacMillan, J. MacMillan, and D. Offord, with the Canadian Task Force on the Periodic Health Examination, Periodic health examination, 1993 update: 1. Primary prevention of child maltreatment, *CMAJ*, 148 (1993): 151–63; H. MacMillan, Preventive health care, 2000 update: prevention of child maltreatment, CMAJ, 163 (2000): 1451–8.

39. *R v Ipeelee*, (2012) SCC 13: 60.

40. *R v John*, (2004) SKCA 13.

41. D. Parkes, D. Milward, S. Keesic, and J. Seymour, *Gladue Handbook: A Resource for Justice System Participants in Manitoba* (Manitoba: University of Manitoba, Faculty of Law, 2012). The Gladue Handbook is updated periodically, and additional relevant materials are to be made available at: http://chrr.info/resources/gladue-projec.

42. *E (Mrs) v. Eve*. (1986), 2 S.C.R.: 388–438.

43. S.Wildeman, The Supreme Court of Canada at the limits of decisional capacity, in J. Downie and E. Gibson (eds.), *Health Law at the Supreme Court of Canada* (Toronto: Irwin Law, 2007), 245–7.

44. B. Dickens, No contraceptive sterilization of the mentally retarded: the dawn of "Eve," *CMAJ*, 137 (1987): 65–7.

45. Wildeman, *op. cit.*, 266–7.

46. D.S. Diekema, Involuntary sterilization of persons with mental retardation: an ethical analysis, *Ment Retard Dev Disabil Res Rev*, 9 (2003): 21–6.

47. J.D. Lantos, Ethics for the pediatrician: the evolving ethics of cochlear implants in children, *Pediatr Rev*, 33 (2012): 323–6.

48. Adapted from D. Gunther and D. Diekama, Attenuating growth in children with profound developmental disability, *Arch Pediatr Adolesc Med*, 160 (2006): 1013–17.

49. A. Solomon. *Far from the Tree: Parents, Children, and the Search for Identity*, (New York: Scribner, 2012).

50. W. Curran, Beyond the best interests of a child: Bone marrow transplantation

among half-siblings, *N Engl J Med*, 324 (1991): 1818–19.

51. L.M. Liao and S.M. Creighton. Requests for cosmetic genitoplasty: how should healthcare providers respond? *BMJ*, 334 (2007): 1090–2.

52. N. Toubia, Female circumcision as a public health issue, *N Engl J Med*, 331 (1994): 712–16; J. Black and G. Debelle, Female genital mutilation in Britain, *BMJ*, 310 (1995): 1590–2; C. Gallard, Female genital mutilation in France, *BMJ*, 310 (1995): 1592–3.

53. B. Nurcombe and D. Partlett, *Child Mental Health and the Law* (New York: The Free Press, 1994), 119–21.

Chapter 8

1. R. Saundby, *Medical Ethics: A Guide to Professional Conduct*, 2nd edn. (London: Charles Griffin & Co, 1907), 2.

2. E. Pellegrino, Medical professionalism: Can it, should it survive? *J Am Board Fam Pract*, 13 (2000): 147–9.

3. F. Hafferty, Professionalism: the next wave, *N Engl J Med*, 355 (2006): 2151–2.

4. R. Cruess, S. Cruess, and S. Johnston, Professionalism and medicine's social contract, *J Bone Joint Surg Am*, 82-A (2000): 1189–94.

5. F. Peabody, The care of the patient, *JAMA*, 88 (1927): 877–82.

6. "Patients clearly and rightly feel doctors should heed minimum standards of courtesy, should acknowledge their patients' human distress, just like anyone else." C. Schneider, *The Practice of Autonomy: Patients, Doctors, and Medical Decisions* (New York: Oxford University Press, 1998), 227. What he says about doctors should apply across the board to all healthcare professionals. Much of the examples of common rudeness in medicine are drawn from this book (see pp. 219–27).

7. N. Ambady, D. LaPlante, T. Nguyen, R. Rosenthal, N. Chaumeton, and W. Levinson, Surgeons' tone of voice: A clue to malpractice history, *Surgery*, 132 (2002): 5–9.

8. Editorial, Evidence-based handshakes, *Lancet*, 370 (2007): 2.

9. M. Lill and T. Wilkinson, Judging a book by its cover: descriptive survey of patients' preferences for doctors' appearance and mode of address, *BMJ* 331 (2005):1524–7.

10. S. Rehman, P. Nietert, D. Cope, and A. Kilpatrick, What to wear today? Effect of doctor's attire on the trust and confidence of patients, *Am J Med*, 118 (2005): 1279–86.

11. R. Reddy, Slippers and a white coat? (Hawai'i physician attire study), *Hawaii Med J*, 68 (2009): 284-5.

12. H. Chung, H. Lee, D.S. Chang, H.S. Kim, H. Lee, H.J. Park, and Y. Chae, Doctor's attire influences perceived empathy in the patient-doctor relationship, *Patient Educ Couns*, 89 (2012): 387–91.

13. Permission to adapt this case from Dr Harriet Van Spall who wrote movingly about the impact the circumstances of her father's death had upon her. H.G.C. Van Spall, When my father died, *Ann Intern Med*, 146 (2007): 893–4.

14. B.Williams, *Moral Luck: Philosophical Papers 1973-1980* (Cambridge, UK: Cambridge University Press, 1981), 18.

15. H. Frankfurt, *The Reasons of Love* (Princeton, NJ: Princeton University Press, 2004): 47.

16. Medical professionalism in the new millennium: A physician's charter, *Lancet*, 359 (2002): 520–2. Simultaneously published in *Ann Intern Med*, 136 (2002): 243–6.

17. C. Cassel, V. Hood and W. Bauer, A Physician Charter: The 10th Anniversary. *Ann Intern Med*, 157 (2012): 290–1.

18. *Norberg v. Wynrib* [1992] 2 SCR 226.

19. D. Winslow, Treating the enemy, *Ann Intern Med*, 147 (2007): 278–9.

20. P. Surdyk, D. Lynch, and D. Leach, Professionalism: identifying current themes, *Curr Opin Anaesthesiol*, 16 (2003): 597–602.

21. D. Healy, *Pharmageddon* (Los Angeles: University of California Press, 2012).

22. M.R. Griffin, C.M. Stein, and W. Ray, Postmarketing surveillance for drug safety: surely we can do better, *Clin Pharmacol Ther*, 75 (2004): 491–4.

23. K.P. Hill, J. Ross, D. Egilman, and H. Krumholz, The ADVANTAGE seeding trial: A review of internal documents, *Ann Intern Med*, 149 (2008): 251–8. See also: H. Sox, and D. Rennie, "Seeding" trials: just say "no." *Ann Intern Med*, 149 (2008): 279–80.

24. Adapted from E.H. Morreim, Conflicts of interest for physician entrepreneurs, in R. Spece, D. Shimm, and A. Buchanan (eds.), *Conflicts of Interest in Clinical Practice and Research* (New York: Oxford University Press, 1996): 251–85.

25. E.G. Campbell, Doctors and drug companies—scrutinizing influential relationships, *N Engl J Med*, 357 (2007): 1796–7.

26. The Pew Trust, *Federal Reporting Requirements on Payments to Physicians: Impact on State Laws* (November 2010). See www.pewtrusts.org/news_room_detail.aspx?id=61812

27. "Medical products are central to modern health care, and academic-industry collaboration is vital for their development. At the same time, it is essential that the use of these products be guided by sound evidence and good science. Every patient deserves the safest, most effective treatment." D. Carlat, Written submission on the Physician Payments Sunshine Act to US Senate Special Committee on Aging. (Sept 12, 2012). Accessed at www.pewhealth.org/uploadedFiles/PHG/Content_Level_Pages/Issue_Briefs/carlat-statement.pdf.

28. Pew Prescription Project, Pharmaceutical Industry Marketing: Fact Sheet. (Jan 28, 2009). Available at: www.pewhealth.org/uploadedFiles/PHG/Supporting_Items/IB_FS_PPP_Pharmaceutical_Industry_Marketing.pdf

29. Canadian Medical Association, Guidelines for Physicians in Interactions with Industry. Approved 2007-Dec-01. http://policybase.cma.ca/dbtw-wpd/Policypdf/ PD08-01.pdf.

30. T. Brennan, D. Rothman, L. Blank, D. Blumenthal, S. Chimonas, J. Cohen, et al., Health industry practices that create conflicts of interest: a policy proposal for academic medical centers, *JAMA*, 295 (2006): 429–33.

31. Institute of Medicine, *Conflict of Interest in Medical Research, Education, and Practice* (Washington: National Academies Press, 2009).

32. *CPSO v. R Devgan*. www.cpso.on.ca/info_public/dis_sum/WEBDISC/2003/DevganR.pdf.

33. CBC News, Turner psychiatrist ordered to pay $10,000, 31 March 2006 www.cbc.ca/canada/newfoundland-labrador/story/2006/03/31/nf-doucet-decision-20060331.html.

34. C. Nadelson and M. Notman, Boundaries in the doctor–patient relationship, *Theor Med Bioeth*, 23 (2002): 191–201.

35. S. Rosenbloom, *Boundary Transgressions in Therapeutic Relationships* (M.Sc. thesis, Virginia State University, 2003), 2–3.

36. L. Lyckholm, Should physicians accept gifts from patients? *JAMA*, 280 (1998):1944–6.

37. S. Spence, Patients bearing gifts: are there strings attached? *BMJ*, 331 (2005): 1527–9.

38. The quotation in Box 8.1 is from T. Miksanek, Should I give money to my patients? *Am Fam Physician*, 67 (2003): 1629; D. Krassner, Gifts from physicians to patients: an ethical dilemma, *Psychiatr Serv*, 55 (2004): 505–6.

39. T. Gutheil and G. Gabbard, Misuses and misunderstandings of boundary theory in clinical and regulatory settings, *Focus*, 1 (2003): 421.

40. A. Smolar, When we give more: reflections on intangible gifts from therapist to patient, *Am J Psychother*, 57 (2003): 300–23.

41. K. Hall, Sexualization of the doctor-patient relationship: is it ever ethically permissible? *Fam Pract*, 18 (2001): 511–15.

42. *Ibid.*

43. The quotation in Box 8.3 is based on the *Regulated Health Professional Act*, S.O., 1991. c. 18, schedule 2, s. 1(3); College of Physicians and Surgeons of Ontario, *The Final Report on the Task Force on Sexual Abuse of Patients* (Toronto, 1991); College of Physicians and Surgeons of British Columbia, *Crossing the Boundaries: The Report of the Committee on Physician Sexual Misconduct* (Vancouver, 1992).

44. CMA, The patient-physician relationship and the sexual abuse of patients, *CMAJ*, 150 (1994): 1884A-F.

45. College of Nurses of Ontario, *Mandatory Reporting of Sexual Abuse* www.cno.org/Global/docs/ih/42006_fsMandReporting.pdf.

46. C. Winchell, Curbside Consultation: The seductive patient, *Am Fam Physician*, 62 (2000): 1196–8.

47. See D. Jewell, I do not love thee Mr Fell, *BMJ*, 297 (1988): 498–9. A children's

limerick: "I do not love thee Mr. Fell/ for what reason I cannot tell/ but this I know very well/ I do not love thee Mr. Fell."

48. The following are the generally accepted conditions for ending the doctor–patient relationship and avoiding allegations of patient "abandonment." In certain circumstances—where there are few alternatives for care or where the patient's care is unique—more time may have to be given for the patient to find alternative care. The practitioner, in removing a patient from his or her list, should: not do so for trivial reasons; not do so in emergencies; provide the patient with a reasonable interval to find a new doctor (perhaps one month, longer if fewer doctors available); make suggestions as to how he or she might find a new doctor; look after the patient's needs until he or she finds a new doctor; and send a registered letter informing the patient of the decision to terminate.

49. J. Davies, P.C. Hébert, and C. Hoffman, *Canadian Patient Safety Dictionary* (Ottawa: RCPSC, 2003).

50. Lord Denning, "We must not condemn as negligence that which is only a misadventure." Quoted in E. Picard and G. Robertson, *Legal Liability of Doctors and Hospitals in Canada*, 3rd edn. (Toronto: Carswell Thomson Canada, 1996), 212.

51. "If the error is one which a reasonable doctor would not have made in similar circumstances, liability will be imposed." *Ibid.*, 281.

52. The quotation in Box 8.5 is taken from *Mahone v. Osborne*, [1939]2 KB 14 at 31 (CA).

53. G.R. Baker, P.G. Norton, V. Flintoft, R. Blais, A. Brown, J. Cox, et al., The Canadian Adverse Events Study: the incidence of adverse events among hospital patients in Canada, *CMAJ*, 170 (2004): 1678–86; R. Wilson, W. Runciman, R. Gibberd, B. Harrison, L. Newby, and J. Hamilton, The Quality in Australian Health Care Study, *Med J Aust*, 163 (1995): 458–71; An Organisation with a Memory, UK Department of Health (2000) www.doh.gov.uk; A. Gawande, E. Thomas, M. Zinner, and T. Brennan, The incidence and nature of surgical adverse events in Colorado and Utah in 1992, *Surgery*, 126 (1999): 66–75.

54. Institute of Medicine, *To Err is Human: Building a Safer Health System* (Washington, DC: National Academy Press, 1999).

55. A. Arriaga, A. Bader, J. Wong, S. Lipsitz, W. Berry, J. Ziewacz, et al., Simulation-based trial of surgical-crisis checklists, *N Engl J Med*, 368 (2013): 246–53.

56. L. Curry, E. Spatz, E. Cherlin, J. Thompson, D. Berg, H. Ting, et al, What distinguishes top-performing hospitals in acute myocardial infarction mortality rates? A qualitative study, *Ann Inter Med*, 154 (2011): 384–90.

57. Centers for Disease Control and Prevention, *Healthcare Associated Infections*. Accessed 15/01/2013 at: http://www.cdc.gov/HAI/

58. Editorial, Medical errors in the USA: human or systemic? *Lancet*, 377 (2011): 1289. "Methods for detecting medical errors . . . are unreliable [and] underestimate the real burden."

59. "Shame is so devastating because it goes right to the core of a person's identity, making them feel exposed, inferior, degraded; it leads to avoidance, to silence." F. Davidoff, Shame: The elephant in the room, *BMJ*, 324 (2002): 623–4.

60. Although there are few "laws" on the books requiring honesty, there is certainly ample case law and the weight of professional opinion to make veracity a standing duty for healthcare professionals. See "The duty to disclose medical mistakes," in Picard and Robertson, *op. cit.*, 170–2.

61. Institute of Medicine, *op. cit.*, 2–3.

62. *Shobridge v. Thomas* [1999] BCJ No 1747 (SC).

63. C. Vincent, M. Young, and A. Phillips, Why do people sue doctors? A study of patients and relatives taking legal action, *Lancet*, 343 (1994): 1609–13.

64. A.B. Witman, D.M. Park, and S.B. Hardin, How do patients want physicians to handle mistakes? A survey of internal medicine patients in an academic setting, *Arch Intern Med*, 156 (1996): 2565–9.

65. L. Iezzoni, S. Rao, C. DesRoches, C. Vogeli, and E. Campbell, Survey shows that at least some physicians are not always open or honest with patients, *Health Aff*, 31 (2012): 383–91.

66. N. Varjavand, L. Bachegowda, E. Gracely and D. Novack, Changes in intern attitudes toward medical error and disclosure, *Med Educ*, 46 (2012): 668–77.

67. T.H. Gallagher, C.R. Denham, L.L. Leape, G. Amori, and W. Levinson, Disclosing unanticipated outcomes to patients: The art and practice, *J Patient Saf*, 3 (2007): 158–65.

68. K.M. Mazor, S.R. Simon, and J.H. Gurwitz, Communicating with patients about medical errors: a review of the literature, *Arch Intern Med*, 164 (2004): 1690–7. See also: Z. R. Wolf, and R. G. Hughes, Error reporting and disclosure, Chapter 35 in R. G. Hughes, *Patient Safety and Quality: An Evidence-Based Handbook for Nurses*, (Rockville (MD): 2008, Agency for Healthcare Research and Quality).

69. S. Kraman and G. Hamm, Risk management: extreme honesty may be the best policy, *Ann Intern Med*, 131 (1999): 963–7.

70. A. Kachalia, S. Kaufman, R. Boothman, S. Anderson, K. Welch, S. Saint, and M. Rogers, Liability claims and costs before and after implementation of a medical error disclosure program, *Ann Intern Med*, 153 (2010); 213–21.

71. D. Hilfiker, Facing our mistakes, *N Engl J Med*, 310 (1984): 118–22. The original classic paper on self-disclosure of harmful error. "Medicine has no place for its mistakes," Hilfiker wrote. How times have changed—at least for some.

72. J. McMurray, Caring for Mr. Gray, *J Gen Intern Med*, 15 (2000): 144–6.

73. A. Wu, Medical error: the second victim. The doctor who makes the mistake needs help too, *BMJ*, 320 (2000): 726–7.

74. R. Boyte, Casey's legacy, *Health Aff*, 20 (2001): 250–4.

75. Canadian Patient Safety Institute (CPSI) *Canadian Disclosure Guidelines: Being Open with Patients and Families* (Edmonton, AB, Canada: CPSI, 2011).

76. The second to fifth bullets in Box 8.6 are from *Wickoff v. James*, 324P2d 441 Cal App (1958); *Lashley v. Koerber*, 156 P2d 441 cal (1945); *Robertson v. La Croix*, 534 P2d 17 Okla App (1975); *A Rest Home & Hospital*, HDC 13293 (1999).

77. M. Castel, The impact of the Canadian Apology Legislation when determining civil liability in Canadian private international law, *Advocates' Quarterly* 39 (2012); 440–51.

78. See , for example, E. Camiré, F. Moyen, and T. Stelfox, Medication errors in critical care: risk factors, prevention and disclosure, *CMAJ*, 180 (2009): 936–43.

79. K. Vicente, *The Human Factor: Revolutionizing the Way We Live with Technology* (Toronto: Vintage Canada Books, 2004).

80. *Braun v. Vaughan* Manitoba Court of Appeal [2000] M.J. No. 63.

81. "Managing test results effectively is vital to quality patient care." CPSO, *Test Results Management*, Policy 11-1 (2011). Available at: http://www.cpso.on.ca/ policies/policies/default.aspx?ID=4698

82. M. Balint, *The Doctor, His Patient and the Illness*, rev. edn. (Madison, CT: International Universities Press, 1988), 69–80.

83. S. Brown, C. Lehman, R. Truog, D. Browning, and T. Gallagher, Stepping out further from the shadows: disclosure of harmful radiologic errors to patients, *Radiology*, 262 (2012): 381–6.

84. C. Garvey and S. Connolly, Radiology reporting—where does the radiologist's duty end? *Lancet*, 367 (2006): 444.

85. L. Berlin, Using an automated coding and review process to communicate critical radiologic findings: One way to skin a cat, *AJR*, 185 (2005): 840–3. The author has written extensively and eloquently on error in radiology and the scope of the radiologist's duty to disclose mistakes to patients. See: L Berlin, *Malpractice Issues in Radiology, 3rd ed.* (Leesburg, VA, USA: ARRS, 2009).

86. T. Alcorn, Meningitis outbreak reveals gaps in US drug regulation, *Lancet,* 380 (2012): 1543–4; J. Perfect, Iatrogenic fungal meningitis: tragedy repeated, *Ann Intern Med,* 157 (2012): 825–6.

87. D. Dudzinski, P.C. Hébert, M.B. Foglia, and T. Gallagher, The disclosure dilemma—large-scale adverse events, *N Engl J Med*, 363 (2010): 978–86.

88. CBC news, Hormone Testing: Judicial inquiry probes faulty breast cancer tests, March 18, 2008 http://www.cbc.ca/news/ background/cancer/inquiry.html

89. Commission of Inquiry on Hormone Receptor Testing at http://www.cihrt.

nl.ca/; http://www.releases.gov.nl.ca/releases/2009/health/CameronInquiry.pdf.

90. M. O'Toole, "Robin Hood doctor" guilty of professional misconduct, *National Post* (Dec 13, 2012), page A1.

91. J. Young, S. Ranji, R. Wachter, C. Lee, B. Niehaus, and A. Auerbach, "July Effect": impact of the academic year-end changeover on patient outcomes: a systematic review, *Ann Intern Med*, 155 (2011): 309–15.

Chapter 9

1. C. Dickens, *A Tale of Two Cities* [1859] (Markham, ON: Penguin Books Canada, 1976), 35.

2. N. Daniels, *Just Health: Meeting Health Needs Fairly* (Cambridge UK; Cambridge University Press, 2008), 99.

3. A. Wildavsky, Doing better, feeling worse: The political pathology of social policy, in A. Wildavsky, *Speaking Truth to Power: The Art and Craft of Policy Analysis* (Boston: Little Brown, 1979), 284–308.

4. *R v Gladue* (1999) 1 S.C.C. 688.

5. *Oxford English Dictionary* [CD-ROM] 2nd edn., Version 3.0 (Oxford: Oxford University Press, 2002).

6. P. Hartzband and J. Groopman, The new language of medicine, *N Engl J Med*, 365 (2011): 1372–3.

7. R. Tallis, *Hippocratic Oaths: Medicine and its Discontents* (London: Atlantic Books, 2004).

8. T. Beam, Medical ethics on the battlefield, in T. Beam and L. Sparacino (eds.), *Military Medical Ethics*, vol. 2 (Washington, DC: Office of the Surgeon General, 2003), 369–402.

9. J. La Puma, *Managed Care Ethics* (New York: Hatherleigh Press, 1998).

10. P. Ubel, *Pricing Life: Why It's Time for Health Care Rationing* (Cambridge, MA: First MIT Press, 2001).

11. H. Brody, From an ethics of rationing to an ethics of waste avoidance. *N Engl J Med*, 366 (2012): 1949–51.

12. N. Daniels, *op. cit.:* 146-8.

13. J. Rawls, Social unity and primary goods, in A. Sen and B. Williams, (eds.) *Utilitarianism and Beyond* (Cambridge UK: Cambridge University Press,1982), 168–9.

14. J. Rawls, *Justice as Fairness: A Restatement* (Cambridge, MA: Harvard University Press, 2001): 9.

15. A. Sen, *The Idea of Justice* (Harvard, Mass: Harvard University Press, 2009).

16. M.C. Nussbaum. *Frontiers of Justice: Disability, Nationality, Species Membership* (Harvard, Mass: Harvard University Press, 2006).

17. M. Balint, *The Doctor, His Patient and the Illness*, rev. edn. (Madison, CT: International Universities Press, 1988): 3–6, 242–8.

18. 2005 SCR 35. [2005] 1 SCR 791 (CanLII) [*Chaoulli* cited to SCR]

19. M. Yeo and C. Lucock, Quality v. Equality: the divided Court in *Chaoulli v. Québec, Health Law J,* 14 (2006): 129–50.

20. *Oxford English Dictionary* [CD-ROM] 2nd edn., Version 3.0 (Oxford: Oxford University Press, 2002).

21. Daniels, *op. cit.*:13.

22. Adapted from: L. Iezzoni, Boundaries: What happens to the disabled poor when insurers draw a line between what's "medically necessary" and devices that can improve quality of life?, *Health Aff*, 18 (1999): 171–6.

23. L. Iezzoni, Eliminating health and health care disparities among the growing population of people with disabilities, *Health Aff*, 30 (2011):1947–54.

24. M. Cabana and S. Jee, Does continuity of care improve patient outcomes? *J Fam Pract*, 53 (2004): 974–80.

25. J. Cheng, Confronting the social determinants of health—obesity, neglect, and inequity, *N Engl J Med* 367 (2012):1976–7.

26. Balint, *op. cit.:* 69–80.

27. D. Hilfiker, *Not All of Us are Saints: A Doctor's Journey with the Poor* (New York: Hill and Wang, 1994).

28. P. Neumann, What we talk about when we talk about health care costs, *N Engl J Med* 366 (2012): 385–6.

29. Adapted from J. McIntyre quoted in M. Jackman, The Canadian Charter as a barrier to unwanted medical treatment of pregnant women in the interests of the foetus, *Health Law Can*, 14/2 (1993): 53.

30. Box 9.1 is taken from Council on Ethical and Judicial Affairs, AMA, Ethical considerations in the allocation of organs and other scarce medical resources among patients, *Arch Intern Med*, 155 (1995): 40.

31. S. Alexander, They decide who lives, who dies, *Life*, 9 Nov. 1962, 102ff.

32. P. Eggers, Medicare's end stage renal disease program, *Health Care Financing Review,* 22 (2000): 55–60.

33. R. Baker, Visibility and the just allocation of health care: A study of age-rationing in the British NHS, *Health Care Anal,* 1 (1993): 139–50.

34. A.Wing, A different view from different countries: UK, in C. Kjellstrand and J. Dossetor (eds.), *Ethical Problems in Dialysis and Transplantation* (Dordrecht: Kluwer Academic, 1992), 205–10.

35. K. Madhan, The epidemic of elderly patients with dialysis-requiring end-stage renal disease in New Zealand, *N Z Med J,* 117 (2004): U912.

36. K. Clarke, D. Gray, N. Keating, and J. Hampton, Do women with acute myocardial infarction receive the same treatment as men? *BMJ,* 309 (1994): 563–6.

37. P. Kaul, W. Chang, C. Westerhout, M. Graham, and P. Armstrong, Differences in admission rates and outcomes between men and women presenting to emergency departments with coronary syndromes, *CMAJ,* 177 (2007): 1193–9.

38. C. Borkhoff, G. Hawker, H. Kreder, R. Glazier, N. Mahomed, and J.Wright, The effect of patients' sex on physicians' recommendations for total knee arthroplasty, *CMAJ* 178 (2008): 681–7.

39. Aristotle, *Nicomachean Ethics.* Book V. (New York: Bobbs-Merrill Publishers, 1962).

40. D. Miller, D. Jahnigan, M. Gorbien, and L. Simbartl, CPR: How useful? Attitudes and knowledge of an elderly population, *Arch Intern Med,* 152 (1992): 578–82.

41. Royal College of Surgeons of England and Age UK, *Access all Ages Report* (2012). Accessed at: http://www.rcseng.ac.uk/publications/docs/access-all-ages

42. S. Schroeder and J. Cantor, On squeezing balloons. Cost control fails again, *N Engl J Med,* 325 (1991): 1099–1100.

43. Cf. ref 9 above.

44. N. Daniels, Is the Oregon rationing plan fair? *JAMA,* 265 (1991): 2232–5. "One of the best avenues to improve accountability is to make decision-making less opaque and more transparent. Unfortunately, health care decisions have been and continue to be made behind closed doors." C. Flood and M. Zimmerman, Judicious choices: Health care resource decisions

and the Supreme Court of Canada, in J. Downie and E. Gibson, (eds.) *Health Law at the Supreme Court of Canada* (Toronto: Irwin Law, 2007): 54.

45. D. Hopkins, Disease eradication, *N Engl J Med,* 368 (2013): 54–63.

46. Polio has been eradicated in 99.9% of the world with only 222 cases reported worldwide (as compared with 350,000 cases in 1988). *PolioInfo,* see: http://www.polioeradication.org.

47. US policy on vaccine allocation, see: http://www.flu.gov/images/reports/pi_vaccine_allocation_guidance.pdf.

48. See the *United Network for Organ Sharing* (UNOS) <www.unos.org>.

49. M. Benjamin, C. Cohen, and E. Grochowski, What transplantation can teach us about health care reform, *N Engl J Med,* 330 (1994): 858–60.

50. N. Daniels, Four unsolved rationing problems. A Challenge, *Hastings Cent Rep,* 24 (July–Aug. 1994): 27–9.

51. R. Gaston, I. Ayres, L. Dooley, and A. Diethelm, Racial equity in renal transplantation: The disparate impact of HLA-based allocation, *JAMA,* 270 (1993): 1352–6.

52. Ubel, *op. cit.,* 84.

53. J. Radcliffe Richards, *The Ethics of Transplants: Why Careless Thought Costs Lives* (Oxford, UK: Oxford University Press, 2012).

54. B. Hippen, Organ sales and moral travails: Lessons from the living kidney vendor program in Iran, *Policy Analysis* No 614, Mar 20, 2008, accessed at www.cato.org/sites/cato.org/files/pubs/pdf/pa-614.pdf

55. N.R. Hicks, Some observations on attempts to measure appropriateness of care, *BMJ,* 309 (1994): 730–3; K. Warren and F. Mosteller (eds.), *Doing More Good Than Harm: The Evaluation of Health Care Interventions* (New York: The New York Academy of Sciences, 1993). See also: C. Phelps, The methodological foundations of studies of the appropriateness of care, *N Engl J Med,* 329 (1993): 1241–5.

56. H. Fineberg, A successful and sustainable health system—how to get there from here, *N Engl J Med,* 366 (2012):1020–7.

57. S .Weinberger, Providing high-value, cost-conscious care: a critical seventh general competency for physicians, *Ann Intern Med,* 155 (2011): 386–8.

58. D. Owens, A. Qaseem, R. Chou and P. Shekelle for the Clinical Guidelines Committee of the ACP, High-value, cost-conscious health care: concepts for clinicians to evaluate the benefits, harms, and costs of medical interventions, *Ann Intern Med* 154 (2011): 174–80.

59. The questions in Box 9.2 are from: C. Laine, High-value testing begins with a few simple questions, *Ann Intern Med,* 156 (2012): 162–3.

60. D. Eddy, Practice policies: What are they? *JAMA,* 263 (1990): 877–80.

61. S. Woolf, Practice guidelines: a new reality for medicine. III. Impact on patient care, *Arch Intern Med,* 153 (1993): 2646–55.

62. D. Ransohoff, M. Pignone and H. Sox, How to decide whether a clinical practice guideline is trustworthy, *JAMA,* 309 (2013): 139–40.

63. K. Warren and F. Mosteller (eds.), *Doing More Good Than Harm: The Evaluation of Health Care Interventions* (New York: The New York Academy of Sciences, 1993).

64. S. Dorr Goold and M. Lipkin Jr, The doctor-patient relationship: challenges, opportunities, and strategies, *J Gen Intern Med,* 14, S1 (1999): 26–33.

65. R. Brook, Implementing medical guidelines, *Lancet,* 346 (1995): 132.

66. P. Oppenheim, G. Sotiropoulos, and L. Baraff, Incorporating patient preferences into practice guidelines: management of children with fever without source, *Ann Emerg Med,* 24 (1994): 836–41.

67. Box 9.3 is adapted from Colloquium Report on *Legal Issues Related to Clinical Practice Guidelines* (Washington, DC: National Health Lawyers Association, 1995).

68. J. O'Meara, R. McNutt, A. Evans, S. Moore, and S. Downs, A decision analysis of streptokinase plus heparin as compared with heparin alone for deep-vein thrombosis, *N Engl J Med,* 330 (1994): 1864–9.

69. J. Wennberg, The paradox of appropriate care, *JAMA,* 258 (1987): 2568–9.

70. "[T]o increase trust, all guidelines should include explicit information about cost-effectiveness to help physicians better assess the objectivity of the recommendations. Cost-effectiveness information enhances the credibility and usefulness of guidelines by showing their reasonableness." E. Hummel and P. Ubel, Cost and clinical practice guidelines: can two wrongs make it right? *Virtual Mentor,* 6/12 (2004) http://virtualmentor.ama-assn.org/2004/12/pfor1-0412.html.

71. J. Swales, Guidelines for management of hypertension. Sticking to guidelines can be expensive, *BMJ,* 308 (1994): 855.

72. *Early v. Newham Health Authority* [1994] 5 Med LR 214.

73. P. Dwyer, Legal implications of clinical practice guidelines, *Med J Aust,* 169 (1998): 292–3.

74. Colloquium Report on *Legal Issues Related to Clinical Practice Guidelines* (Washington, DC: National Health Lawyers Association, 1995): 20; E. Hirshfeld, Should ethical and legal standards for physicians be changed to accommodate new models for rationing health care? *Univ PA Law Rev,* 140 (1992): 1809.

75. D. Sulmasy, Physicians, cost control and ethics, *Ann Intern Med,* 116 (1992): 920–6.

76. J. Kassirer, Managed care and the morality of the marketplace, *N Engl J Med,* 333 (1995): 50–2.

77. E. Oshima Lee, and E.E. Emanuel, Shared decision making to improve care and reduce costs, *N Engl J Med,* 368 (2013): 6–8.

78. R. Faden, and K. Chalkidou, Determining the value of drugs—the evolving British experience, *N Engl J Med,* 364 (2011):1289-91.

79. La Puma, *op. cit.,* 166.

80. Daniels, *op. cit.,* 243–7.

81. Colloquium Report on *Legal Issues Related to Clinical Practice Guidelines* (Washington, DC: National Health Lawyers Association, 1995): 16.

82. *Law Estate v. Simice,* [1994] B.C.J. No. 979.

83. D. Mechanic, Dilemmas in rationing health care services: the case for implicit rationing, *BMJ,* 310 (1995): 1655–9.

84. *R. v. Gladue,* [1999] 1 S.C.R. 688. *R. v. Ipeelee* [2012] SCC 13: "The sentencing judge has a statutory duty, imposed by s. 718.2(e) of the *Criminal Code,* to consider the unique circumstances of Aboriginal offenders."

85. D. Parkes, D. Milward, S. Keesic, and J. Seymour, *The Gladue Handbook* (Manitoba, University of Manitoba, Faculty of Law, 2013). This handbook provides guidelines for taking the

social circumstances of the offender into account. Updated periodically, and additional relevant materials will be made available, at http://chrr.info/resources/gladue-projec.

86. N. Biller-Andorno and T.H. Lee, Ethical physician incentives—from carrots and sticks to shared purpose, *N Engl J Med*, 368 (2013): 980–2.

87. D. DeLillo, *Mao II* (New York: Viking Penguin, 1991), 16.

88. E. Campbell, S. Regan, R. Gruen, T. Ferris, S. Rao, P. Cleary, and D. Blumenthal, Professionalism in medicine: results of a national survey of physicians, *Ann Intern Med*, 147 (2007): 795–802.

89. L. Snyder and R. Neubauer for the American College of Physicians Ethics, Professionalism and Human Rights Committee, Pay-for-performance principles that promote patient-centered care: an ethics manifesto, *Ann Intern Med*, 147 (2007): 792–4.

90. For the real case from the 1880s, see: B. Simpson, *Cannibalism and the Common Law: The Story of the Tragic Last Voyage of the Mignonette and the Strange Legal Proceedings to Which it gave Rise* (Chicago: University of Chicago Press,1984). In this real-life case from the 1880s, the name of the unfortunate cabin boy was Richard Parker, the same name as the lifeboat tiger in Yan Martel's popular novel *The Life of Pi*.

Chapter 10

1. *Dobson v. Dobson* 1999 2 SCC per C.J. Lamer.

2. *Reference re Assisted Human Reproduction Act*, 2010 SCC per CJ. McLachlin

3. G.W.F. Hegel, *The Philosophy of History*, Trans. J. Sibree (New York: Dover Publications, 1956), 40.

4. A. Templeton and D. Grimes, A request for abortion, *N Engl J Med*, 365 (2011): 2198–204.

5. J.J. Thomson, A defense of abortion, *Philosophy & Public Affairs*, 1/1 (Fall 1971). Reprinted in R. Munson (ed.), *Intervention and Reflection: Basic Issues in Medical Ethics*, 5th ed. (Belmont, CA: Wadsworth, 1996), 69–80.

6. B. Sneiderman, Issues in reproductive choice: Part 2, in B. Sneiderman, J. Irvine, and P. Osborne (eds.), *Canadian*

Medical Law: An Introduction for Physicians, Nurses and Other Health Care Professionals, 3rd edn. (Toronto: Thomson Carswell, 2003), 347.

7. *R. v. Morgentaler* (1988), 44 D.L.R. (4th) 385 (S.C.C.), 402.

8. *Roe v. Wade* (No. 70-18) 314 F. Supp. 1217, aff'd in part and rev'd in part.

9. M. Greene and J. Ecker, Abortion, health and the law, *N Engl J Med*, 350 (2004): 184–6.

10. T.R. Berger, *One Man's Justice: A Life in the Law* (Vancouver; Douglas & McIntyre; 2002): 272-98.

11. *Ximena Renaerts v. Vancouver Gen. Hosp.*, (1998) B.C.T.C. Lexis 2214 (B.C.S.C. Dec. 4, 1998), No. C937086.

12. The statistics and recommendations in this paragraph are from A. Jefferies and H. Kirpalani, The Canadian Paediatric Society, Fetus and Newborn Committee, Counselling and management for anticipated extremely preterm birth, *Paediatr Child Health*, 17 (2012): 443.

13. See B. Farlow, A child like Annie, in S. McIver, and R. Wyndham, eds., *After the Error: Speaking Out About Patient Safety to Save Lives* (Toronto: ECW Press, 2013): 3–17.

14. G. Sedgh, S. Henshaw, S. Singh, E. Ahman, and I. Shah, Induced abortion: estimated rates and trends worldwide, *Lancet*, 370 (2007): 1338–45.

15. B. Dickens and R. Cook, The scope and limits of conscientious objection, *Int J Gynaecol and Obstet*, 71 (2000): 71–7.

16. H. Fernandez Lynch, *Conflicts of Conscience in Health Care: An Institutional Compromise* (Cambridge MA; MIT Press, 2008): 51.

17. R. A. Charo, The partial death of abortion rights, *N Engl J Med*, 356 (2007): 2125–8.

18. "[T]he majority of ART programs believe that they have the right and responsibility to screen candidates before providing them with ART to conceive a child. The key value that seems to guide programs' screening practices is ensuring a prospective child's safety and welfare and not risking the welfare of the prospective mother." A. Gurmankin, A. Caplan, and A. Braverman, Screening practices and beliefs of ART programs, *Fertil Steril*, 83 (2005): 61–7.

19. R.A. Charo, The celestial fire of conscience—refusing to deliver medical care, *N Engl J Med*, 352 (2005): 2471–3.

20. *Tremblay v. Daigle*, [1989] 2 S.C.R. 530.
21. *Ibid.*
22. S. Rodgers and J. Downie, Abortion: ensuring access, *CMAJ*, 175 (2006): 9.
23. M. Day, Abortion should be made easier, charity says, *BMJ*, 333 (2006): 1139.
24. A. Cheng, Chinese couple sue over forced abortion. One child policy: Citizens push their rights in first case of its kind, *National Post*, 29 Aug. 2007, A16.
25. "It is inappropriate and contrary to good medical practice to use ultrasound only to…determine the gender of the fetus." CPSO. Fetal ultrasound for non-medical reasons. Policy Statement #4-10. Published in *Dialogue* (Issue 2; 2010).
26. Sneiderman, *op. cit.*, 323.
27. C.A. Kent, *Medical Ethics: The State of the Law* (Toronto: LexisNexis Canada, 2005), 215.
28. E. Picard and G. Robertson, *Legal Liability of Doctors and Hospitals in Canada*, 3rd edn. (Toronto: Carswell Thomson Canada, 1996), 213.
29. *Jones (Guardian ad litem of) v. Rostvig.* [2003] B.C.J. No. 1840 2003 BCSC 1222.
30. A. Solomon, *Far from the Tree: Parents, Children, and the Search for Identity* (New York: Scribner, 2012).
31. I. Bretherton, The origins of attachment theory: John Bowlby and Mary Ainsworth, *Developmental Psychology*, 28 (1992): 759–75.
32. R. Mukherjee, N. Eastman, J. Turk, and S. Hollins, Fetal alcohol syndrome: law and ethics, *Lancet*, 369 (2007): 1149–50.
33. *Tremblay v. Daigle*, [1989] 2 S.C.R. 530. The quotation in Box 10.1 is from Kent, *op. cit.*, 161.
34. J. Cantor, Court-ordered care—a complication of pregnancy to avoid, *N Engl J Med*, 366 (2012): 2237–40.
35. PGD is a powerful technique that can be used on an embryo prior to womb implantation to determine its precise chromosomal makeup—including its sex and inherited characteristics such as genetic disorders.
36. G. Rivard and J. Hunter, *The Law of Assisted Human Reproduction* (Toronto: LexisNexis Canada, 2005), 125.
37. *Potter v. Korn* [1995] BCCHRD No 20.
38. *Korn v. Potter* [1996] BCJ No 692.
39. The Ethics Committee of the American Society for Reproductive Medicine, Access to fertility treatment by gays, lesbians, and unmarried persons, *Fertil Steril*, 92 (2009): 1190–3.
40. Discrimination is defined in Chapter 9 on justice.
41. Rivard and Hunter, *op. cit.*, 11.
42. Solomon, *op. cit.*, 115.
43. The Ethics Committee of the American Society for Reproductive Medicine Child-rearing and the provision of fertility services, *Fertil Steril*, 92 (2009): 864–7.
44. Rivard and Hunter, *op. cit.*, 11.
45. C. Boorse, On the distinction between disease and illness, in M. Cohen, T. Nagel, and T. Scanlon (eds.), *Medicine and Moral Philosophy* (Princeton, NJ: Princeton University Press, 1981), 3–48.
46. *Cameron v. Nova Scotia (ag)* [1999] NSJ No 297 para 170.
47. A. Wolfberg, Genes on the web—direct-to-consumer marketing of genetic testing, *N Engl J Med*, 355 (2006): 543–5.
48. The quotation in Box 10.2 is from Rivard and Hunter, *op. cit.*, 21.
49. *Ibid.*, 31.
50. The Ethics Committee of the American Society for Reproductive Medicine, Preconception gender selection for nonmedical reasons, *Fertil Steril*, 75 (2001): 861–4.
51. The US is much more liberal as regards payment for components, allowing up to $10,000 payment for oocyte donation alone as a recompense for "time, inconvenience, and discomfort." It is recognized that the higher the payment, the more likely donors will discount the risks. The Ethics Committee of the American Society for Reproductive Medicine, Financial compensation of oocyte donors, *Fertil Steril*, 88 (2007), 305–9.
52. *Reference re Assisted Human Reproduction Act* SCC [2010] 3 S.C.R. 457 per SJ MacLachlin.
53. *Reference re Assisted Human Reproduction Act* SCC [2010] 3 S.C.R. 457.
54. R.S.C. 1985, c. F-27.
55. See http://www.hfea.gov.uk/112.html.
56. *Pratten v. BC (Attorney General)*. (2011) Carswell BC 1231, 2011 BCSC 656 (B.C. S.C.)
57. S. Zomorodi. Should s. 7 Charter rights impose positive state obligations in the context of donor anonymity? *Reg Offenses and Compliance Newsletter*, 40; (Sept., 2011): 1–5.

58. G. Annas, Assisted reproduction – Canada's Supreme Court and the "global baby." *N Engl J Med*, 365 (2011): 459–63.

59. J. Slack, *Stem Cells: A Very Short Introduction* (Oxford, UK: Oxford University Press, 2012): 87.

60. R. Bolli, A. Chugh, D. D'Amario, H. Loughran, M. Stoddart, S. Ikram, G. Beache, et al., Cardiac stem cells in patients with ischaemic cardiomyopathy (SCIPIO): initial results of a randomized phase 1 trial, *Lancet*; 378 (2011): 1847–57.

61. R. Makkar, R. Smith, K. Cheng, K. Malliaras, L. Thomson, D. Berman, L. Czer, et al., Intracoronary cardiosphere-derived cells for heart regeneration after myocardial infarction (CADUCEUS): a prospective, randomized phase 1 trial. *Lancet*; 379 (2012): 895–904.

62. L Ptaszek, M Mansour, J Ruskin, and K Chien, Towards regenerative therapy for cardiac disease, *Lancet*, 379 (2012): 933–42.

63. P. White, Cure or hoax in China? Stem cell therapy: "Some get miracles"; others are skeptical, *National Post*, 23 Aug. 2007, L1, 3.

64. S. Laidlaw, Battle lines being drawn for new war over stem cells, *Toronto Star*, 25 Aug. 2007, ID6.

65. Slack, *op. cit.*, 32–3.

66. R. Blendon, M. Kim, and J. Benson, The public, political parties, and stem-cell research, *N Engl J Med* 365 (2011):1853–6.

67. The Ethics Committee of ASRM, Financial compensation of oocyte donors, *Fertil Steril*, 88 (2007): 305–9.

68. I. Kant, *Groundwork of the Metaphysic of Morals* [1785] (New York: Harper & Row, 1956), 96.

69. R. Clark, Bone marrow donation by mentally incapable adults, *Lancet*, 352 (1998): 1847–8.

70. C. Tauer, International policy failures: cloning and stem cell research, *Lancet*, 364 (2004): 209–14.

Chapter 11

1. T. Hobbes, *Leviathan* [1651] (New York: Collier Books, 1977), 100.

2. *Criminal Code of Canada*, s. 215c.

3. *Ibid.*, s. 217.

4. *Nancy B. v. Hôtel-Dieu de Québec et al.* (1992), 86 D.L.R. (4th) 385–95 (Q.S.C.).

5. The quotation in Box 11.1 is from the US case, *Brophy v. New England Sinai Hospital*, [1986] Sup Jud Ct Mass 497 NE 2d 626.

6. *Criminal Code of Canada*, s. 216.

7. *Ibid.*, s. 219

8. L. Glantz quoted in G. Snider, Withholding and withdrawing life-sustaining therapy, *Am J Respir Crit Care Med*, 151 (1995): 279.

9. *Ibid.*, 279–81.

10. The quotation in Box 11.2 is from *In the Matter of Claire Conroy*, 486 A.2d 1209, NJ, 1985.

11. C. von Gunten, F. Ferris, and L. Emanuel, The patient-physician relationship. Ensuring competency in end-of-life care: communication and relational skills, *JAMA*, 284 (2000): 3051–7.

12. L. Crawley, P. Marshall, B. Lo, and B. Koenig for the End-of-Life Care Consensus Panel, Strategies for culturally effective end-of-life care, *Ann Intern Med*, 136 (2002): 673–9.

13. S. Baumrucker, J. Sheldon, G. Morris, M. Stolick, G. Carter, and D. Harrington, Withdrawing treatment for the "wrong" reasons, *Am J Hosp Palliat Care*, 24 (2008): 509–14.

14. C. Rodgers, H. Field, and E. Kunkel, Countertransference issues in termination of life support in acute quadriplegia, *Psychosomatics*, 36 (1995): 305–9.

15. Thanks to Monica Branigan for this point.

16. C. Kjellstrand, Practical aspects of stopping dialysis and cultural differences, in J. Dossetor and C. Kjellstrand (eds.), *Ethical Problems in Dialysis and Transplantation* (Boston: Kluwer Academic, 1992), 103.

17. ESRD Network of New England, *2001 Annual Report to the Centers for Medicare and Medicaid Services* (New Haven, CT: Tyco Printers, 2002), 60–3.

18. A. Turgeon, F. Lauzier, J. Simard, D. Scales, K. Burns, L. Moore, D. Zygun, et al., Mortality associated with withdrawal of life-sustaining therapy for patients with severe traumatic brain injury, *CMAJ*, 183 (2011): 1581–8.

19. D. Cook, G. Rocker, J. Marshall, P. Sjokvist, P. Dodek, L. Griffith, et al., Withdrawal of mechanical ventilation in anticipation of death in the ICU, *N Engl J Med*, 349 (2003): 1123–32.

20. S. Bok, Personal directions for care at the end of life, *N Engl J Med*, 295 (1976): 367–9.

21. D. Wendler and A. Rid, Systematic review: the effect on surrogates of making treatment decisions for others, *Ann Intern Med*, 154 (2011): 336–46.

22. The SUPPORT Principal Investigators, The SUPPORT study: A controlled trial to improve care for seriously ill hospitalized patients: the Study to Understand Prognoses and Preferences for Outcomes and Risks of Treatments (SUPPORT), *JAMA*, 274 (1995): 1591–8.

23. P. Gozalo, J. Teno, S. Mitchell, J. Skinner, J. Bynum, D. Tyler, and V. Mor, End-of-life transitions among nursing home residents with cognitive issues, *N Engl J Med*, 365 (2011): 1212–21.

24. A. Kelley, S Ettner, R. Morrison, Q. Du, N. Wenger, and C. Sarkisian, Determinants of medical expenditures in the last 6 months of life, *Ann Intern Med*, 154 (2011): 235–42.

25. H. Perkins, Controlling death: the false promise of advance directives, *Ann Intern Med*, 147 (2007): 51–7.

26. M. Silveira, S. Kim, and K. Langa, Advance directives and outcomes of surrogate decision making before death, *N Engl J Med*, 362 (2010): 1211–18.

27. L. Castillo, B. Williams, S. Hooper, C. Sabatino, L. Weithorn, and R. Sudore, Lost in translation: the unintended consequences of advance directive law on clinical care, *Ann Intern Med*, 154 (2011): 121–28.

28. T. Thompson, R. Barbour, and L. Schwartz, Adherence to advance directives in critical care decision making: vignette study, *BMJ*, 327 (2003): 1011.

29. T. Hope and J. McMillan, Advance directives, chronic mental illness, and everyday care, *Lancet*, 377 (2011): 2076–7.

30. K. Marx, *The 18th Brumaire of Louis Napoleon* (1852); In: *The Collected Works of Marx and Engels*, Vol 11 (New York, International Publishers, 1979): 103.

31. J. Weeks, P. Catalano, A. Cronin, M. Finkelman, J. Mack, N. Keating, and D. Schrag, Patients' expectations about effects of chemotherapy for advanced cancer, *New Engl J Med*, 367 (2012); 1616–25.

32. L. Allen, J. Yager, M. Funk, W. Levy, J. Tulsky, M. Bowers, et al., Discordance between patient-predicted and model-predicted life expectancy among ambulatory patients with heart failure, *JAMA*, 299 (2008): 2533–42.

33. L. Zier, P. Sottile, S. Hong, L. Weissfield, and D. White, Surrogate decision makers' interpretation of prognostic information: a mixed-methods study, *Ann Intern Med*, 156 (2012): 360–6.

34. "Code" is the code word for CPR (Cardio-Pulmonary Resuscitation) which is called and, hopefully, performed when a patient suffers a cardiac arrest. CPR will, generally be performed on a patient unless a "No CODE" order is written on the patient's chart.

35. *Sawatsky v. Riverview Health Centre Inc.* (1998), 167 D.L.R. (4th) 359 at 362 (Man. Q.B.).

36. M. Zeytinoglu, Talking it out: helping our patients live better while dying, *Ann Intern Med*, 154 (2011): 830–2.

37. CMPA, End-of-life care: support, comfort, and challenging decisions, (Sept, 2011) P1103-4-E.

38. P. Chan, B. Nallamothu, H, Krumholz, J. Spertus, Y. Li, B. Hammill, et al., Long-term outcomes of elderly survivors of in-hospital cardiac arrest, *N Engl J Med*, 368 (2013): 1019–26. This study of the long-term survival of elderly patients who did have a cardiac arrest in hospital *and* survived to discharge showed that, one year after discharge 60%, were still alive. Survival correlated with "younger" old age and better neurologic status at discharge.

39. Ed., End-of-life care: the neglected core business of medicine, *Lancet*, 379 (2012): 1171.

40. CMA, CHA, CHAC, Joint Statement on Resuscitative Interventions, *CMAJ*, 151 (1994): 1176A–C.

41. CPSO, *Decision-Making for the End-of-life*. Policy Statement #1-06, (2011

42. J.R. Curtis, What is the "right" intensity of care at the end of life and how do we get there? *Ann Intern Med*, 154 (2011): 283–4.

43. T. Quill, R. Arnold, and F. Platt, "I wish things were different": expressing wishes in response to loss, futility, and unrealistic hopes, *Ann Intern Med*, 135 (2001): 551–5.

44. *Re Child and Family Services of Central Manitoba v. Lavallee* (1997), 154 D.L.R. (4th) 409 at 413 (Man. C.A.).

45. *Scardoni v. Hawryluck*, (2004) CanLII 34326 (ON S.C.), http://canlii.ca/t/1gcdr retrieved on 2013-02-14.

46. *Scardoni v. Hawryluck* (2004), CanLII 34326 (ON S.C.).

47. PVS refers to a state of the absence of awareness and the irreversible loss of higher brain function. Such patients go through sleep-wake cycles but have no purposive movements or communication and must be artificially fed and sometimes artificially ventilated. B. Jennett, *The Vegetative State. Medical Facts, ethical and legal dilemmas* (Cambridge, UK: Cambridge University Press, 2002).

48. *In re Quinlan* [1976] 137 NJ Sup 227, 348 A2d 801, modified, 70 NJ 10, 335A 2d 647 cert denied, 429 US 922.

49. *In the matter of Claire Conroy*, [1985] 98 NJ 32; *Brophy v. New England Sinai Hospital*, [1986] Sup Jud Ct Mass 497 NE 2d 626; *Cruzan v. Director, Missouri Dept of Health*, [1990] 110 S, Ct, 2841.

50. G. Annas, "Culture of Life" politics at the bedside—the case of Terri Schiavo, *N Engl J Med*, 352 (2005): 1710–15.

51. *Re a Ward of the Court* [1995] 2ILRM 401 (Ir Sup Ct); *Airedale NHS Trust v. Bland* [1993] Appeal Cases 789.

52. D. Cruse, S. Chennu, C. Chatelle, A. Beckinschtein, D. Fernandez-Espejo, J. Pickard, et al., Bedside detection of awareness in the vegetative state: a cohort study, *Lancet*, 378 (2011): 2088–94.

53. A. Goldfine, J. Bardin, Q. Noirhomme, J. Fins, N. Schiff, and J. Victor, Reanalysis of "Bedside detection of awareness in the vegetative state: a cohort study," *Lancet*, 381 (2013): 289–91.

54. *Rasouli v. Sunnybrook Health Sciences Centre and Cuthbertson*, 2011 ONSC 1500.

55. H. Young, Why withdrawing life-sustaining treatment should not require "Rasouli consent," *McGill J Law Health*, 6 (2012): 54–104.

56. A. Smith, B. Williams, and B. Lo, Discussing overall prognosis with the very elderly, *N Engl J Med, 365* (2011): 2149–51.

57. Box 11.5 is adapted from S. Goold, B. Williams, and R. Arnold, Conflicts regarding decisions to limit treatment: a differential diagnosis, *JAMA,* 283 (2000): 909–14.

58. Manitoba College of Physicians and Surgeons. Withholding and Withdrawal of Life-Sustaining Treatment. Policy Statement 1602 (2010). Acccessed on 14-02-2013 at: http://cpsm.mb.ca/cjj39alckF30a/wp-content/uploads/st1602.pdf. This policy appears currently inaccessible (as of 21-10-2013) and may be under review as a result of *Cuthbertson v Rasouli, infra.*

59. *Cuthbertson v Rasouli,* [2013] SCC 53.

60. *Cuthbertson v Rasouli,* [2013] SCC 53: 72.

61. T. Smith and D. Longo, Talking with patients about dying, *N Engl J Med*, 367 (2012): 1651–2.

62. C. Lilly and B. Daly, The healing power of listening in the ICU, *N Engl J Med*, 356 (2007): 513–15.

63. M. Vierra, Death panels, *Ann Intern Med,* 156 (2012): 394–5.

64. K. Swetz and A. Kamal, In the Clinic: Palliative Care. *Ann Intern Med,* 156 (2012): ITC2-1.

65. The quotation in Box 11.6 is from the *Criminal Code of Canada*, s. 241(b).

66. R. Portenoy, U. Sibirceva, R. Smout, S. Horn, S. Connor, R. Blum, et al., Opioid use and survival at the end of life: a survey of a hospice population, *J Pain Symptom Manage*, 32 (2006): 532–40.

67. *Rodriguez v. B.C.* (A.G.) [1993] 3 S.C.R.: 519–632.

68. *Rodriguez. Ibid.*

69. *Carter v AG (Canada)* [2012] BCSC 886.

70. *Carter v. Canada (Attorney General)* [2013] BCCA 435.

71. The UK report has testimony from many sources. Accessed on 21-10-2013 at: http://www.commissiononassisteddying.co.uk.

72. Collège des Médecins du Québec, *Physicians, Appropriate Care and the Debate on Euthanasia: A Reflection* (October 2009) Available at www.cmq.org.

73. *The Royal Society of Canada Expert Panel: End-of-Life Decision Making*; (RSC, Ottawa, Nov 2011). Available at rsc-src.ca/en/expert-panels/rsc-reports/end-life-decision-making.

74. S.J. Genuis, S.K. Genuis, and W.C. Chang, Public attitudes toward the right to die, CMAJ, 150 (1994): 701–8.

75. M. Angell, et al., Why do Americans balk at euthanasia laws? *New York Times*, April 10, 2012. Accessed on 23-04-2013 at: http://www.nytimes.com/roomfordebate/2012/04/10/why-do-americans-balk-at-euthanasia-laws

76. D. Kinsella and M. Verhoef, Alberta euthanasia survey: 1. Physicians' opinions

about the morality and legalization of active euthanasia, CMAJ, 148 (1993): 1921–26; D. Kinsella, and M. Verhoef, Alberta euthanasia survey: 2. Physicians' opinions about the acceptance of active euthanasia as a medical act and the reporting of such practice, CMAJ, 148 (1993): 1929–33.

77. D. Meier, C.A. Emmons, S. Wallenstein, T. Quill, R. Morrison, and C. Cassell, A national survey of physician-assisted suicide and euthanasia in the US, N Engl J Med, 338 (1998): 1193–201.

78. E. Emanuel, D. Fairclough, B. Clarridge, D. Blum, E. Bruera, W. Penley, et al., Attitudes and practices of US oncologists regarding euthanasia and physician-assisted suicide, Ann Intern Med, 133 (2000): 527–32.

79. L. Hart, T. Norris, and D. Lishner, Attitudes of family physicians in Washington state toward physician-assisted suicide, J Rural Health, 19 (2003): 461–9.

80. Cancerview, In Memory of Dr Donald Low. Video available at You Tube, posted Sept 24 and accessed Sept 25, 2013.

81. M. Lee, and S. Tolle, Oregon's plans to legalise suicide assisted by a doctor, BMJ, 310 (1995): 613–14.

82. J. Griffiths, H. Weyers, and M. Adams, Euthanasia and Law in Europe (Oxford: Hart Publishing, 2008).

83. A. Gawande, D. Denno, R. Truog, and D. Waisel, Physicians and executions—highlights from a discussion of lethal injection, N Engl J Med, 358 (2008): 448–51.

84. Carter v. the Attorney-General of Canada, 2012 BCSC 886. At 247, 253.

85. E. Emanuel, Euthanasia and physician-assisted suicide: a review of the empirical data from the US, Arch Intern Med, 162 (2002): 142–52.

86. G. Kasting, The nonnecessity of euthanasia, in J. Humber, R. Almeder, and G. Kasting (eds.), Physician-Assisted Death (New Jersey: Humana Press, 1994), 25–46.

87. T. Quill, B. Lee, and S. Nunn, Palliative treatments of last resort: choosing the least harmful alternative, Ann Intern Med, 132 (2000): 488–93.

88. T. Quill, Death and dignity: A case of individualized decision making, N Engl J Med, 324 (1991): 691–4.

89. J Prokopetz and L. Lehmann, Redefining physicians' role in assisted dying, N Engl J Med, 367 (2012): 97–9.

90. S. Wolf, Confronting physician-assisted suicide and euthanasia: my father's death, Hastings Cent Rep, 38 (2008): 23–6.

91. The quotation in Box 11.7 is from Oregon Death with Dignity Act. Or Rev Stat 127. 800–127.897 (1994).

92. L. Ganzini, H. Nelson, T. Schmidt, D. Kraemer, M. Delorit, and M. Lee, Physicians' experiences with the Oregon Death with Dignity Act, N Engl J Med, 342 (2000): 557-63.

93. S. Okie, Physician-assisted suicide—Oregon and beyond, N Engl J Med, 352 (2005): 1627–30.

94. A. Sullivan, K. Hedberg, and D. Fleming, Legalized physician-assisted suicide in Oregon—the second year, N Engl J Med, 342 (2000): 598–604.

95. E.T. Loggers, H. Starks, M. Shannon-Dudley, A. Back, F. Appelbaum, and F. Steward, Implementing a Death with Dignity program at a comprehensive cancer center, N Engl J Med, 368 (2013): 1417–24.

96. B Onwuteaka-Philipsen, A. Brinkman-Stoppelenburg, C. Penning, G. de Jong-Krul, J. van Delden, and A. van der Heide, Trends in end-of-life practices before and after the enactment of the euthanasia law in the Netherlands from 1990 to 2010: a repeated cross-sectional survey, Lancet, 380 (2012): 908–15.

97. Lord Browne-Wilkenson quoted in C. Franklin, Elm Road and Hillsborough: tragedy, the law and medicine, Intensive Care Med, 19 (1993): 307–8.

98. "Death is not an event in life . . ." L. Wittgenstein, Tractatus Logico-Philosophicus [1921] (London: Routledge & Kegan Paul, 1961), 147.

99. N. Brown, Life against Death: The Psychoanalytical Meaning of History (Middletown, CT: Wesleyan University Press, 1959), 101–6.

100. L. Snyder, and D. Sulmasy, Physician-assisted suicide, Ann Intern Med, 135 (2001): 209–16.

Chapter 12

1. R. Macklin, Against Relativism: Cultural Diversity and the Search for Ethical Universals in Medicine (Oxford: Oxford University Press, 1999): 37.

2. D. Parfit, On What Matters, Vol. 1(Oxford: Oxford University Press, 2011): 418.

3. A. Sen, *Identity and Violence: The Illusion of Destiny* (New York: W.W. Norton, 2006).

4. Indigenous Physician's Association of Canada, First Nations, Inuit, Métis Health Core Competencies (Ottawa: The Association of Faculties of Medicine of Canada April, 2009). Available at: http://www.afmc.ca/pdf/CoreCompetenciesEng.pdf

5. C. Lévi-Strauss, *The Savage Mind* (London: Weidenfeld and Nicolson, 1968): 16–17. A bricolage is a "heterogeneous repertoire" of elements and practices that is taken to refer to "primitive" cultures, but could refer to aspects of any culture. A "bricoleur" is the one who creates the assemblage.

6. A. Sen, *op. cit.*: 13.

7. A. Fadiman, *The Spirit Catches You and You Fall Down: A Hmong Child, her American Doctors, and the Collision of Cultures* (New York: Noonday Press, Farrar, Straus and Giroux, 1997).

8. A. Padela and B. Punekar, Emergency medical practice: advancing cultural competence and reducing healthcare disparities, *Acad Emerg Med*, 16 (2009): 69–75.

9. This list is adapted from A. Kleinman, in A. Fadiman. *op. cit.*: 260–1.

10. A. Kleinman, Moral experience and ethical reflection: can ethnography reconcile them? A quandary for the "new bioethics," *Daedalus*, 128 (1999): 70; C.L. Tait, Ethical programming: Towards a community-centred approach to mental health and addiction programming in aboriginal communities, *Pimatisiwin: A Journal of Aboriginal and Indigenous Community Health*, 6 (2008): 29–60.

12. J. Oram and P. Murphy, Diagnosis of death, *Contin Educ Anaesth, Crit Care Pain*, 11 (2011): 77–81.

13. "Policies may include specific accommodations, such as the continuation of artificial respiration under certain circumstances, as well as guidance on limits to accommodation." *New York State Guidelines for Determining Brain Death Statute;* 10 N.Y.C.R.R. § 400.16 (2005): 2–3. Available at: http://www.health.ny.gov/professionals/doctors/guidelines/determination_of_brain_death/docs/determination_of_brain_death.pdf.

14. R. Olick, E. Braun, and J. Potash, Accommodating religious and moral objections to neurological death, *J Clin Ethics*, 20 (2009): 183–91.

15. J. Bugge, Brain death and its implications for management of the potential organ donor, *Acta Anaesthesiol Scand*; 53 (2009): 1239–50.

16. "Ultimately, the heart stops in brain death . . . despite full cardiovascular support, 97% of . . . brain-dead bodies developed asystole in a week." E.F.M. Wijdicks and J.L.D. Atkinson, Pathophysiologic responses to brain death, in E.F.M. Wijdicks (ed.), *Brain Death* (Philadelphia: Lippincott Williams & Wilkins, 2001), 35. Of course, just how long one can prolong circulation in a (brain) dead person may depend on how hard one tries and on the advance of medical science. Such perfusion never reverses the sequence of inexorable circulatory decline.

17. D. Powner and I. Bernstein, Extended somatic support for pregnant women after brain death, *Crit Care Med*, 31 (2003): 1241–9.

18. A. Brett and P. Jersild, "Inappropriate" treatment near the end of life: conflict between religious convictions and clinical judgment, *Arch Intern Med*, 163 (2003): 1645–9.

19. P.D.N. Hébert, A. Cywinska, S.L. Ball, and J.R. deWaard, Biological identifications through DNA barcodes, *Proc R Soc Lond B*, 270 (2003): 313–321. Also see: http://www.ibol.org.

20. G. Ginsberg and H Willard, The foundations of genomic and personalized medicine. In: G. Ginsberg, and H. Willard, eds., *Essentials of Genomic and Personalized Medicine* (San Diego Calif., Elsevier Pub., 2010): 1–10. See: http://www.sciencedirect.com/science/book/9780123749345.

21. N. Houchens, G. Dhaliwal, F. Askari, B. Kim, and S. Saint, Clinical problem-solving. The essential element, *N Engl J Med*, 368 (2013): 1345–51.

22. Adapted from W .C. Leung, E. Mariman, J.C. van der Wouden, H. van Amergongen, and C. Weijer, Ethical debate: Results of genetic testing: when confidentiality conflicts with a duty to warn relatives, *BMJ*, 321 (2000): 1464–6.

23. A. Lucassen and M. Parker, Confidentiality and sharing genetic information with relatives, *Lancet*, 375 (2010): 1507–9.

24. See: http://www.unesco.org/new/en/social-and-human-sciences/themes/bioethics/bioethics-and-human-rights/

25. Dr J. Sadler. Quoted in Z. Qadir, Genomic future beckons for cancer management, *Lancet*, 378 (2011): 1838.

26. L. Wang, H. McLeod, and R. Weinshilboum, Genomics and drug response, *N Engl J Med*, 364 (2011): 1144–53.

27. K. Hudson, Genomics, health care, and society, *N Engl J Med*, 365 (2011): 1033–41.

28. T. Manolio, Genomewide association studies and assessment of the risk of disease, *N Engl J Med*, 363 (2010): 166–76.

29. R. Coupland, S. Martin, and M.T Dutli. Protecting everybody's genetic data, *Lancet*, 365 (2005): 1754–6.

30. *Havasupai Tribe of Havasupai Reservation v Arizona Board of Regents*, 204 P.3d 1063 (Ariz App Div 1 2008).

31. *Tri-Council Policy Statement (TCPS 2). Ethical Conduct for Research Involving Humans* (Ottawa, 2010): 107.

32. Tait, *op. cit.,* 31.

33. Hudson, *op. cit.,* 1034.

34. R. Coupland, S. Martin, and M.T. Dutli, *op. cit.,* 1754–6.

35. A. Gaw, Exposing unethical human research: the transatlantic correspondence of Beecher and Pappworth, *Ann Intern Med*, 156 (2012): 150–5.

36. D. Macrae, The Council for International Organizations and Medical Sciences (CIOMS) guidelines on ethics of clinical trials, *Proc Am Thorac Soc*, 4 (2007): 176–9.

37. B. Freedman, Equipoise and the ethics of clinical research, *N Engl J Med*, 317 (1987): 141–5.

38. See Tri-Council Policy Statement, *op. cit.*

39. "No one—and certainly not researchers, can claim a monopoly of relevant wisdom in discussions about what deserves attention in health research." I. Chalmers, What do I want from health research and researchers when I am a patient? *BMJ*, 310 (1995): 1315–18.

40. R. Skloot, *The Immortal Life of Henrietta Lacks* (New York: Crown Publishers, 2010).

41. C. Cheung, B. Martin, and S. Asa, Defining diagnostic tissue in the era of personalized medicine, CMAJ, 185 (2013): 135–9.

42. S.F. Gibson, *The Washington University v. Catalona:* Determining ownership of genetic samples, *Jurimetrics J*, 48 (2008): 167–91.

43. J. Limbaugh *Catalona v Washington University*, (2006) as quoted in C Schmidt, Tissue banks trigger worry about ownership, JNCI 98 (2006): 1174–5.

44. Adapted from: M. Mello, and L. Wolf, The Havasupai Indian tribe case—lessons for research involving stored biologic samples, *N Engl J Med*, 363 (2010): 204–7.

45. "Tissues are held in trust for the donors by a trustee who oversees uses in accordance with the wishes of the beneficiaries of the trust; in this case the general public." C. Emerson, P.A. Singer, and R. Upshur, access and use of human tissues from the developing world: ethical challenges and a way forward using a tissue trust, *BMC Med Ethics*, 12 (2011): 2.

46. J. Burns, British council bars doctor who linked vaccine with autism, *NY Times* (May 24, 2010). Accessed at: http://www.nytimes.com/2010/05/25/health/policy/25autism.html.

47. A. Gutmann, Safeguarding children—pediatric research on medical countermeasures, *N Engl J Med*, 368 (2013): 1171–3.

48. N. Kass, P. Pronovost, J. Sugarman C. Goeschel, L. Lubomski, and R. Faden, Controversy and quality improvement: lingering questions about ethics, oversight, and patient safety oversight, *Jt Comm J Qual Patient Saf*, 34 (2008): 349–53.

49. A collection of US Regulations for Drug Studies, the Code of Federal Regulations, and European Directives on Good Clinical Practice is usefully found in one book, *Selected Regulations & Guidance for Drug Studies* (Philadelphia: Clinical Research Resources, 2012).

50. G. Silberman and K. Kahn, Burdens on research imposed by institutional review boards: the state of the evidence and its implications for regulatory reform, *Milbank Q*, 89 (2011): 599–627.

51. K. Ormond, Medical ethics for the genome world, *J Mol Diagn,* 10 (2008): 377–82.

52. E. Emanuel in J. Lavery, C. Grady, E. Wahl, and E. Emanuel (eds.), *Ethical Issues in International Biomedical Research: A Casebook,* (Oxford: Oxford University Press, 2007): 192–4.

53. S. Kharawala and J. Dalal, Challenges in conducting psychiatry studies in India, *Perspect Clin Res,* 2 (2011): 8–12.

54. S. Glickman, J. McHutchison, E. Peterson, C. Cairns, R. Harrington, R. Califf, and K. Schulman, Ethical and scientific implications of the globalization of clinical research, *N Engl J Med,* 360 (2009): 816–23.

Conclusion

1. C. Hedges, *The World As It Is: Dispatches on the Myth of Human Progress* (New York: Nation Books, 2013).

2. D. Irvine, *The Doctors' Tale: Professionalism and Public Trust* (Oxford: Radcliffe Medical Press, 2003). These themes pervade the influential "CanMEDS" roles for doctors in Canada. C. Whitehead, D. Martin, N. Fernandez, M. Younker, R. Kouz, J. Frank and A. Boucher, *Integration of CanMEDS Expectations and Outcomes* (Members of the FMEC PG consortium, 2011). http://www.afmc.ca/pdf/fmec/15_Whitehead_CanMEDS.pdf

3. R. Tamblyn, M. Abrahamowicz, D. Dauphinee, E. Wenghofer, A. Jacques, D. Klass, et al., Physician scores on a national clinical skills examination as predictors of complaints to medical regulatory authorities, *JAMA,* 298 (2007): 993–1001.

4. T. Beauchamp and J. Childress, *Principles of Biomedical Ethics,* 6th edn. (New York: Oxford University Press, 2007).

5. A. Jonsen, M. Siegler, and W. Winslade, *Clinical Ethics,* 5th edn. (New York: McGraw-Hill, 2002).

6. R. Ashcroft, A. Dawson, H. Draper and J. MacMillan, (eds.) *Principles of Health Care Ethics,* 2nd edn. (New York: John Wiley & Sons, Ltd, 2007).

7. P.A. Singer and A.M. Viens, (eds.) *The Cambridge Textbook of Bioethics* (New York: Cambridge University Press, 2008).

8. S. Post, (ed) *Encyclopedia of Bioethics,* 3rd edn. (Farmingham, MI: MacMillan Reference Library, Gale Publ., 2003).

9. T. Beam and M. Sparacino (eds.), *Military Medical Ethics* (Washington, DC: Office of the Surgeon General, 2003).

10. The British Medical Association, *Medical Ethics Today: The BMA's Handbook of Ethics and Law,* 3rd edn. (London: BMJ Publishing Group, 2010).

11. J. Sugarman and D. Sulmasy, *Methods in Medical Ethics,* 2nd edn. (Washington, DC: Georgetown University Press, 2010).

12. S. Blackburn, *Think: A Compelling Introduction to Philosophy* (Oxford: Oxford University Press, 1999); S. Blackburn, *Being Good: A Short Introduction to Ethics* (Oxford: Oxford University Press, 2001).

13. H. Frankfurt, *The Reasons of Love* (Princeton, NJ: Princeton University Press, 2004); H. Frankfurt, *The Importance of What We Care About: Philosophical Essays* (Cambridge MA: Cambridge University Press, 2005).

14. R. Amdur and E. Bankert, *Institutional Review Board: Management and Function,* 2nd edn. (Mississauga, ON: Jones and Bartlett Publishers Canada, 2006).

15. J. Rawls, *Justice as Fairness: A Restatement* (Cambridge, MA: Harvard University Press, 2001).

16. M. Nussbaum, The Frontiers of Justice: Disability, Nationality, *Species Membership* (Cambridge, MA: Belknap Books, 2006).

17. N. Daniels, *Just Health: Meeting Health Care Needs Fairly* (Cambridge: Cambridge University Press, 2012).

18. A. Sen, *Identity and Violence: The Illusion of Destiny* (New York: WW Norton & Co, 2006).

19. P. Ford and D. Dudzinski, eds, *Complex Ethics Consutations: Cases that Haunt Us* (New York: Cambridge University Press, 2008).

20. J. Lavery, C. Grady, E. Wahl, E. Emanuel, eds, *Ethical Issues in International Biomedical Research: A Casebook* (New York: Oxford University Press, 2007).

21. P. Appelbaum, *Almost a Revolution: Mental Health Law and the Limits of Change* (New York: Oxford University Press, 1994).

22. M. Balint, *The Doctor, His Patient and the Illness,* rev. edn. (Madison, CT: International Universities Press, 1988).

23. J. Berger, *A Fortunate Man: The Story of a Country Doctor* (New York: Pantheon Books, 1967).

24. R. Tallis, *Hippocratic Oaths: Medicine and Its Discontents* (London: Atlantic Books, 2004).

25. D. Orfi, *Medicine in Translation: Journeys with My Patients* (Boston: Beacon Press, 2010).

26. A. Gawande, *Better: A Surgeon's Notes on Performance* (New York: Metropolitan Books, 2007).

27. J. Groopman, *How Doctors Think* (Boston: Houghton Mifflin, 2007).

28. O. Sacks, *A Leg to Stand On* (New York: Summit Books, 1984).

29. A. Solomon, *Far From the Tree: Parents, Children, and the Search for Identity* (New York: Scribner, 2012).

30. N. Dubler and C. Liebman, *Bioethics Mediation: A Guide to Shaping Shared Silutions*, 2nd edn. (Nashville: Vanderbilt U Press, 2011).

31. I. Abuelaish, *I Shall Not Hate: A Gaza Doctor's Journey on the Road to Peace and Human Dignity* (New York: Walker and Co., 2011).

32. R. Skloot, *The Immortal Life of Henrietta Lacks* (New York: Crown Publishers, 2010).

33. E. Topol, *The Creative Destruction of Medicine: How the Digital Revolution Will Create Better Health Care* (New York: Basic Books, 2012).

34. R. Porter, *The Greatest Benefit to Mankind: A Medical History of Humanity* (New York: Norton & Co., 1997), 717–18.

Index